T0310104

Oral
Dermatology

In memory of our colleague and friend,
Newell Walter Johnson CMG

Oral Dermatology

A practical guide for dermatologists and medical practitioners

S R Prabhu

BDS, MDS (Oral Path), FFDRCSIre (Oral Med),
FDS RCS (Eng), FDS RCS (Edin), FDSRCPS (Glas),
FFGDP RCS (UK), FICD
Honorary Associate Professor (Oral Pathology/
Oral Medicine), School of Dentistry,
University of Queensland, Australia

Amanda Oakley

CNZM, MBChB, PGDipHealInf, FRACP,
FNZDS, IFAAD
Honorary Professor, Department of Medicine,
University of Auckland, New Zealand

Sue-Ching Yeoh

BDS (Hons), MDSc (Oral Med Oral Path), MPhil,
FRACDS, FRACDS (Oral Med), FICD, FPFA, FDS
RCPS (Glas), FOMAA
Associate Professor, Sydney Dental School,
University of Sydney, Australia

Scion

© **Scion Publishing Ltd, 2024**

First published 2024

All rights reserved. No part of this book may be reproduced or transmitted, in any form or by any means, without permission.

A CIP catalogue record for this book is available from the British Library.

ISBN 9781914961410

Scion Publishing Limited

The Old Hayloft, Vantage Business Park, Bloxham Road, Banbury OX16 9UX, UK

www.scionpublishing.com

Important Note from the Publisher

The information contained within this book was obtained by Scion Publishing Ltd from sources believed by us to be reliable. However, while every effort has been made to ensure its accuracy, no responsibility for loss or injury whatsoever occasioned to any person acting or refraining from action as a result of information contained herein can be accepted by the authors or publishers.

Readers are reminded that medicine is a constantly evolving science and while the authors and publishers have ensured that all dosages, applications and practices are based on current indications, there may be specific practices which differ between communities. You should always follow the guidelines laid down by the manufacturers of specific products and the relevant authorities in the country in which you are practising.

Although every effort has been made to ensure that all owners of copyright material have been acknowledged in this publication, we would be pleased to acknowledge in subsequent reprints or editions any omissions brought to our attention.

Registered names, trademarks, etc. used in this book, even when not marked as such, are not to be considered unprotected by law.

Typeset in India by DataWorks

Printed in the UK

Last digit is the print number: 10 9 8 7 6 5 4 3 2

CONTENTS

Foreword   xv
Preface   xvi
About the authors   xvii
Acknowledgements   xix
Terminology   xx
Abbreviations   xxi

1 Anatomical features and variants of the oral cavity   **1**

1.1   Overview   1
     1.1.1   The oral mucosa   1
     1.1.2   Anatomic variations   2

1.2   Lips   3
     1.2.1   Vascular supply   4
     1.2.2   Innervation   4
     1.2.3   Anatomic variations   4

1.3   Cheeks   5
     1.3.1   Vascular supply   6
     1.3.2   Innervation   6
     1.3.3   Anatomic variations   7

1.4   The tongue and the floor of the mouth   7
     1.4.1   Glossal papillae   7
     1.4.2   Vascular supply   8
     1.4.3   Innervation   8
     1.4.4   Anatomic variations   8

1.5   The hard palate, soft palate, and uvula   10
     1.5.1   Hard palate   10
     1.5.2   Soft palate   10
     1.5.3   Vascular supply   10
     1.5.4   Innervation   10

1.6   Maxilla and the mandible   11
     1.6.1   Maxilla   11
     1.6.2   Mandible   11
     1.6.3   Anatomic variations   11

1.7   Temporomandibular joint   13
     1.7.1   Innervation   13

1.8   Maxillary sinuses   13
     1.8.1   Vascular supply   13
     1.8.2   Innervation   13

1.9   Lymph nodes   14
     1.9.1   Lymphoid tissue   14

2 Diagnostic procedures for diseases of the oral mucosa   17

2.1   Introduction   17

2.2   Clinical evaluation   17
    2.2.1   Dermoscopy   17
    2.2.2   Clinical photography   17
    2.2.3   Diascopy   18
    2.2.4   The Nikolsky sign   18
    2.2.5   *In vivo* toluidine blue staining   18
    2.2.6   Samples for microbial culture   18
    2.2.7   Smear for cytology   19
    2.2.8   Biopsy for histopathology   19
    2.2.9   Fine-needle aspiration   19

2.3   Laboratory processes   20
    2.3.1   Histopathology   20
    2.3.2   Immunofluorescent and immunohistochemical staining   20
    2.3.3   Molecular pathology   21
    2.3.4   Haematology   21
    2.3.5   Biochemistry   21
    2.3.6   Immunology/serology   22
    2.3.7   Salivary diagnostic tests   22

2.4   Diagnostic imaging   22
    2.4.1   Diagnostic imaging of oral soft tissues   22
    2.4.2   Sialography   23

3 The differential diagnosis of oral mucosal lesions   25

Classification based on the clinical appearance   25

3.1   White lesions of the oral mucosa   25
    3.1.1   Key points   25

3.2   Red and purple lesions of the oral mucosa   27
    3.2.1   Key points   27

3.3   Pigmented lesions of the oral mucosa   29
    3.3.1   Key points   29

3.4   Papillary and verrucous lesions of the oral mucosa   30
    3.4.1   Key points   30

3.5   Non-neoplastic oral soft tissue swellings   31
    3.5.1   Key points   32

3.6   Oral vesicles and bullae   33
    3.6.1   Key points   33

3.7   Oral erosions and ulcers   34
    3.7.1   Key points   34

Classification of common oral symptoms 36

3.8   Dry mouth   36
       3.8.1   Key points   36

3.9   Halitosis   37
       3.9.1   Key points   37

Diseases of specific oral sites 38

3.10   Diseases affecting the lips – cheilitis   38
       3.10.1   Key points   38

3.11   Diseases affecting the gingivae   41

Desquamative gingivitis   41
       3.11.1   Key points   41

Gingival enlargement   42
       3.11.2   Key points   42

3.12   Diseases affecting the tongue   43
       3.12.1   Key points   44

3.13   Mucocutaneous disorders   46
       3.13.1   Key points   46

3.14   Oral diseases associated with systemic disorders   49
       3.14.1   Key points   49

4   Reactions of the oral mucosa to local or exogenous factors 51

4.1   Dental and oral hygiene   51
       4.1.1   Adults   51
       4.1.2   Children   52
       4.1.3   Patients with oral mucositis due to radiotherapy or
                chemotherapy   52

4.2   Debris   52
       4.2.1   Hairy tongue   52
       4.2.2   Materia alba   54

4.3   Acute injury   54
       4.3.1   Traumatic ulceration   54
       4.3.2   Extravascular blood   54
       4.3.3   Traumatic haemorrhagic bulla   56
       4.3.4   Mucosal burn   57
                Thermal burn   57
                Chemical burn   58
                Chemotherapy-induced oral mucositis   59
                Radiation mucositis   60

| | 4.3.5 | Traumatic neuroma | 62 |
| | 4.3.6 | Pyogenic granuloma / vascular epulis | 62 |

4.4	Chronic repetitive injury		63
	4.4.1	Fibroepithelial polyp and fibrous epulis	64
	4.4.2	Giant cell epulis	65
	4.4.3	Denture-induced hyperplasia	66
	4.4.4	Papillary hyperplasia	66
	4.4.5	Peripheral ossifying fibroma of the gingiva	67
	4.4.6	Frictional keratoses	68
	4.4.7	Verruciform xanthoma	71
	4.4.8	Contact stomatitis	71

4.5	Toxins		73
	4.5.1	Areca nut	73
		Oral submucous fibrosis	73
		Oral verrucous hyperplasia	75
	4.5.2	Smokeless tobacco keratosis	76
	4.5.3	Tobacco smoking	78
		Leukokeratosis nicotina palati	78
		Smoker's melanosis	79

4.6	Adverse drug reaction		80
	4.6.1	Chemical burn	82
	4.6.2	Aphthous-like ulceration	83
	4.6.3	Fixed drug eruption	83
	4.6.4	Lichenoid drug eruption	83
	4.6.5	Lupus-like reaction	84
	4.6.6	Immunobullous reaction	84
	4.6.7	Drug-induced gingival hyperplasia	85
	4.6.8	Stevens–Johnson syndrome / toxic epidermal necrolysis	86

4.7	Reaction to infection or vaccination		88
	4.7.1	Infection-related mucositis	88
	4.7.2	Erythema multiforme	88

4.8	Pigment		90
	4.8.1	Amalgam tattoo	90
	4.8.2	Cosmetic tattoo	91
	4.8.3	Drug-induced pigmentation	91
	4.8.4	Postinflammatory pigmentation	92
	4.8.5	Heavy metal pigmentation	92

4.9	Reaction to an underlying disease		93
	4.9.1	Acanthosis nigricans	93
	4.9.2	Plummer–Vinson syndrome	94
	4.9.3	Mouth ulcers due to underlying bowel disease	95

4.10	Reactive gingival hyperplasia		95
	4.10.1	Localized juvenile spongiotic gingival hyperplasia	95
	4.10.2	Hormone-related gingivitis	95

5 Oral mucosal diseases of developmental and genetic origin — 97

5.1	Congenital disorders	97
	5.1.1 Congenital macroglossia	97
	5.1.2 White sponge naevus	98
	5.1.3 Vascular malformation	100
	Port wine stain	100
	5.1.4 Lymphatic malformation	100
	5.1.5 Ectodermal dysplasia	103
	5.1.6 Focal dermal hypoplasia	103
	5.1.7 Cystic fibrosis	105
5.2	Disorders usually diagnosed in childhood	105
	5.2.1 Darier disease	105
	5.2.2 Dyskeratosis congenita	108
	5.2.3 Epidermolysis bullosa	110
	5.2.4 Fanconi anaemia	112
	5.2.5 Hereditary benign intraepithelial dyskeratosis	113
	5.2.6 Hereditary gingival fibromatosis	114
	5.2.7 Ligneous gingivitis	114
	5.2.8 McCune–Albright syndrome	115
	5.2.9 Pachyonychia congenita	115
	5.2.10 Peutz–Jeghers syndrome	117
	5.2.11 Multiple endocrine neoplasia type 2B	118
	5.2.12 Cowden syndrome	120
	5.2.13 Lipoid proteinosis	122
5.3	Disorders usually diagnosed in adult life	123
	5.3.1 Fordyce spots	123
	5.3.2 Hereditary haemorrhagic telangiectasia	123
	5.3.3 Laugier–Hunziker syndrome	125
	5.3.4 Leukoedema	126
	5.3.5 Venous lake	126

6 Oral mucosal infections — 129

6.1	Fungal infections	129
	6.1.1 *Candida albicans* infections	129
	Pseudomembranous candidosis	129
	Oral erythematous candidosis	132
	Denture-related stomatitis	132
	Chronic hyperplastic candidosis	134
	Chronic mucocutaneous candidosis	136
	Median rhomboid glossitis	138
	6.1.2 Deep mycoses	139

		Aspergillosis	139
		Mucormycosis	139
		Histoplasmosis	139
		Cryptococcosis	139
		Blastomycosis	140
		Paracoccidioidomycosis	140
6.2	Viral infections		140
	6.2.1	Herpes simplex	140
		Primary herpetic gingivostomatitis	140
		Herpes labialis	142
		Recurrent oral mucosal herpes	143
	6.2.2	Varicella-zoster infection	144
		Varicella	144
		Herpes zoster	145
	6.2.3	Infectious mononucleosis	146
	6.2.4	Cytomegalovirus	147
	6.2.5	Enterovirus	148
		Hand, foot, and mouth disease	148
		Herpangina	149
	6.2.6	Measles	150
	6.2.7	Mumps	152
	6.2.8	Human immunodeficiency virus	153
		Hairy leukoplakia	153
		Linear gingival erythema	154
		HIV-associated oral melanotic hyperpigmentation	155
	6.2.9	Human papillomavirus	156
		Viral warts	156
		Multifocal epithelial hyperplasia	159
	6.2.10	Molluscum contagiosum	160
6.3	Bacterial infections		161
	6.3.1	Staphylococcal infections	161
		Impetigo	161
		Staphylococcal scalded skin syndrome	163
	6.3.2	Streptococcal infections	164
		Streptococcal pharyngitis	165
	6.3.3	Dental plaque (biofilm)	166
		Gingivitis and periodontitis	166
		Necrotizing periodontal diseases	168
		Gingival and periodontal abscess	169
	6.3.4	Gonococcal stomatitis	170
	6.3.5	Strawberry tongue	171
	6.3.6	Syphilis	171
		Syphilitic leukoplakia	173
	6.3.7	Tuberculosis	173

6.4   Mixed infections   174
       6.4.1   Angular cheilitis   174

7 Oral mucosal inflammatory diseases and conditions   177

7.1   Recurrent aphthous ulcer   177

7.2   Lichenoid disorders   179
       7.2.1   Oral lichen planus   179
       7.2.2   Oral lichenoid reaction   183
       7.2.3   Desquamative gingivitis   184
       7.2.4   Graft-versus-host disease   186
       7.2.5   Lupus erythematosus   188
       7.2.6   Chronic ulcerative stomatitis   189

7.3   Granulomatous disorders   190
       7.3.1   Granulomatous gingivitis   190
       7.3.2   Orofacial granulomatosis   191
       7.3.3   Sarcoidosis   193

7.4   Immunobullous diseases   193
       7.4.1   Epidermolysis bullosa acquisita   193
       7.4.2   Pemphigoid   195
                Mucous membrane pemphigoid   195
                Bullous pemphigoid   197
                Pemphigoid gestationis   198
                Linear IgA bullous dermatosis   199
       7.4.3   Pemphigus   199
                Pemphigus vulgaris   199
                Paraneoplastic pemphigus   202
       7.4.4   Dermatitis herpetiformis   203

7.5   Other inflammatory diseases localized to the mouth   204
       7.5.1   Geographic tongue   204
       7.5.2   Lingual papillitis   205
       7.5.3   Glandular cheilitis   206
       7.5.4   Plasma cell gingivitis/cheilitis   207

8 Oral mucosal non-inflammatory disorders and conditions   209

8.1   Endogenous pigmentation   209
       8.1.1   Racial pigmentation   209
       8.1.2   Oral melanotic macule   210
       8.1.3   Addison disease   210

8.2   Cysts   211
       8.2.1   Cysts of minor salivary glands   211
       8.2.2   Gingival odontogenic cyst   212

8.2.3   Eruption cyst   213
8.2.4   Dermoid and epidermoid cysts   213
8.2.5   Lymphoepithelial cyst   215
8.2.6   Nasolabial cyst   216
8.2.7   Thyroglossal duct cyst   216

8.3   Oral mucinosis   217

9   Oral mucosal manifestations of systemic diseases   219

9.1   Atrophic glossitis   219

9.2   Vitamin deficiencies   220
9.2.1   Riboflavin (vitamin B2) deficiency   220
9.2.2   Niacin (vitamin B3) deficiency   221
9.2.3   Pyridoxine (vitamin B6) deficiency   221
9.2.4   Biotin (vitamin B7) deficiency   221
9.2.5   Folate (vitamin B9) deficiency   222
9.2.6   Cyanocobalamin (vitamin B12) deficiency   222
9.2.7   Tocopherol (vitamin E) deficiency   222
9.2.8   Vitamin K deficiency   223
9.2.9   Ascorbic acid (vitamin C) deficiency   223

9.3   Angioedema   224

9.4   Hypothyroidism   226

9.5   Thrombocytopenic purpura   227

9.6   Leukaemia   228

9.7   Coeliac disease   230

9.8   Inflammatory bowel disease   230
9.8.1   Non-specific oral lesions   231
9.8.2   Oral lesions specific to Crohn disease   231
9.8.3   Pyostomatitis vegetans   232

9.9   Oral manifestations of diabetes mellitus   233

9.10   Vasculitis   234
9.10.1   Cutaneous small vessel vasculitis   234
9.10.2   Giant cell arteritis   235
9.10.3   Granulomatosis with polyangiitis   236

9.11   Cushing syndrome   237

9.12   Acromegaly   238

9.13   Parathyroid disease   239

9.14   Sickle cell anaemia   239

9.15   Amyloidosis   240

9.16   Drug-induced osteonecrosis of the jaw   241

9.17   Psychogenic oral disease   242
    9.17.1   Burning mouth syndrome   243
    9.17.2   Atypical odontalgia   244
    9.17.3   Oral dysaesthesia   244
    9.17.4   Halitophobia   244
    9.17.5   Phantom bite syndrome   244
    9.17.6   Odontophobia   245

10 Oral neoplastic lesions: benign, potentially malignant, and malignant   247

10.1   Benign lesions of the oral mucosa   247
    10.1.1   Melanocytic naevus   247
    10.1.2   Melanotic neuroectodermal tumour of infancy   248
    10.1.3   Lipoma   249
    10.1.4   Peripheral nerve sheath tumours   250
            Neurofibroma   251
            Schwannoma   252
            Granular cell tumour   253
            Mucosal neuroma   254
    10.1.5   Haemangioma   255
            Infantile haemangioma   256
    10.1.6   Angioleiomyoma   257
    10.1.7   Rhabdomyoma   257
    10.1.8   Peripheral ameloblastoma   257
    10.1.9   Rare odontogenic tumours   258

10.2   Benign salivary gland tumours   258
    10.2.1   Pleomorphic adenoma   258
    10.2.2   Warthin tumour   260
    10.2.3   Sialadenoma papilliferum   261
    10.2.4   Other benign salivary gland tumours   262

10.3   Oral potentially malignant disorders   262
    10.3.1   Actinic keratosis of the lip   263
    10.3.2   Leukoplakia   266
    10.3.3   Erythroplakia   269
    10.3.4   Reverse smoker's palate   270

10.4   Malignant lesions of the oral mucosa   271
    10.4.1   Squamous cell carcinoma   272
            Oral verrucous carcinoma   274
            Oral carcinoma cuniculatum   275
    10.4.2   Melanoma   276
    10.4.3   Kaposi sarcoma   278

	10.4.4	Lymphoma	279
	10.4.5	Leukaemia	280
	10.4.6	Other primary malignant tumours	280
	10.4.7	Metastases	280
10.5	Malignant salivary gland tumours		281
	10.5.1	Acinic cell carcinoma	281
	10.5.2	Mucoepidermoid carcinoma	281
	10.5.3	Adenoid cystic carcinoma	282
	10.5.4	Other malignant salivary gland tumours	284
Index			287

FOREWORD

It has been a pleasure and an honour to be asked to write a foreword to this new publication, *Oral Dermatology: A practical guide for dermatologists and medical practitioners*, a reference book primarily targeted at dermatologists.

Often, dermatologists encounter patients with oral mucosal diseases. In some cases, the presenting oral lesion may be the sole clinical presentation. A range of oral lesions may also appear as the only or early manifestations of underlying mucocutaneous diseases. In such circumstances, dermatologists may be uncertain of diagnosing and managing oral mucosal and mucocutaneous presentations. Diagnosing and managing mucosal or mucocutaneous disease demands logical structuring of clinical information. It is also important not to miss an oral cancer at its first presentation. *Oral Dermatology* provides a systematic approach to address these challenging issues.

Oral Dermatology contains ten chapters, offering readers in-depth information about oral mucosal disease encountered in dermatology practice or in primary care. It begins with chapters discussing anatomical structures of the oral cavity and variants of the oral mucosa, diagnostic procedures for evaluating diseases of the oral mucosa, differential diagnosis of the oral lesions, reactions of the oral mucosa to local or exogenous factors, oral mucosal disease of developmental and genetic origin, infections of the oral mucosa, oral mucosal inflammatory diseases and conditions, oral mucosal non-inflammatory diseases and conditions, oral mucosal manifestations of systemic diseases, and oral neoplastic lesions: benign, potentially malignant, and malignant. This book offers essential knowledge to understand the aetiology, clinical features, and differential diagnosis and management protocol of oral mucosal diseases. The book provides clear advice to arrive at a working diagnosis. It includes over 200 clinical images to aid in complementing the text.

This book is a welcome addition to the available resources in dermatology and medicine. I highly recommend this valuable reference book to every dermatologist, primary care physician, postgraduate student of dermatology and medicine, and any other physician who deals with oral and skin care.

This book is authored jointly by internationally reputed oral medicine experts and a dermatologist. I wish to congratulate Professors S R Prabhu, Amanda Oakley, and Sue-Ching Yeoh for compiling this thorough and easy-to-read book that covers all significant aspects of oral mucosal and mucocutaneous diseases.

Saman Warnakulasuriya OBE
BDS, FDSRCS, FDSRCPS, PhD, DSc, FKC
Emeritus Professor of Oral Medicine and Experimental Oral Pathology
King's College London, UK

PREFACE

The idea for this book was conceived in 2021 by Oral Medicine Specialist and Honorary Associate Professor S R Prabhu (University of Queensland), who recognized a gap in the market for an up-to-date guide to oral diseases targeted at dermatologists and medical practitioners. He soon co-opted Dermatologist, Adjunct Associate Professor Amanda Oakley (now Honorary Professor, University of Auckland) and a practising Oral Medicine Specialist, Associate Professor Sue-Ching Yeoh (Sydney), to help with the task.

We recognized that often patients with oral mucosal diseases and conditions consult a dermatologist or a family doctor, who are frequently unfamiliar with acute and chronic mucosal disorders and lesions within the oral cavity. In this book, we start with a chapter about oral anatomical features and another containing a brief outline of investigations and procedures available. Our readers should find *Chapter 3* particularly helpful, where we have assembled lists of diseases and conditions and their key points according to their morphology or location. *Chapters 4* to *10* provide greater detail about individual topics and are accompanied by clinical illustrations. Many of these illustrations come from the authors' own collections or their institutions (in particular, Health New Zealand | Te Whatu Ora – Waikato). Others have been acquired from Open Access online resources or published works, after gaining permission for copyrighted works. We have tried to acknowledge the copyrighted material for the images used. If copyright infringement has occurred unintentionally, we wish to tender our apologies.

Our goal is to provide an easy-to-read textbook where readers can quickly find what they need to confidently assess symptoms and signs of lesions within and around the mouth.

S R Prabhu
Amanda Oakley
Sue-Ching Yeoh

ABOUT THE AUTHORS

Professor S R Prabhu is an Honorary Associate Professor at the University of Queensland School of Dentistry, Brisbane. His expertise is in Oral and Maxillofacial Pathology and Oral Medicine, with a special interest in tropical oral diseases. Professor Prabhu formerly held academic positions in Oral Medicine and Oral Pathology at university dental schools in India, Kenya, Sudan, Trinidad and Tobago, Malaysia, Saudi Arabia, and the UAE and administrative positions as Director and Dean of Dental Schools in Trinidad and Tobago West Indies, and the UAE, respectively. Professor Prabhu is a Fellow of the dental faculties Royal Colleges of Surgeons in the UK and Ireland and the International College of Dentists. He was an external examiner for the Royal College of Surgeons of Edinburgh, UK dental membership examinations. He received the Commonwealth Medical Scholarship awarded by the British Council and the Rotary Foundation award for teaching in developing countries. Professor Prabhu has conducted workshops on HIV/AIDS for oral healthcare professionals in several countries in the Asian and Caribbean regions. He has published numerous papers in refereed journals, edited/co-edited, and authored/co-authored over fifteen books. Prominent among these include *Oral Diseases in the Tropics*, *Textbook of Oral Medicine*, *Textbook of Oral Anatomy Histology and Embryology*, *Textbook of Oral Diagnosis*, *Oral Diseases for Medical Practitioners* (all with Oxford University Press), *HIV/AIDS for Dental Practice* (Dental Council of India), *Clinical Diagnosis in Oral Medicine* (Jaypee Bros Medical Publishers), *Handbook of Oral Pathology and Oral Medicine* (John Wiley & Sons), and *Sexually Transmissible Oral Diseases* (John Wiley & Sons). Professor Prabhu is on the editorial board of the *International Dental Journal* (IDJ), published by the FDI World Dental Federation, Geneva.

Professor Amanda Oakley is an experienced medical dermatologist in Hamilton, New Zealand. She is Head of the Department of Dermatology at Health New Zealand | Te Whatu Ora – Waikato and an Honorary Professor for the Department of Medicine of the University of Auckland. Her research interests include artificial intelligence, teledermatology and dermoscopy, aiming to improve the equity of dermatological care to patients in New Zealand and worldwide. Professor Oakley is passionate about medical education, authoring several textbooks, including *Dermatology Made Easy*, publishing numerous papers in peer-reviewed dermatological journals, writing a regular column for the primary care medical magazine *New Zealand Doctor Rata Aotearoa,* and contributing to several online resources. She serves on several Editorial Boards and medical committees. Dr Oakley was Editor in Chief of DermNet for 25 years, for which she received several Honorary Memberships and awards, including the Companion of New Zealand Order of Merit in 2018. She has been President of Waikato Postgraduate Medical Incorporated (1999–2004), New Zealand Dermatological Society Incorporated (2011–13), Australian and New Zealand Vulvovaginal Society (2011–13), and the International Society of Teledermatology (2020–3).

Professor Sue-Ching Yeoh is an Associate Professor at Sydney Dental School, University of Sydney and maintains an Oral Medicine specialist practice with a clinical appointment at the Royal Prince Alfred Hospital and Chris O'Brien Lifehouse. Associate Professor Yeoh is the Head of Training in Oral Medicine at the University of Sydney. She is a Fellow of the Royal Australasian College of Dental Surgeons (General and Special Fields Stream), the International College of Dentists, the Pierre Fauchard Academy and the Royal College of Physicians and Surgeons of Glasgow.

Associate Professor Yeoh is currently the President of the Oral Medicine Academy of Australasia (OMAA) and the Chair of the Australian Dental Association Therapeutics Committee and is a contributing author to the *Therapeutic Guidelines: Oral and Dental V3* (2019). She is committed to continuing professional development and has been a frequently invited speaker for the Australian Dental Association CPD programme. Associate Professor Yeoh has presented nationally and internationally at various conferences, generated publications in peer-reviewed journals, and contributed to and edited several oral medicine textbooks. Associate Professor Yeoh's clinical interests include oral mucosal disease, odontogenic pathology, salivary gland pathology, orofacial pain, and temporomandibular dysfunction. Her current research focus is the autoimmune vesiculobullous disease.

ACKNOWLEDGEMENTS

AIPDerm (www.aipderm.com) utilized its expertise in computer vision techniques based on pixel interpolation to enhance certain images within this book (these are clearly indicated in the figure legend). These images were manipulated individually and without utilizing external images for deep learning AI. Subsequently all images were deleted to prevent unintentional usage or incorporation into deep learning databases in the future. AIPDerm is a company headquartered in Europe which is striving to transform dermatology care through its proprietary AI and technology platform.

Editorial assistance from Jonathan Ray of Scion Publishing is gratefully acknowledged.

TERMINOLOGY

The following terms describe mucosal lesions based on their clinical appearance.

Bulla (plural **bullae**): a bulla is a blister containing clear fluid >1cm in diameter.

Erosion: erosion is a partial-thickness loss of epithelium. Typically, erosions follow the rupture of vesicles or bullae, or are due to trauma. Mucosal erosions may also result from an inflammatory disease of infection.

Macule: a macule is flat and is noticeable because of its difference in colour from normal skin or mucosa. Macules may be red due to increased vascularity or inflammation, or pigmented due to melanin, haemosiderin, or foreign material.

Nodule: a nodule develops within the deep mucosa and may protrude above the mucosa, forming a dome-shaped structure. A nodule is >1cm in diameter.

Papule: a papule is raised above the mucosal surface and is <1cm in diameter. Papules may be dome-shaped or flat-topped.

Plaque: a plaque is a raised or thickened lesion >1cm in diameter, often composed of coalescing papules.

Purpura: purpura is a reddish-purple discolouration caused by blood leaking into the connective tissue. They do not blanch when pressure is applied. They are classified by size as petechiae (<0.3cm), purpura (0.4–0.9cm), or ecchymoses (>1cm).

Pustule: pustules are blisters containing purulent material. They appear turbid and yellow.

Ulcer: an ulcer is a well-circumscribed, full-thickness epithelial defect covered by a fibrin membrane, resulting in a yellow-white depressed centre.

Vesicle: vesicles are small blisters that contain clear fluid, each <1cm in diameter.

ABBREVIATIONS

ACTH	adrenocorticotrophic hormone
ANCA	antineutrophil cytoplasmic antibodies
CBC	complete blood count
CMV	cytomegalovirus
CN	cranial nerve
CT	computerized tomography
DIF	direct immunofluorescence
EB	epidermolysis bullosa
EBA	epidermolysis bullosa acquisita
EBV	Epstein–Barr virus
ELISA	enzyme-linked immunosorbent assay
EM	erythema multiforme
ESR	erythrocyte sedimentation rate
GvHD	graft-versus-host disease
HAART	highly active antiretroviral therapy
HHV	human herpesvirus
HIV	human immunodeficiency virus
HPV	human papillomavirus
HSV	herpes simplex virus
IBD	inflammatory bowel disease
IHC	immunohistochemistry
IIF	indirect immunofluorescence
LE	lupus erythematosus
MEN	multiple endocrine neoplasia
MRI	magnetic resonance imaging
NHL	non-Hodgkin lymphoma
NSAID	non-steroidal anti-inflammatory drug
OLP	oral lichen planus
OPMD	oral potentially malignant disorder
PCR	polymerase chain reaction
PET	positron emission tomography
SCC	squamous cell carcinoma
SJS/TEN	Stevens–Johnson syndrome / toxic epidermal necrolysis
SSSS	staphylococcal scalded skin syndrome
TB	tuberculosis
TMJ	temporomandibular joint
UV	ultraviolet
VZV	varicella-zoster virus

CHAPTER 1

ANATOMICAL FEATURES AND VARIANTS OF THE ORAL CAVITY

1.1 Overview

The oral cavity is bounded by the lips anteriorly, the cheeks laterally, and the oropharynx posteriorly. It encloses the tongue, palates, gingivae, floor of the mouth, and teeth (see *Fig. 1.1*).

- The oral cavity begins at the junction of the vermilion border of the lips and the mucosa lining the inside of the lips. It extends posteriorly to the palatoglossal folds or arch.
- Beyond the palatoglossal folds are the palatopharyngeal folds and the beginning of the oropharynx. The oropharynx comprises the soft palate, the uvula, the anterior and posterior pillars (or fauces), the posterior pharyngeal wall, the palatine tonsils, and the base of the tongue.
- The nasal cavity is separated from the oral cavity anteriorly by the hard palate and posteriorly by the soft palate. The soft palate seals the oropharynx from the nasopharynx during swallowing and speech.

1.1.1 The oral mucosa

The mucous membrane lining of the oral cavity extends from the vermilion border of the lips to the anterior pillars of the fauces.

- The oral mucous membrane consists of an outermost stratified squamous epithelium and underlying fibrous connective tissue (lamina propria) separated by a basement membrane (basal lamina). It is contiguous with the submucosa.
- The deeper layer of the epithelium forms undulating projections (rete pegs), which interdigitate with papillary projections of the lamina propria.
- The submucosa contains neurovascular structures, lymphatic vessels, adipose tissue, and minor salivary glands.

The oral mucosa is classified as lining, masticatory, and specialized mucosa.

- Lining mucosa is found over mobile structures such as the soft palate, cheeks, lips, vestibular sulci, the floor of the mouth, and inferior and ventral surfaces of the tongue.
- Masticatory mucosa covers the free and attached gingiva and the hard palate, which is tightly bound by dense connective tissue to the underlying bone and the dorsum of the tongue. The epithelium of the masticatory mucosa is keratinized.

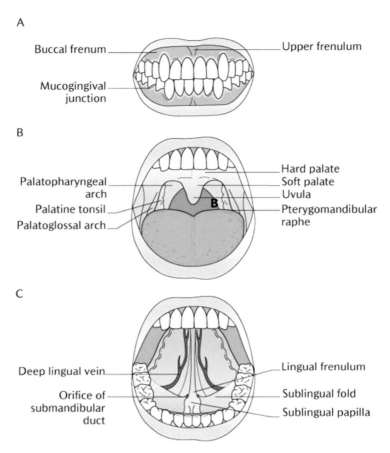

Figure 1.1. The anatomical features of the oral cavity. (A) The vestibule, (B) the oral cavity with the tongue lowered, and (C) the oral cavity proper with the tongue raised.

Reproduced with permission from *Pocket Dentistry* (Chapter 25; www.pocketdentistry.com).

- Specialized mucosa adapted for taste sensation is found on the dorsum of the tongue.

1.1.2 Anatomic variations

- Diffuse symmetrical physiological pigmentation is commonly seen in individuals of colour, particularly of African descent (see *Fig. 1.2*). It may mimic pigmentation of Addison disease, smoker's melanosis, and drug-induced oral pigmentation.
- Leukoedema (see *Section 5.3.4* for further details) is a bilateral diffuse milky white translucent whitening of the buccal mucosa or, less often, the soft palate, tongue, and floor of the mouth, due to intercellular oedema. It fades on stretching the mucosa. Leukoedema is commonly seen in individuals of African descent (see *Fig. 1.3*).

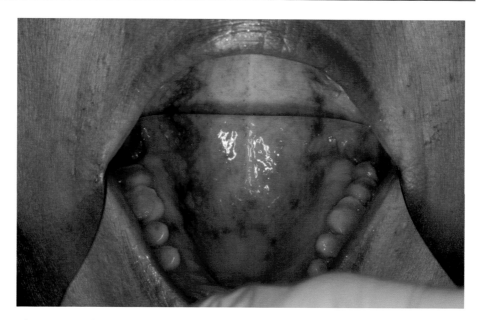

Figure 1.2. Physiological pigmentation of the gingiva and palatal mucosa.

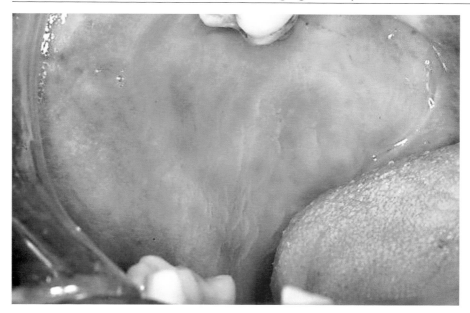

Figure 1.3. Leukoedema shows translucent whitening of the buccal mucosa.

Reproduced from *Diagnosis and Management of Oral Lesions and Conditions: A resource handbook for the clinician;* Eds: CA Migliorati and FS Panagakos (http://dx.doi.org/10.5772/57597) under CC BY 3.0 licence. © 2014 InTech.

1.2   Lips

The upper and lower lips have vermilion and cutaneous surfaces joined by the labial commissures. The principal muscle of the lips is the circumferential orbicularis oris, a sphincter for the oral aperture.

- The upper lip connects to the gums by the superior labial frenulum.
- The lower lip connects to the gums by the inferior labial frenulum.
- The lips are lined inside the mouth by non-keratinizing epithelium.

1.2.1 Vascular supply

- The facial artery branches into superior and inferior labial arteries about 1cm lateral to the angles of the mouth.
- The facial vein drains the lip via the superior and inferior labial veins.
- Lymph from the upper lip and lateral aspects of the lower lip drains into the ipsilateral submandibular lymph nodes.

1.2.2 Innervation

- Sensory innervation of the upper lip is via the infraorbital branch of the maxillary division of the trigeminal nerve (cranial nerve (CN) V2).
- Sensory innervation of the lower lip is via the mental nerve derived from the mandibular division of the trigeminal nerve (CN V3).
- Motor innervation to the orbicularis oris and elevators of the lip and lip angle is via the buccal branch of the facial nerve (CN VII).

1.2.3 Anatomic variations

- Fordyce spots (see *Section 5.3.1* for further details) of lips are white or yellow papules formed by ectopic/heterotopic sebaceous glands (see *Fig. 1.4*).

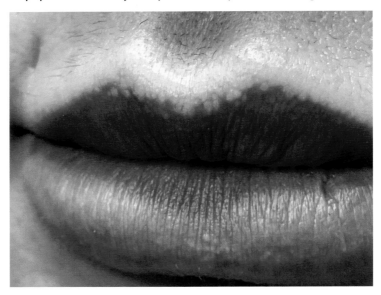

Figure 1.4. Fordyce spots on the upper lip.

Reproduced from Health NZ – Waikato (www.waikatodhb.health.nz) with permission.

- A venous lake (see *Section 5.3.5* for further details) is a dilated venule. It is often seen on the lower lip (see *Fig. 1.5*).

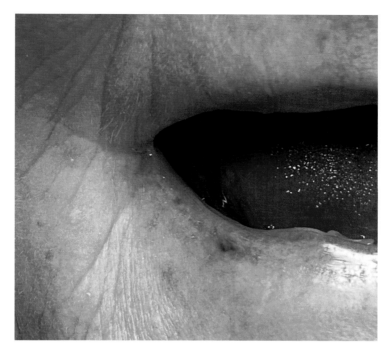

Figure 1.5. Venous lake on the lower lip.

Reproduced from Health NZ – Waikato (www.waikatodhb.health.nz) with permission.

1.3 Cheeks

Cheeks are bounded by vestibular fornices. The principal muscle is the buccinator.
- The mucosa of the cheek is lined by non-keratinized epithelium tightly attached to the buccinator.
- A fold of mucosa containing the pterygomandibular raphe extends from the upper to the lower alveolus in the retromolar region anterior to the pillars of the fauces.
- A groove is located between the pterygomandibular raphe and the ramus of the mandible.
- The parotid duct drains into the cheek opposite the maxillary second molar tooth.
- Its opening may be covered by a small fold of mucosa called the parotid papilla (see *Fig. 1.6*).

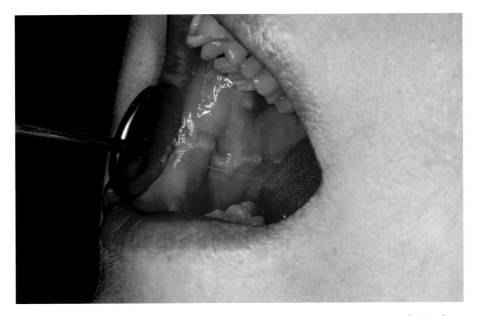

Figure 1.6. Parotid papilla. Note the small, elevated round mucosal fold of buccal mucosa opposite the maxillary molars.

1.3.1   Vascular supply

- The buccinator muscle receives its arterial blood supply mainly from the buccal artery, a branch of the maxillary artery, and some branches of the facial artery.
- Tortuous veins are common in older people.

1.3.2   Innervation

- Sensory innervation to the cheek is via the buccal branch of the mandibular division of the trigeminal nerve (CN V).
- Motor innervation of the buccinator muscle is via the buccal branch of the facial nerve (CN VII).

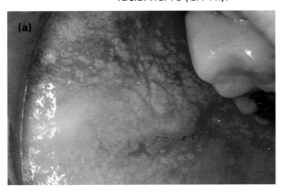

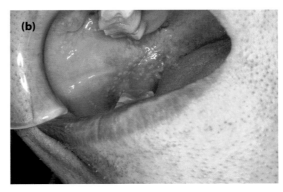

Figure 1.7 (a and b). Fordyce spots of the buccal mucosa.

(a) Reproduced from *Diagnosis and Management of Oral Lesions and Conditions: A resource handbook for the clinician;* Eds: CA Migliorati and FS Panagakos (http://dx.doi.org/10.5772/57597) under CC BY 3.0 licence. © 2014 InTech. (b) Reproduced with permission from Professor Nagamani Narayana, University of Nebraska Medical Centre, NE, USA.

1.3.3 Anatomic variations

Fordyce spots (see *Section 5.3.1*) of buccal mucosa (see *Fig. 1.7*).

1.4 The tongue and the floor of the mouth

The tongue is a muscle divided into anterior two-thirds (the oral tongue) and posterior one-third (the base of the tongue) (see *Fig. 1.8*).

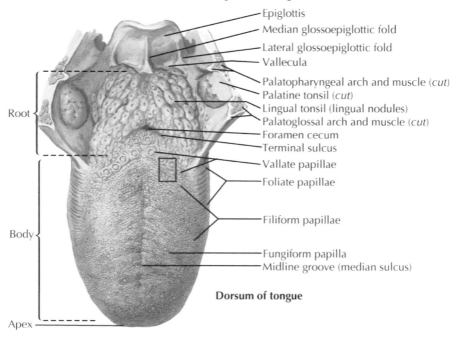

Figure 1.8. Anatomical features of the dorsum of the tongue.

Reproduced with permission from *Pocket Dentistry* (Chapter 14; www.pocketdentistry.com).

- The terminal sulcus is a V-shaped groove that runs laterally and anteriorly from a small central pit (the foramen cecum) and forms the boundary between the anterior two-thirds and the posterior one-third of the tongue.
- The lingual frenulum joins the centre of the ventral surface of the tongue to the floor of the mouth.
- The sublingual caruncle is a fold of tissue on either side of the lingual frenulum.
- Each sublingual caruncle contains an orifice for the submandibular salivary gland duct (Wharton duct).
- Folds of sublingual tissue run from the sublingual caruncles posteriorly toward the base of the tongue. These contain multiple small ducts from the sublingual salivary gland that drain into the floor of the mouth.

1.4.1 Glossal papillae

- Eight to twelve prominent dome-shaped vallate or circumvallate papillae separate the anterior two-thirds of the dorsal tongue from its posterior one-third.

- Many cone-shaped filiform papillae and fewer, more peripheral, mushroom-shaped fungiform papillae are located on the anterior two-thirds of the dorsum of the tongue.
- The vallate and fungiform papillae contain taste buds.

1.4.2   Vascular supply

- The lingual artery, a branch of the external carotid artery, provides most of the tongue's blood supply.
- Tortuous, purple-coloured lingual veins drain both sides of the lingual frenulum and may become more apparent with age (see *Fig. 1.9*).

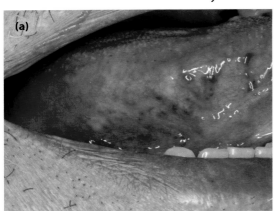 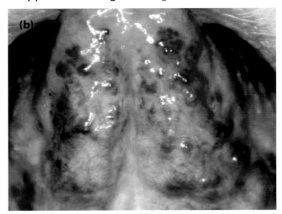

Figure 1.9 (a and b). Lingual varicosities. Tortuous, purple-coloured dilated lingual veins in an older individual.

(b) Reproduced from *Diagnosis and Management of Oral Lesions and Conditions: A resource handbook for the clinician;* Eds: CA Migliorati and FS Panagakos (http://dx.doi.org/10.5772/57597) under CC BY 3.0 licence. © 2014 InTech.

1.4.3   Innervation

- Motor innervation of the intrinsic and extrinsic muscles of the tongue is via the hypoglossal nerve (CN XII), except for the palatoglossus muscle, which is innervated by the vagus nerve (CN X).
- General sensory innervation to the anterior two-thirds of the tongue is via the lingual nerve, a branch of the mandibular branch of the trigeminal nerve (CN V3).
- Taste in the anterior two-thirds of the tongue is via the chorda tympani nerve, a branch of the facial nerve (CN VII).
- General sensory innervation and taste to the posterior one-third of the tongue are via the glossopharyngeal nerve (CN IX).
- General sensory innervation and taste to the epiglottic region of the tongue are via the internal laryngeal branch of the vagus nerve (CN X).

1.4.4   Anatomic variations

The plicated tongue, also known as a fissured tongue or lingua plicata, is characterized by longitudinal crevices in the midline (see *Fig 1.10a*) or extending from the midline to the sides of the tongue (see *Fig. 1.10b*). Although it is often

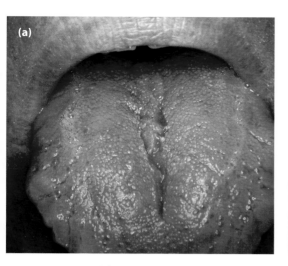
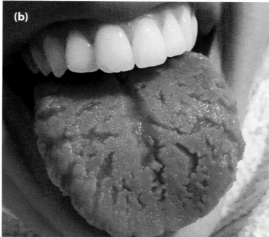

Figure 1.10 (a and b). Plicated tongue (fissured tongue). (a) A longitudinal crevice in the midline; (b) fissures extending from the midline to the sides of the tongue.

(b) Reproduced from Wikimedia Commons under a CC BY_SA 4.0 licence (image by Laila – own work; https://commons.wikimedia.org/w/index.php?curid=43208530.

not associated with other conditions, it is common in patients with trisomy 21 syndrome and orofacial granulomatosis (see *Section 7.3.2* for further details).
- Although usually asymptomatic, a plicated tongue may become sore due to food particles lodging in the fissures. Remind the patient to keep their tongue clean.
- Foliate papillae. These are leaf-like vertical folds and grooves on the posterolateral borders of the tongue (see *Figs 1.8* and *1.11*).

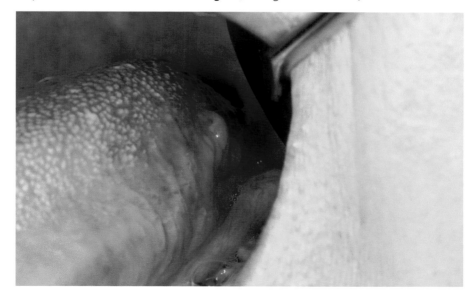

Figure 1.11. Foliate papillae. Note the leaf-like structures on the lateroventral surface of the tongue.

1.5   The hard palate, soft palate, and uvula

The palate is composed of the hard palate, soft palate, and uvula. The palatal mucosa is pink and tightly attached to the mucoperiosteum.

1.5.1   Hard palate

- The anterior hard palate has rugae (transverse ridges) on either side of the median incisive papilla.
- The posterior hard palate includes several minor salivary glands.
- The underlying bony structure of the hard palate comprises palatine processes of the maxilla and the horizontal plates of the palatine bones.
- The main foramina in the hard palate are the incisive canal in the anterior midline, which transmits the nasopalatine nerve; the greater palatine foramen medial to the third molar tooth, which transmits the greater palatine nerve and vessels; and the lesser palatine foramen in the pyramidal process of the palatine bone, which transmits the lesser palatine nerve.

1.5.2   Soft palate

- The soft palate is posterior to the hard palate.
- The posterior border of the soft palate is free and has a central process – the uvula.
- Two arches bind the palate to the tongue and pharynx: the palatoglossal arches anteriorly and the palatopharyngeal arches posteriorly. Between these two arches lie the palatine tonsils.
- The muscles in the soft palate are tensor veli palatini, levator veli palatini, palatoglossus, palatopharyngeus, and musculus uvulae.

1.5.3   Vascular supply

- The palate receives arterial supply primarily from the greater palatine arteries, which run anteriorly from the greater palatine foramen.
- Venous drainage is into the pterygoid venous plexus.

1.5.4   Innervation

- Sensory innervation to the palate is via the maxillary branch of the trigeminal nerve (CN V).
- The greater palatine nerve innervates most of the glandular structures of the hard palate.
- The nasopalatine nerve innervates the mucous membrane of the anterior hard palate.
- The lesser palatine nerves innervate the soft palate.
- The medial pterygoid nerve (a branch of CN V3) innervates tensor veli palatini.
- The pharyngeal branch of the vagus nerve (CN X) innervates the other muscles.

1.6 Maxilla and the mandible

1.6.1 Maxilla

The maxillae are a pair of symmetrical bones joined at the midline. Each maxilla contains a maxillary sinus and bears the maxillary tooth-bearing alveolar processes.

- The maxilla has anterior, infratemporal, orbital, and nasal surfaces and zygomatic, frontal, and palatine processes.
- The maxilla articulates with frontal, ethmoid, nasal, zygomatic, lacrimal, middle nasal concha, inferior nasal concha, palatine, and vomer bones.
- The palatine process forms the anterior three-quarters of the hard palate. It contains two posterolateral grooves that transmit the greater palatine vessels and nerves, incisive fossa behind the incisor teeth, intermaxillary suture, and two lateral incisive canals.

1.6.2 Mandible

The mandible is a single bone, and each side articulates with the temporal bone at the temporomandibular joint.

- The body of the mandible is curved, with two surfaces and two borders. The mandibular symphysis is in the midline.
- The mental foramen is inferior to the second premolar tooth on the external surface of each side of the mandible.
- The internal surface of the mandible has mental spines to attach to the geniohyoid and genioglossus muscles and the mylohyoid line to attach to the mylohyoid muscle.
- The medial surface of the ramus includes the mandibular foramen, the opening of the mandibular canal, and the lingula, a sharp ridge in front of the mandibular canal, to attach the sphenomandibular ligament.

1.6.3 Anatomic variations

- Exostosis is an extra bony growth that extends outwards from an existing bone. Torus palatinus is a solitary or lobulated exostosis in the midline of the palate (see *Fig. 1.12*).

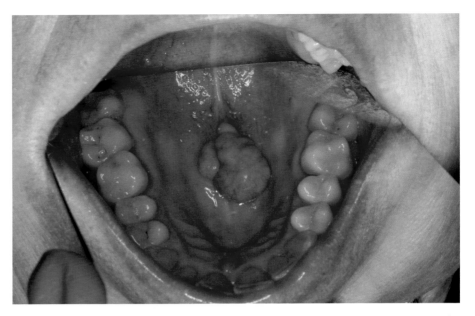

Figure 1.12. Torus palatinus. Note the lobulated exostosis on the midline of the palate.

- Torus mandibularis is an exostosis in the lingual alveolus above the attachment of mylohyoid muscle in the premolar region of the mandible (see *Fig. 1.13*).
- Occasionally exostoses on the maxillary facial surfaces occur (see *Fig. 1.14*).

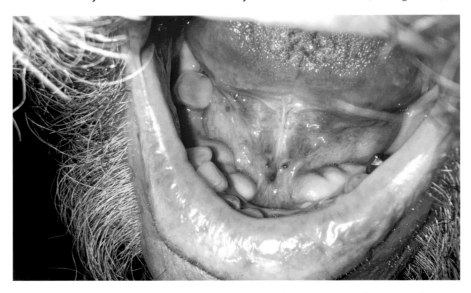

Figure 1.13. Torus mandibularis. Note bilateral exostoses in the premolar region on the lingual surface of the mandible.

Reproduced from Health NZ – Waikato (www.waikatodhb.health.nz) with permission.

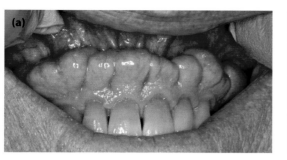
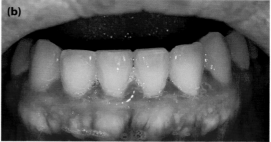

Figure 1.14 (a and b). Exostoses in the (a) anterior maxillary region and (b) mandibular region.

(a) Reproduced with permission from Professor Nagamani Narayana, University of Nebraska Medical Centre, NE USA. (b) Reproduced from Health NZ – Waikato (www.waikatodhb.health.nz) with permission.

- Exostoses and tori are occasionally subjected to trauma which may cause mucosal ulceration or infection.
- It may be necessary to remove exostoses and tori surgically to fabricate mandibular dentures.

1.7 Temporomandibular joint

The temporomandibular joint (TMJ) is formed by the insertion of the mandibular condyle into the glenoid fossa of the temporal bone. It is a complex synovial system comprising two joints separated by the articular disc.
- The TMJ includes the four primary muscles of mastication: the masseter, temporalis, medial, and lateral pterygoid muscles.
- The TMJ includes three extracapsular ligaments. The lateral ligament runs from the beginning of the articular tubule to the mandibular neck to prevent posterior dislocation of the joint. The sphenomandibular ligament originates from the sphenoid spine and attaches to the mandible. The stylomandibular ligament supports the weight of the jaw along with the facial muscles.

1.7.1 Innervation

Sensory innervation to the TMJ comes from the third division of the trigeminal nerve (CN V3), including the auriculotemporal and masseteric nerves.

1.8 Maxillary sinuses

The maxillary sinuses are the largest of the paranasal sinuses. They drain into the nasal cavity at the hiatus semilunaris under the frontal sinus opening.

1.8.1 Vascular supply

The maxillary sinus blood supply comes from branches of the maxillary artery, the posterior superior alveolar artery, the infraorbital artery, and the descending palatine artery.

1.8.2 Innervation

Innervation of the maxillary sinuses is via the maxillary nerve (CN V2).

1.9 Lymph nodes

The lymph nodes of the head include facial, occipital, post-auricular, pre-auricular, parotid, submental, and submandibular nodes.

- Submental nodes collect lymph from the central lower lip, the floor of the mouth, and the apex of the tongue.
- Submandibular nodes collect lymph from the cheeks, the lateral aspects of the nose, the upper lip, lateral parts of the lower lip, gums, the anterior tongue, and the submental and facial lymph nodes.
- The superficial anterior cervical and the posterior lateral superficial cervical lymph nodes in the neck collect lymph from the neck's superficial anterior and posterior surfaces.
- The superior and inferior deep cervical groups of lymph nodes in the neck collect lymph from the head and neck directly or indirectly via the superficial lymph nodes.

1.9.1 Lymphoid tissue

Reddish lymphoid tissue or tonsils may occur anywhere within the oral cavity, especially within the Waldeyer ring, which includes the oropharynx, lateral tongue (see *Fig. 1.15*), soft palate, and the floor of the mouth.

- The palatine tonsils are in the tonsillar fauces between the palatoglossal and palatopharyngeal folds.
- The pharyngeal tonsils are also known as adenoids.
- Lingual tonsils cover the dorsal surface of the base of the posterior tongue extending from the circumvallate papillae to the root of the epiglottis (see *Fig. 1.8*). They are best examined with the tongue protruded (see *Fig. 1.15*).

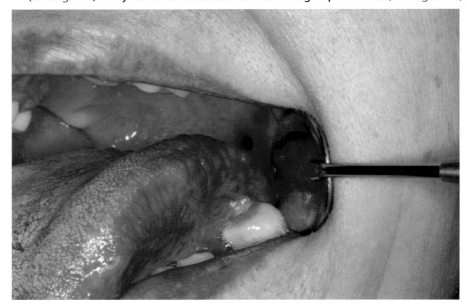

Figure 1.15. Lingual tonsil on the dorsolateral surface of the tongue.

- Oral lymphoid aggregates may become hyperplastic, inflamed and tender with an upper respiratory viral or bacterial infection. Inflammatory episodes are typically self-limiting or resolve after the management of the infection (see *Fig. 1.16*). Often these lymphoid aggregates mimic cancerous growth.

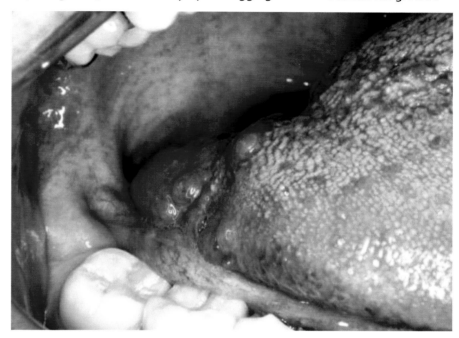

Figure 1.16. Lymphoid aggregate on the lateroventral surface of the tongue.

Reproduced from *Diagnosis and Management of Oral Lesions and Conditions: A resource handbook for the clinician;* Eds: CA Migliorati and FS Panagakos (http://dx.doi.org/10.5772/57597) under CC BY 3.0 licence. © 2014 InTech.

CHAPTER 2

DIAGNOSTIC PROCEDURES FOR DISEASES OF THE ORAL MUCOSA

2.1 Introduction

The definitive diagnosis of an oral disease often depends on a combination of the following:
- The clinical findings and differential diagnosis
- Adjunctive clinic-based procedures
- The results of biopsy/histopathology
- Laboratory tests
- Diagnostic imaging.

Clinical and laboratory-based diagnostic procedures relevant to diagnosing oral mucosal disease are briefly described in this chapter.

2.2 Clinical evaluation

2.2.1 Dermoscopy

The clinical examination of the oral mucosa needs good lighting and magnification. A hand-held dermatoscope is used to evaluate the overall pattern, local structures, colours, and vascularity of the skin (dermoscopy) and oral inflammatory mucosal lesions and tumours (mucoscopy), improving the accuracy of diagnosis by trained observers compared with visual inspection alone. Polarized devices help visualize subepithelial components. Photographs of the mucoscopy views are referred to as digital mucoscopy and are useful for the clinical record, follow-up, and referral.

2.2.2 Clinical photography

Clinical photographs intended for documentation are also used for:
- referral, particularly for remote consultation or case-sharing
- the health professional to gain experience
- clinicopathological correlation
- teaching and publication
- clinical audit and research
- medico-legal and insurance purposes.

It is best to obtain written consent for photography, establishing which purposes (clinical, education, publication, audit, research, and other) the patient agrees to.

Photographs of the oral lesions/conditions are performed:
- on presentation
- before and after a diagnostic or therapeutic procedure
- at follow-up.

Although images of excellent quality can be captured using the latest model of smartphone, intraoral photography can be challenging without the assistance of a professional medical photographer and specialist equipment such as:
- digital single-lens reflex camera with macro lens and ring/twin flash
- a cheek retractor (T- or C-shaped)
- an intraoral mirror with a defogger
- flexible contraster.

Follow-up images should aim to use similar camera settings for consistency.

2.2.3   Diascopy

Diascopy uses pressure from transparent glass or plastic to see a lesion blanch. It is used to see if red or purple is due to erythema or purpura or to exclude blood flow in a pigmented or scaly lesion.

2.2.4   The Nikolsky sign

In a blistering disease, elicit the Nikolsky sign by applying tangential/lateral pressure by a thumb or finger in the perilesional skin or mucous membrane, which dislodges the upper layers of the epidermis from the lower layers.
- It differentiates intraepidermal blisters, which extend on lateral pressure, from subepidermal blisters, which do not.
- The Nikolsky sign is positive in conditions such as pemphigus, toxic epidermal necrolysis, and staphylococcal scalded skin syndrome (see *Sections 7.4.3, 4.6.8, and 6.3.1*, respectively).

2.2.5   *In vivo* toluidine blue staining

Toluidine blue is a thiazine metachromatic dye that binds with DNA, revealing the cell nucleus. It selectively stains potentially malignant and malignant mucosal lesions. It also stains the normal papillae on the dorsum of the tongue, the pores of seromucinous glands in the hard palate, and inflammatory lesions.

Toluidine blue staining can be used to:
- determine the extent of a potentially malignant lesion
- assess its margins
- select the site for the biopsy.

A positive test must be followed by tissue biopsy and histopathological evaluation.

2.2.6   Samples for microbial culture

Microbial culture is often unnecessary, as an infection is usually apparent clinically (for more, see *Chapter 6*). The following methods confirm severe or resistant infection (for example, methicillin-resistant *Staphylococcus aureus*, mixed infection of candida and staphylococci in angular cheilitis or acute necrotizing gingivitis). Gram staining is no longer routinely performed. Before transport, store the specimen at refrigerator temperature.

- Aspirated pus or a sample of infected tissue can be sent in a pot for culture.
- A bacterial swab (Amies gel) can reveal pathogenic bacteria and yeasts in the mucosa or the fitting surface of a denture.
- An oral rinse can quantitatively assess candida in oral microflora.
- A viral swab (viral transport medium) identifies herpes simplex virus (HSV), varicella-zoster virus (VZV), or enterovirus by polymerase chain reaction (PCR) (see *Sections 6.2.1, 6.2.2,* and *6.2.5*, respectively).
- Specialized swabs collect samples for sexually transmitted infections (STIs) such as gonorrhoea (see *Section 6.3.4*).

The laboratory can also conduct susceptibility testing by exposing a standardized concentration of the cultured bacteria, fungus, or virus to specific concentrations of antimicrobial drugs.

2.2.7 Smear for cytology

Exfoliative cytology is a rapid screening test. Results are inferior to biopsy, with varying reports of sensitivity and specificity.

The Tzanck test, also known as the Tzanck smear, is undertaken by scraping the base of an ulcer or blister, smearing the tissue onto a glass slide, air drying, and applying a fixative. The smear is stained with Giemsa or toluidine blue; an experienced histopathologist or cytologist should confirm the findings.

- Tzanck cells are acantholytic round cells characteristically found in pemphigus vulgaris.
- Multinucleated giant cells indicate herpes simplex or varicella-zoster (see *Sections 6.2.1* and *6.2.2*).

Brush cytology is used to distinguish potentially malignant disorders.
- Cytology specimens are usually stained with haematoxylin–eosin.
- They must be examined by an oral pathologist experienced in cytology.

2.2.8 Biopsy for histopathology

Soft tissue biopsy is performed on a wide range of oral mucosal lesions (see *Chapter 10* for more; look also for specific topics in the index).
- Incisional or punch biopsy samples a large lesion (usually >1cm in diameter).
- Excisional biopsy is used to surgically excise a small lesion or a confirmed malignancy of any size.
- Scalpel blade, biopsy punch, cutting laser, or electrosurgical methods are used.

2.2.9 Fine-needle aspiration

Fine-needle aspiration (FNA) is a specialist technique for collecting a specimen from a major salivary gland, an enlarged lymph node, or a lump in the neck when suspicious of malignancy.

2.3 Laboratory processes

2.3.1 Histopathology

Histopathology is the microscopic diagnosis of inflammatory disease and suspected malignancy.

The tissue specimen undergoes five stages of preparation before the slides are viewed by a histopathologist.
1. Formalin fixation
2. Processing
3. Embedding
4. Sectioning
5. Staining, primarily haematoxylin–eosin.

Different stains and tests may be applied to the specimen or slides when the initial diagnosis is unclear.

A frozen section can be examined for immediate diagnosis of epithelial malignancy during a surgical procedure, but it is less accurate than the evaluation of paraffin-embedded tissue.

2.3.2 Immunofluorescent and immunohistochemical staining

Immunofluorescence reveals an antigen or antibody and investigates an autoimmune bullous disorder (see the named topics in *Chapter 7*).

Direct immunofluorescence (DIF)

The antigen in the freshly frozen, unfixed biopsy sample reacts directly with a fluorescein-conjugated antibody. DIF is positive in:
- mucosal pemphigus
- bullous pemphigoid
- benign mucous membrane pemphigoid
- dermatitis herpetiformis
- lupus erythematosus
- lichen planus
- some forms of vasculitis.

Indirect immunofluorescence (IIF)

IIF identifies specific antibodies circulating in the patient's plasma. IIF is positive in:
- mucosal pemphigus
- bullous pemphigoid
- systemic lupus erythematosus
- primary syphilis (see *Section 6.3.6*).

Immunohistochemistry

Immunohistochemistry (IHC) uses an antibody to label a protein and then a secondary antibody to reveal it by staining the protein brown or showing a fluorescence pattern.

IHC stains are often used on paraffin-fixed or frozen tissue to classify a tumour. Tissue-specific markers include epithelial, lymphoid, and vascular stains. There are numerous options.

2.3.3   Molecular pathology

Molecular pathology applies the principles of basic molecular biology to the investigation of human diseases, including:
- screening for genetic abnormalities (see *Chapter 5*)
- identifying bacteria and viruses (see *Chapter 6*).

Polymerase chain reaction (PCR)

PCR is a highly specific and sensitive technique by which minute quantities of specific DNA or RNA segments are enzymatically amplified to detect various genetic and microbial nucleic acids. PCR is most used for oral disease in the diagnosis of viral infection (see *Chapter 6*).

In situ hybridization and fluorescent *in situ* hybridization

In situ hybridization (ISH) or fluorescent *in situ* hybridization (FISH) is used to detect specific chromosomal changes (such as translocations) found in:
- viral infections including cytomegalovirus, Epstein–Barr virus (EBV), human papillomavirus (HPV) type 16 and intracellular human herpesvirus 8 (see *Chapter 6*)
- salivary tumours (see *Chapter 10*).

2.3.4   Haematology

Oral manifestations can be the result of or associated with haematological disorders, such as:
- anaemia
- bleeding disorders
- clotting disorders
- leukaemia.

Standard haematological tests include:
- complete blood count (CBC)
- international normalized ratio (INR) in a patient on an anticoagulant
- coagulation tests.

2.3.5   Biochemistry

Biochemical investigations are not commonly needed in the diagnosis of oral mucosal lesions. However, they may be ordered for an underlying systemic disease or to monitor treatment. Some examples include:
- renal function tests (e.g. renal failure or haemodialysis patients who also present with oral mucosal disease)
- liver function tests (e.g. for patients with suspected hepatitis, cirrhosis or alcohol-related disorders presenting with oral mucosal disease)

- glycosylated haemoglobin (HbA1c) and glucose (e.g. for patients with suspected or uncontrolled diabetes presenting with oral mucosal disease or complications)
- serum calcium, phosphorus (e.g. for patients with calcium/phosphorus metabolism disorders presenting with oral mucosal disease)
- uric acid (e.g. for patients presenting with oral mucosal complications of cancer chemotherapy or kidney disease)
- electrolytes such as sodium, potassium, and chloride (e.g. for patients suspected of renal disease presenting with oral mucosal disease).

2.3.6 Immunology/serology

Immunological investigations in oral dermatology may be requested in patients with:
- potential viral infections (see *Chapter 6*), including serology of herpes simplex (rarely needed), varicella-zoster (if contemplating immune-suppressing drugs), herpangina, enteroviral stomatitis, and human immunodeficiency virus (HIV)
- syphilis (see *Section 6.3.6*)
- autoimmune disorders such as lupus erythematosus or Sjögren syndrome (see *Chapter 7*).

2.3.7 Salivary diagnostic tests

Like the serum, saliva contains hormones, antibodies, growth factors, enzymes, microbes, and their products.

Salivary diagnostic tests are non-invasive, accurate, easy to use, and cost-effective.

Salivary biomarkers may be used to diagnose a range of diseases and infections. Some examples include testing saliva for:
- SARS-CoV-2 virus (the cause of Covid-19) by PCR or rapid antigen testing
- pathogens that contribute to periodontitis
- genetic profiling
- oral cancer screening by detection of HPV
- drug detection
- HIV infection
- proteomics in Sjögren syndrome
- pH and electrolyte changes in cystic fibrosis
- biomarkers associated with cardiovascular diseases.

2.4 Diagnostic imaging

2.4.1 Diagnostic imaging of oral soft tissues

Conventional radiographs, computerized tomography (CT), ultrasound, magnetic resonance imaging (MRI), and positron emission tomography (PET) examinations are commonly employed in the preoperative staging of head and neck cancer to determine:

- the extent or progression of the tumour
- infiltration of large vessels
- the presence of bone marrow and lymph node metastasis.

Clinical imaging may also be used to investigate oral infection or inflammatory disease.

2.4.2   Sialography

Sialography is a radiographic technique used to demonstrate the salivary duct network and glandular architecture.
- A radiopaque dye (contrast medium) is injected into the salivary duct.
- Radiographs of the area are taken within 2–4 minutes of injecting the dye.
- In Sjögren syndrome, sialography of the parotid gland typically shows a snowstorm appearance characteristic of sialectasia.

Salivary gland ultrasonography can yield valuable information on salivary gland stones and ductal obstruction.

CHAPTER 3

THE DIFFERENTIAL DIAGNOSIS OF ORAL MUCOSAL LESIONS

This chapter summarizes the key points and classifies oral mucosal lesions depending on their clinical appearance, location, symptoms, and aetiology.

A careful history and clinical examination are necessary to diagnose oral diseases, as a broad spectrum of conditions can have similar characteristics. A histopathological evaluation may be required.

Classification based on the clinical appearance

3.1 White lesions of the oral mucosa

Oral white lesions may be reactive, developmental/genetic, infective, inflammatory, or neoplastic.

3.1.1 Key points

- White lesions appear clinically white because of increased epithelial thickness, abnormal production of surface keratin, deposition of exogenous material, necrosis of surface tissue, lack of vascularity, intraepithelial oedema, submucosal collection of ectopic sebaceous glands, inflammation, and viral or fungal infections.
- Most white lesions are asymptomatic and acquired; a few are congenital, with or without a genetic basis.
- Shades of white may be paper-white, yellowish-white, pale, cloudy, or blanched.
- White lesions may be solitary (focal) or multiple and can occur on any part of the oral mucosa.
- White lesions may be macules, patches, papules, plaques, or nodules with smooth, rough, warty, or corrugated surfaces.
- Keratotic white lesions cannot be wiped off the mucosal surface; superficial white lesions can be wiped with gauze or cotton swabs.
- Some white lesions may be associated with red or pigmented lesions or backgrounds.
- Their morphological features provide clues to diagnosis. For example:
  - multiple curd-like white papules and plaques due to *Candida albicans*
  - lace-like white striations, papules, and plaques in lichen planus
  - diffuse filmy whitish-grey areas of the buccal mucosa in leukoedema
  - specific dermoscopic features.

Table 3.1 Aetiological classification of oral white lesions

Reactions to local and exogenous factors (see *Chapter 4*)

• Materia alba
• Hairy tongue
• Mucosal burn
  ◦ thermal burn
  ◦ chemical burn
  ◦ radiation mucositis
• Frictional keratoses
  ◦ alveolar ridge keratosis
  ◦ linea alba
  ◦ chronic cheek biting
  ◦ excessive tooth brushing
• Effects of tobacco
  ◦ smokeless tobacco keratosis
  ◦ leukokeratosis nicotina palati
• Effects of areca nut
  ◦ oral submucous fibrosis

Developmental or genetic origin (see *Chapter 5*)

• Non-hereditary
  ◦ Fordyce spots
  ◦ leukoedema
• Hereditary
  ◦ white sponge naevus
  ◦ Darier disease
  ◦ dyskeratosis congenita
  ◦ hereditary benign intraepithelial dyskeratosis
  ◦ pachyonychia congenita

Infections (see *Chapter 6*)

• Candida infection
  ◦ pseudomembranous candidosis
  ◦ chronic hyperplastic candidosis
  ◦ chronic mucocutaneous candidosis
• Viral infection
  ◦ EBV: hairy leukoplakia
  ◦ HPV: oral warts
  ◦ molluscum contagiosum
• Bacterial infection
  ◦ syphilitic leukoplakia

Inflammatory diseases and conditions (see *Chapter 7*)

• Lichenoid inflammation
  ◦ lichen planus
  ◦ oral lichenoid reaction
  ◦ graft-versus-host disease
  ◦ lupus erythematosus

Neoplastic lesions: benign, potentially malignant, malignant (see *Chapter 10*)

• A potentially malignant lesion
  ◦ actinic keratosis of the lip
  ◦ leukoplakia
  ◦ proliferative verrucous leukoplakia
  ◦ reverse smoker's palate
• A malignant lesion
  ◦ squamous cell carcinoma
  ◦ verrucous carcinoma

3.2 Red and purple lesions of the oral mucosa

Oral red and purple lesions may be reactive, developmental/genetic, infective, inflammatory, non-inflammatory, or neoplastic.

3.2.1 Key points

- Red and purple lesions are common in the mouth.
- A red or purple lesion may be caused by trauma, infection, immune disorder, a haematological disorder, vascular malformation, a potentially malignant disorder, or neoplasia.
- Lesions may be solitary (focal) or multiple and can occur on any part of the oral mucosa.
- Red and purple lesions may present as macules, patches, papules, plaques, or nodules.
- They may have a smooth, rough, warty, or corrugated surface.

Table 3.2 Aetiological classification of oral red and purple lesions

Reactions to local or exogenous factors (see *Chapter 4*)

• Extravascular blood
• Traumatic oral haemorrhagic bulla
• Mucosal burn
  ◦ thermal burn
  ◦ cold burn
  ◦ chemical burn

- Chemotherapy-induced mucositis
- Radiation-induced mucositis
- Contact stomatitis
- Hormone-related gingivitis (e.g. pregnancy)
- Pyogenic granuloma
- Erythema multiforme, Stevens–Johnson syndrome / toxic epidermal necrolysis

Developmental or genetic origin (see *Chapter 5*)

- Vascular malformation
- Port wine stain
- Lymphatic malformation
- Hereditary haemorrhagic telangiectasia
- Venous lake

Oral infections (see *Chapter 6*)

- Candida
  ◦ erythematous candidosis
  ◦ median rhomboid glossitis
  ◦ linear gingival erythema (in patients with HIV infection)
- Viral infection
  ◦ infectious mononucleosis
- Bacterial infection
  ◦ gonococcal stomatitis
  ◦ strawberry tongue due to scarlet fever
- Mixed infection
  ◦ angular cheilitis
  ◦ denture stomatitis

Inflammatory diseases and conditions (see *Chapter 7*)

- Lichenoid inflammation
  ◦ lichen planus
  ◦ oral lichenoid reaction
  ◦ lupus erythematosus
  ◦ desquamative gingivitis, graft-versus-host disease
- Granulomatous inflammation
  ◦ granulomatous gingivitis
  ◦ granulomatosis with polyangiitis
- Geographic tongue
- Plasma cell gingivitis / cheilitis
- Vasculitis
  ◦ small vessel vasculitis
  ◦ giant cell vasculitis

Non-inflammatory diseases and conditions (see *Chapter 8*)

• Nutritional and haematological disease
    ◦ atrophic glossitis
    ◦ thrombocytopenic purpura
    ◦ leukaemia

Systemic diseases (see *Chapter 9*)
• Angioedema • Petechiae associated with vasculitis
Neoplastic lesions: benign, potentially malignant, malignant (see *Chapter 10*)

• Non-malignant lesion
    ◦ infantile proliferative haemangioma
• Potentially malignant lesion
    ◦ erythroplakia
    ◦ reverse smoker's palate
• Malignant lesion
    ◦ Kaposi sarcoma

3.3 Pigmented lesions of the oral mucosa

An oral pigmented lesion may include any localized or diffuse black, brown, or dark blue area. It may be due to melanocytic proliferation, increased melanin production by a usual number of melanocytes, or the deposition of endogenous or exogenous pigment or foreign material.

3.3.1 Key points

- Mucosal pigmented lesions may be black, brown, or dark blue macules, or plaques, or present as diffuse pigmentation of endogenous or exogenous origin.
- Endogenous pigment (melanin) is produced by melanocytes within the basal layer of the lining epithelia.
- Normal physiological variations in mucosal colour observed in many races are due to increased melanin production rather than an increased number of melanocytes.
- Melanocytic naevi are hamartomas in which the proliferation of melanocytic naevus cells in mucosal lesions is mainly in the lamina propria.
- Focal exogenous pigmentation can be due to an accidental amalgam tattoo or deliberate cosmetic tattoo using a variety of pigments.
- Diffuse pigmentation can be due to the deposition of heavy metals or increased melanin production caused by various drugs.

Table 3.3 Aetiological classification of oral pigmented lesions

Reactions to local and exogenous factors (see *Chapter 4*)
• Hairy tongue • Amalgam tattoo • Cosmetic tattoo • Drug-induced pigmentation • Postinflammatory pigmentation • Heavy metal pigmentation • Smoker's melanosis • Acanthosis nigricans
Developmental or genetic origin (see *Chapter 5*)
• Laugier–Hunziker syndrome • McCune–Albright syndrome • Peutz–Jeghers syndrome
Infections (see *Chapter 6*)
• Viral infection   ◦ melanotic hyperpigmentation (HIV infection)
Non-inflammatory (see *Chapter 8*)
• Racial (physiological) pigmentation • Oral melanotic macule • Addison disease
Neoplastic lesions: benign, potentially malignant, malignant (see *Chapter 10*)

• Benign lesion
   ◦ melanocytic naevus
   ◦ neuroectodermal tumour of infancy
• Malignant lesion
   ◦ melanoma
   ◦ metastasis

3.4 Papillary and verrucous lesions of the oral mucosa

Verrucopapillary oral cavity lesions may be reactive, benign, potentially malignant, or malignant.

3.4.1 Key points

- Verrucopapillary lesions present with exophytic, pointed, finger-like pedunculated projections (papillary lesions) or blunt, sessile elevations (papular and polypoid lesions).
- Most of them are white due to keratinization.
- Most verrucopapillary lesions are associated with human papillomavirus (HPV).

- Some are potentially malignant or are frankly malignant at presentation.
- Verrucopapillary lesions often pose a diagnostic challenge, and biopsy is essential for diagnosis.

Table 3.4 Aetiological classification of papillary and verrucous lesions of the oral mucosa

Reactions to local or exogenous factors (see *Chapter 4*)
• Oral verruciform xanthoma • Oral papillary hyperplasia • Oral acanthosis nigricans • Oral verrucous hyperplasia
Developmental or genetic origin (see *Chapter 5*)
• Fordyce spots • Cobblestone oral papules in Darier disease • Mucosal neuromas in multiple endocrine neoplasia type 2B • Fibroepithelial papules and papillomatosis in Cowden syndrome • Dental deformities in focal dermal hypoplasia
Infections (see *Chapter 6*)

• Viral infection – HPV
  ◦ squamous papilloma
  ◦ verruca vulgaris
  ◦ condyloma acuminatum
  ◦ multifocal epithelial hyperplasia

Inflammatory diseases and conditions (see *Chapter 7*)
• Oral Crohn disease
Neoplastic lesions: benign, potentially malignant, malignant (see *Chapter 10*)

• Benign
  ◦ sialadenoma papilliferum
• Potentially malignant
  ◦ proliferative verrucous leukoplakia
• Malignant
  ◦ verrucous carcinoma (carcinoma cuniculatum)

3.5   Non-neoplastic oral soft tissue swellings

Non-neoplastic oral soft tissue swellings in the mouth can be due to traumatic, inflammatory, hereditary, developmental, infectious, or hormonal causes.

See also benign neoplastic lesions (*Chapter 10*): melanocytic naevus (*Section 10.1.1*), neurofibroma (*Section 10.1.4*), lipoma (*Section 10.1.3*), schwannoma (*Section 10.1.4*), and pleomorphic adenoma (*Section 10.2.1*).

3.5.1 Key points

- Oral soft tissue swellings may be derived from mucosal epithelium, connective tissue, or minor salivary glands.
- Acute swelling usually has a traumatic, inflammatory, or infectious cause and is painful and tender.
- Chronic swelling may have a developmental or traumatic cause and is usually painless.
- Developmental swellings mostly occur early in life.
- Localized swellings are pedunculated or sessile; firm, fibrous, fluid-filled; round, oval, dome-shaped; with a papillary or verrucous surface.
- Oral soft tissue swellings may be the same colour as the surrounding mucosa or red, blue, or purple.
- Fibrous lumps are most often caused by chronic irritation.

Table 3.5 Aetiological classification of non-neoplastic oral soft tissue swellings

Reactions to local or exogenous factors (see *Chapter 4*)
<ul><li>Traumatic haemorrhagic bulla</li><li>Traumatic neuroma</li><li>Fibroepithelial polyp</li><li>Giant cell epulis</li><li>Denture-induced gingival hyperplasia</li><li>Peripheral ossifying fibroma</li></ul>
Developmental or genetic origin (see *Chapter 5*)
<ul><li>Hereditary gingival fibromatosis</li></ul>
Infections (see *Chapter 6*)
<ul><li>Bacteria or mixed infection<ul><li>gingival abscess</li><li>periodontal abscess</li></ul></li></ul>
Inflammatory diseases and conditions (see *Chapter 7*)
<ul><li>Pyogenic granuloma, including pregnancy tumour (vascular epulis)</li><li>Cheilitis glandularis</li><li>Orofacial granulomatosis, including granulomatous cheilitis</li></ul>
Non-inflammatory diseases and conditions (see *Chapter 8*)
<ul><li>Oral mucinosis</li><li>Cyst<ul><li>mucus extravasation cyst (mucocele, ranula)</li><li>mucus retention cyst</li><li>gingival cyst</li><li>eruption cyst</li><li>dermoid and epidermoid cyst</li></ul></li></ul>

> ◦ lymphoepithelial cyst
> ◦ nasolabial cyst
> ◦ thyroglossal duct cyst
>
> **Systemic diseases** (see *Chapter 9*)
>
> - Angioedema
> - Drug-induced gingival hyperplasia
> - Gingival enlargement in leukaemia

3.6 Oral vesicles and bullae

Oral vesicles and bullae may be reactive, developmental/genetic, infective, or inflammatory.

See also oral erosions and ulcers (*Section 3.7*).

3.6.1 Key points

- A vesicle has a diameter of <5mm; a bulla is larger.
- A vesiculobullous disease may be localized or affect multiple sites.
- Blistering due to an immunological or infectious cause tends to be widespread and painful.
- Blisters may appear transparent or haemorrhagic.
- Oral mucosal vesicles often rupture, leaving painful erosions or ulcers.
- A positive Nikolsky sign (expansion of a blister with lateral pressure) demonstrates a loss of coherence between epithelial cells.

Table 3.6 Aetiological classification of oral vesicles and bullae

Reactions to local or exogenous factors (see *Chapter 4*)
<ul><li>Mucosal burn</li><li>Traumatic oral haemorrhagic bulla</li><li>Erythema multiforme</li><li>Stevens–Johnson syndrome / toxic epidermal necrolysis</li></ul>
Developmental or genetic origin (see *Chapter 5*)
<ul><li>Epidermolysis bullosa</li></ul>
Infections (see *Chapter 6*)
<ul><li>Viral infection<ul><li>herpes simplex</li><li>varicella-zoster infection</li><li>enteroviral infection</li><li>herpangina</li></ul></li><li>Bacterial infection<ul><li>staphylococcal scalded skin syndrome</li></ul></li></ul>

Inflammatory diseases and conditions (see *Chapter 7*)

- Bullous oral lichen planus
- Immunobullous diseases
  - epidermolysis bullosa acquisita
  - bullous pemphigoid
  - pemphigus vulgaris

3.7 Oral erosions and ulcers

Oral erosions and ulcers may be reactive, infective, inflammatory, or neoplastic.

See also oral vesiculobullous lesions (*Section 3.6*).

3.7.1 Key points

- An erosion is characterized by partial loss of the epithelium, with an intact basement membrane.
- An ulcer is characterized by full-thickness loss of the epithelium exposing the underlying connective tissue.
- Erosions and ulcers may be localized or affect multiple sites in the oral mucosa.
- They tend to be painful and may affect the patient's ability to eat and speak.

Table 3.7 Aetiological classification of oral erosions and ulcers

---

Reactions to local or exogenous factors (see *Chapter 4*)

- Trauma
  - an iatrogenic injury such as surgery or dental procedure
  - factitial injury
- Mucosal burn
  - thermal burn
  - chemical burn
  - radiation burns
- Drug-induced stomatitis
  - chemotherapy-induced mucositis
  - fixed drug eruption
  - Stevens–Johnson syndrome / toxic epidermal necrolysis
- Contact stomatitis
  - irritant contact stomatitis
  - allergic contact stomatitis
- Erythema multiforme
  - minor
  - major
- Ulcers associated with systemic disease

Infections (see *Chapter 6*)

- Fungal infection
  - candidosis
  - deep mycoses
    - aspergillosis
    - mucormycosis
    - histoplasmosis
    - cryptococcosis
    - blastomycosis
    - paracoccidioidomycosis
- Viral infection
  - herpes simplex
  - varicella-zoster infection
  - herpangina
  - cytomegalovirus
  - HIV infection
- Bacterial infection
  - necrotizing ulcerative gingivitis / periodontitis
  - tuberculosis
  - syphilis

Inflammatory diseases and conditions (see *Chapter 7*)

- Recurrent aphthous stomatitis
  - major
  - minor
- Lichenoid inflammation
  - lichen planus
  - oral lichenoid reaction
  - lupus erythematosus
  - desquamative gingivitis
  - graft-versus-host disease
  - chronic ulcerative stomatitis
- Behçet disease
- Granulomatous inflammation
  - Crohn disease
- Acute febrile neutrophilic dermatosis (Sweet syndrome)
- Periodic fever, aphthous stomatitis, pharyngitis, adenitis (PFAPA)
- Necrotizing sialometaplasia

Systemic diseases (see *Chapter 9*)

- Coeliac disease
- Inflammatory bowel disease
  - Crohn disease
  - ulcerative colitis

> - Granulomatosis with polyangiitis
> - Haematological disease
>   - cyclic neutropenia
>
> **Neoplastic lesions: benign, potentially malignant, malignant** (see *Chapter 10*)
>
> - Malignant lesion
>   - squamous cell carcinoma
>   - lymphoma
>   - leukaemia
>   - sarcoma
>   - salivary gland tumour

Classification of common oral symptoms

Often patients complain of oral symptoms such as dry mouth and halitosis. Key points and aetiological classification of these conditions are given below.

3.8 Dry mouth

A dry mouth is also known as xerostomia. It is a subjective perception affecting 10–46% of the population. A dry mouth may be due to salivary gland hypofunction, in which salivary flow is reduced, and there may be an altered chemical composition of saliva.

3.8.1 Key points

- Symptoms of xerostomia include increased thirst and the need to constantly sip or drink water, difficulty eating and swallowing dry foods, altered sense of taste (dysgeusia), difficulty in wearing dentures, halitosis, a constantly sore mouth (burning mouth syndrome), and a hoarse voice or the inability to speak continuously.
- Xerostomia can increase the risk of dental caries and contribute to periodontal diseases and oral infections such as candidosis.
- Polypharmacy is commonly linked to xerostomia.
- Xerostomia in Sjögren syndrome is associated with increasing dryness of the eyes. Systemic anti-inflammatory and immunosuppressive therapy may be required.
- Profound, often permanent, salivary hypofunction leading to xerostomia is seen in almost all patients after radiotherapy for malignant head and neck tumours. A preventive programme to minimize dental caries is essential, including regular dental visits, dietary and oral hygiene assessment and advice, and topical fluoride.
- Management of xerostomia includes using artificial saliva, oral moisturizing gels, sugar-free lozenges or gums, secretagogue drugs (cevimeline, pilocarpine), chlorhexidine mouthwash, and treatment of candida (nystatin, clotrimazole).

Table 3.8 Aetiological classification of dry mouth

Reactions to local or exogenous factors (see *Chapter 4*)
• Mouth breathing • Drugs: antidepressants, anticholinergics, and antihistamines • Radiotherapy for malignant head and neck tumours
Infections (see *Chapter 6*)
• Dental caries
Inflammatory diseases and conditions (see *Chapter 7*)
• Sjögren syndrome • Parotid disease
Systemic diseases (see *Chapter 9*)
• Diabetes mellitus • Hypothyroidism • Diabetes insipidus

3.9 Halitosis

Halitosis (foetor oris) refers to disagreeable, foul, or unpleasant odours emanating from the mouth.

3.9.1 Key points

- Halitosis affects more than 50% of the general population.
- In 90%, the origin is the oral cavity; in 9%, it is the respiratory, gastrointestinal, or urinary systems, and in 1%, halitosis is caused by diet or drugs.
- Halitosis most often results from the fermentation of food particles by anaerobic Gram-negative bacteria in the mouth. The bacteria degrade organic substrates such as glucose, mucins, peptides, and proteins in saliva, crevicular fluid, soft tissue, and retained debris, and produce odorous compounds.
- Decreased salivary flow and stagnation, and increased salivary pH also cause halitosis.
- One-quarter of those seeking professional advice on bad breath have an exaggerated concern, known as halitophobia or delusional halitosis.
- If halitosis is due to an oral cause, the patient should be referred to a dentist for professional cleaning and treatment of gingival, periodontal disease and dental caries.
- Home oral care involves thorough flossing, tooth brushing, and brushing the tongue with a toothbrush or a tongue scraper. Mouthwash provides only brief benefits.

Table 3.9 Aetiological classification of halitosis

Reactions to local or exogenous factors (see *Chapter 4*)
• Poor oral or denture hygiene • Recent tooth extraction • Smoking • Alcohol • Drugs: anticholinergics • Ingested foods with a volatile component (such as garlic)
Infections (see *Chapter 6*)
• Dental caries • Periodontal disease • Gingivitis • Chronic sinusitis • Chronic caseous tonsillitis
Inflammatory diseases and conditions (see *Chapter 7*)
• Oral ulceration • Decreased salivary flow due to Sjögren syndrome or parotid disease
Systemic diseases (see *Chapter 9*)
• Diabetes mellitus • Renal failure • Depression and obsessive–compulsive disorder

Diseases of specific oral sites

3.10   Diseases affecting the lips – cheilitis

Diseases of the lips are common. Aetiology includes local/exogenous causes, developmental defects, inflammatory and immunological local and systemic diseases, and neoplasms.

Cheilitis, or inflammation of the lips, may be acute or chronic, primarily involving the vermilion zone. Cheilitis may extend to the surrounding skin externally and the labial mucosa inside the mouth.

3.10.1   Key points

- Eczematous cheilitis is due to contact with irritants and allergens or endogenous factors. It is characterized by the loss of plasticity, delayed hypersensitivity, or atopy.
- Angular cheilitis is a moist, fissured, acute or chronic inflammation of the skin and adjacent labial mucosa at the angles of the mouth. It results from saliva and secondary infection with *Candida albicans*, *Staphylococcus aureus*, or both.

- Actinic keratosis (actinic cheilitis) is chronic irregular scaling and inflammation due to sun exposure.
- Drug-induced cheilitis is often due to systemic retinoids, which cause dryness, erythema, scaling, and fissuring of the lips and labial commissures.
- Glandular cheilitis results from inflammation and fibrosis around the salivary glands.
- Granulomatous cheilitis is persistent, non-tender granulomatous inflammation resulting from long-standing oedema and perivascular inflammation of lip and facial tissue.

Table 3.10 Aetiological classification of diseases affecting the lip

Reactions to local or exogenous factors (see *Chapter 4*)
<ul><li>Trauma: physical, mechanical</li><li>Burns: thermal, chemical, radiation</li><li>Contact irritant cheilitis<ul><li>lip licking dermatitis</li><li>chapped lips</li></ul></li><li>Contact allergic cheilitis</li><li>Drug-induced cheilitis</li><li>Mucocele/ranula (see *Chapter 8*)</li></ul>
Developmental or genetic origin (see *Chapter 5*)
<ul><li>Lip pits</li><li>Double lip</li><li>Cleft lip</li><li>Median lip fissure</li><li>Macrocheilia</li><li>Peutz–Jeghers syndrome</li><li>Cobblestone papules in lipoid proteinosis</li><li>Venous lake</li></ul>
Infections (see *Chapter 6*)
<ul><li>Candida infection</li><li>Herpes simplex (herpes labialis)</li><li>Herpes zoster (shingles)</li><li>Viral warts</li><li>Primary syphilis (chancre)</li><li>Tuberculosis</li><li>Angular cheilitis (mixed infection and irritant dermatitis)</li></ul>
Inflammatory diseases and conditions (see *Chapter 7*)
<ul><li>Eczematous cheilitis</li><li>Exfoliative cheilitis</li><li>Contact cheilitis (see *Chapter 4*)</li><li>Angular cheilitis (see *Chapter 6*)</li></ul>

- Lichenoid cheilitis
  - lichen planus
  - oral lichenoid reaction
  - lupus erythematosus
- Granulomatous cheilitis
  - Miescher cheilitis
  - orofacial granulomatosis (Melkersson–Rosenthal syndrome)
- Cheilitis glandularis
- Plasma cell cheilitis
- Recurrent aphthous stomatitis
- Erythema multiforme
- Stevens–Johnson syndrome / toxic epidermal necrolysis

Oral mucosal non-inflammatory disorders and conditions (see *Chapter 8*)

- Mucocele/ranula

Systemic diseases (see *Chapter 9*)

- Angioedema
- Angular cheilitis
  - with fissured lips and granulomatous cheilitis in Crohn disease
  - with atrophic glossitis with nutritional deficiency
- Granulomatous cheilitis due to sarcoidosis
- Cystic fibrosis

Neoplastic lesions: benign, potentially malignant, malignant (see *Chapter 10*)

- Benign lesion
  - fibroma
  - peripheral nerve sheath tumour
  - papilloma
  - haemangioma
  - pleomorphic adenoma (upper lip)
- Potentially malignant lesion
  - submucous fibrosis (see *Chapter 4*)
  - actinic keratosis of the lip (actinic cheilitis)
  - squamous cell carcinoma *in situ*
  - leukoplakia
  - erythroplakia
  - lichen planus (see *Chapter 7*)
- Malignant lesion
  - squamous cell carcinoma
  - basal cell carcinoma (cutaneous, not mucosal)
  - adenocarcinoma
  - adenoid cystic carcinoma
  - angiosarcoma
  - Merkel cell carcinoma
  - melanoma

3.11 Diseases affecting the gingivae

Desquamative gingivitis

The most common inflammatory disease of the gingival tissues is plaque-induced gingivitis. Non-plaque-induced gingival diseases, including desquamative gingivitis, are less common and are often manifestations of systemic immunological conditions.

Desquamative gingivitis is a descriptive term for a specific clinical sign (see *Chapter 7*).

3.11.1 Key points

- Desquamative gingivitis is characterized by sloughing of the gingival epithelium and exposure of a bright red gingival surface after rupturing a subepithelial or intraepithelial vesicle.
- Symptoms are mucosal sloughing, gingival bleeding, and oral discomfort, especially when consuming acidic or spicy foods or beverages.
- About 80% of cases are due to lichen planus or an immunobullous disorder.
- Histopathologic and immunofluorescence studies are required for diagnosis.

Table 3.11 Aetiological classification of desquamative gingivitis

Reactions to local or exogenous factors (see *Chapter 4*)
• Adverse reaction to a drug
Infections (see *Chapter 6*)
• Linear gingival erythema (HIV infection)   • Plaque-induced gingivitis   • Necrotizing ulcerative gingivitis
Inflammatory diseases and conditions (see *Chapter 7*)

• Oral lichen planus
 • Graft-versus-host disease
 • Lupus erythematosus
 • Granulomatous gingivitis
 • Immunobullous diseases
   ◦ epidermolysis bullosa acquisita
   ◦ pemphigoid
     - mucous membrane pemphigoid
     - bullous pemphigoid
     - pemphigoid gestationis
     - linear IgA bullous dermatosis
   ◦ pemphigus
     - pemphigus vulgaris
     - paraneoplastic pemphigus
 • Plasma cell gingivitis

Gingival enlargement

Gingival enlargement is characterized by the increased size of the gingival tissue. Lesions on the periodontium are related to dental plaque, infection, periodontal disease, a drug, localized or generalized inflammatory disease, or a neoplasm.

3.11.2 Key points

- Periodontal and gingival abscesses result in localized acute enlargement of the gingival tissue.
- Chronic inflammatory gingival enlargement is often caused by tissue oedema associated with prolonged bacterial plaque.
- Risk factors include mouth breathing, poor oral hygiene, and physical irritation of the gingiva by restorative and orthodontic appliances.
- Conditioned gingival enlargement occurs in pregnancy, during puberty, and with vitamin C deficiency.
- Immunosuppressants, phenytoin, and calcium channel blockers can cause gingival enlargement.
- Gingival enlargement can be due to leukaemia and granulomatous diseases.
- Benign neoplasms that cause localized gingival enlargement include fibroma, papilloma, and giant cell granuloma.
- Malignant neoplasms presenting with gingival enlargement include squamous cell carcinoma, Kaposi sarcoma, and melanoma.
- False gingival enlargement may arise from an underlying bony exostosis.
- A biopsy of gingival enlargement may show cellular hypertrophy, hyperplasia, oedema, fibrosis, or neoplastic cellular infiltration on histology.
- Gingivectomy is recommended for gingival fibromatosis.

Table 3.12 Aetiological classification of gingival enlargements

Reactions to local or exogenous factors (see *Chapter 4*)
• Traumatic haematoma • Gingival fibroepithelial polyp • Pyogenic granuloma • Giant cell epulis • Peripheral ossifying fibroma • Localized juvenile spongiotic gingival hyperplasia • Drug-induced gingival hyperplasia • Hormone-related gingival hyperplasia
Developmental or genetic origin (see *Chapter 5*)
• Hereditary gingival fibromatosis (and associated syndromes) • Ligneous gingivitis (plasminogen deficiency)

Infections (see *Chapter 6*)

- Viral infection
  - HIV infection
  - multifocal epithelial hyperplasia (HPV)
- Bacterial infection
  - abscess
  - tuberculosis

Inflammatory diseases and conditions (see *Chapter 7*)

- Granulomatous inflammation
  - granulomatous gingivitis
  - orofacial granulomatosis
  - sarcoidosis
  - Crohn disease
  - granulomatosis with polyangiitis
- Plasma cell gingivitis
- Pyostomatitis vegetans
- Cushing syndrome
- Acromegaly

Non-inflammatory diseases and conditions (see *Chapter 8*)

- Scurvy (vitamin C deficiency)
- Odontogenic cysts

Neoplastic lesions: benign, potentially malignant, malignant (see *Chapter 10*)

- Benign lesion
  - odontogenic tumour
  - haemangioma
- Malignant lesion
  - squamous cell carcinoma
  - melanoma
  - Kaposi sarcoma
  - lymphoma
  - leukaemia
  - metastases within the gingivae

3.12 Diseases affecting the tongue

Tongue disease can be reactive to local or exogenous causes, an infection, or a neoplasm. Glossitis describes an inflamed tongue. The tongue is also affected by systemic disease.

3.12.1   Key points

- Linea alba presents as a thin white line of thickened epithelium on the lateral surface of the tongue.
- Hairy tongue shows hypertrophy of filiform papillae, often with discolouration (white, yellow, brown, black).
- Oral hairy leukoplakia presents as a white hairy lesion on the lateral surface of the tongue. It is associated with the Epstein–Barr virus and is usually seen in an immunocompromised individual.
- Loss of filiform papillae results in atrophic glossitis: a smooth, atrophic, erythematous tongue surface, with or without erosions. Patients may complain of lingual pain (glossodynia) or a burning sensation (glossopyrosis). Causes of atrophic glossitis include lichen planus, iron deficiency, pernicious anaemia, vitamin B deficiencies, and candida infections.
- Median rhomboid glossitis describes a rhomboid atrophic area at the junction of the anterior two-thirds with the posterior third of the tongue.
- Geographic tongue (migratory glossitis, erythema migrans) describes the appearance and disappearance of red, depapillated patches on the dorsal tongue surrounded by a serpiginous raised border.
- Chronic dry mouth or Sjögren syndrome results in a smooth cobblestoned tongue surface.
- Lingual papillitis describes eruptive and transient, inflamed, enlarged fungiform papillae on the tip of the dorsum of the tongue.
- Lichen planus manifests as a reticular, white lacy pattern on the dorsal surface of the tongue or as erythematous erosions or ulcerations.
- Fissured tongue manifests as deep grooves on the dorsal and sometimes lateral surfaces of the tongue.
- Macroglossia refers to a generalized tongue enlargement with a scalloped lateral margin.
- Ankyloglossia (tongue-tie) is characterized by shortened lingual frenulum that limits tongue protrusion.
- Glossodynia (burning tongue) is characterized by daily pain in the tongue that commonly worsens throughout the day. The tongue appears normal.
- Traumatic fibroma (irritational fibroma, fibroepithelial polyp) appears along the bite line as a focal, thickened area typically dome-shaped, pink, and smooth.
- A papilloma is a single, isolated pedunculated or sessile lesion with finger-like projections associated with human papillomavirus (HPV 6 and 11) infection.
- A lingual thyroid nodule appears as a smooth nodular mass of tissue located in the midline of the posterior dorsal surface of the tongue, reflecting the failure of the thyroid tissue to descend into the neck during development.
- Leukoplakia, a potentially malignant disorder, can present as a white adherent patch or plaque. Erythroleukoplakia is a lesion that shows a combined red and white patch.
- Squamous cell carcinoma of the tongue can present as thickened white or red plaque, a cauliflower-like exophytic mass, or an ulcer with indurated rolled margins.

Table 3.13 Aetiological classification of conditions affecting the tongue

Reactions to local or exogenous factors (see *Chapter 4*)

- Trauma
  - traumatic/irritational fibroma
  - linea alba
- Hairy tongue
- Mucosal burn
  - thermal burn
  - chemical burn
  - radiation mucositis
- Chemotherapy-induced mucositis

Developmental or genetic origin (see *Chapter 5*)

- Macroglossia (large tongue)
- Ankyloglossia (tongue-tie)
- Bifid tongue
- Vascular malformations
  - port wine stain
- Lymphatic malformation
- Darier disease
- Dyskeratosis congenita
- Hereditary benign intraepithelial dyskeratosis
- Oral leukokeratosis due to pachyonychia congenita
- Oral papillomatosis due to Cowden syndrome
- Cobblestone tongue in lipoid proteinosis
- Telangiectasia in hereditary haemorrhagic telangiectasia
- Pigmented macules in Laugier–Hunziker syndrome

Infections (see *Chapter 6*)

- Candidosis
  - acute or chronic candidosis
  - median rhomboid glossitis
- Viral infections
  - herpes simplex
  - hairy leukoplakia (HIV/EBV)
  - viral wart (HPV)
- Bacterial infection
  - strawberry tongue (group A streptococci in scarlet fever)
  - gonococcal stomatitis
  - tertiary syphilis

Inflammatory diseases and conditions (see *Chapter 7*)

- Lichenoid inflammation
  - lichen planus
  - oral lichenoid reaction
  - lupus erythematosus
- Transient lingual papillitis
- Glossitis
  - atrophic glossitis
  - benign migratory glossitis

Non-inflammatory diseases and conditions (see *Chapter 8*)

- Thrombocytopenic purpura

Systemic diseases (see *Chapter 9*)

- Angioedema
- Macroglossia associated with acromegaly or amyloidosis
- Atrophic glossitis due to iron-deficiency anaemia, pernicious anaemia, vitamin B deficiencies

Neoplastic lesions: benign, potentially malignant, malignant (see *Chapter 10*)

- Benign lesion
  - peripheral nerve sheath tumour
  - other benign tumours
- Potentially malignant lesion
  - leukoplakia
  - squamous cell carcinoma *in situ*
- Malignant lesion
  - squamous cell carcinoma

3.13 Mucocutaneous disorders

Disorders that simultaneously affect the skin and the oral mucosa and other mucous membranes may be acute or chronic.

3.13.1 Key points

- An acute illness involving skin and mucosal surfaces is often related to infection or a drug and is often accompanied by fever and malaise.
- A chronic mucocutaneous disorder is most often immunological in origin.

Table 3.14 Aetiological classification of mucocutaneous disorders

Reactions to local or exogenous factors (see *Chapter 4*)

- Erythema multiforme major
- Drug
  - Stevens–Johnson / toxic epidermal necrolysis
  - drug hypersensitivity syndrome
  - lichenoid drug eruption (see *Chapter 7*)

Developmental or genetic origin (see *Chapter 5*)

- Ectodermal dysplasia
- Darier disease
- Dyskeratosis congenita
- Epidermolysis bullosa
- Fanconi anaemia
- Hereditary benign intraepithelial dyskeratosis
- McCune–Albright syndrome
- Pachyonychia congenita
- Peutz–Jeghers syndrome
- Multiple endocrine neoplasia type 2B
- Cowden syndrome
- Lipoid proteinosis
- Hereditary haemorrhagic telangiectasia
- Laugier–Hunziker syndrome

Infections (see *Chapter 6*)

- Fungal infection
  - candida infection
    - chronic mucocutaneous candidosis
  - deep mycosis
- Viral infection
  - herpes simplex
  - varicella-zoster infection
    - varicella
    - herpes zoster
  - infectious mononucleosis
  - cytomegalovirus
  - enterovirus
    - hand, foot, and mouth disease
  - measles
  - HIV

- Bacterial infection
  - gonococcal stomatitis
  - streptococcal infection
    - scarlet fever
    - toxic shock-like syndrome
  - staphylococcal infection
    - staphylococcal scalded skin syndrome
    - toxic shock syndrome
  - syphilis
  - tuberculosis

Inflammatory diseases and conditions (see *Chapter 7*)

- Lichenoid diseases
  - lichen planus
  - lichenoid drug reaction
  - graft-versus-host disease
  - lupus erythematosus
- Granulomatous disorders
  - Crohn disease
  - sarcoidosis
- Immunobullous diseases
  - epidermolysis bullosa acquisita
  - pemphigoid
    - mucous membrane pemphigoid
    - bullous pemphigoid
    - pemphigoid gestationis
    - linear IgA bullous dermatosis
  - pemphigus
    - pemphigus vulgaris
    - paraneoplastic pemphigus
  - dermatitis herpetiformis

Non-inflammatory diseases and conditions (see *Chapter 8*)

- Pigmentation due to Addison disease

Systemic diseases (see *Chapter 9* and *Section 3.14*)

Neoplastic lesions: malignant (see *Chapter 10*)

- Kaposi sarcoma
- Lymphoma
- Leukaemia
- Metastasis

3.14 Oral diseases associated with systemic disorders

Oral manifestations may lead to a diagnosis of a congenital, infectious, immunological, and malignant systemic disease (see *Chapter 9*).

3.14.1 Key points

- Systemic lupus erythematosus may present with oral mucosal disease including desquamative gingivitis.
- Sjögren syndrome is a connective tissue disease in which xerostomia and sialadenitis are associated with dry eyes, dry skin, tiredness, myalgia, and arthralgia.
- Erythema multiforme major presents with oral blisters and erosions and cutaneous target lesions; it may be triggered by a local or systemic infection or vaccination.
- Stevens–Johnson syndrome / toxic epidermal necrolysis is a severe cutaneous and systemic adverse reaction to various systemic medications, in which oral and lip ulceration is prominent.
- Behçet disease gives rise to recurrent aphthous ulcers; the diagnosis is made when there is a multisystem illness in which there is also genital ulceration, uveitis, erythema nodosum, and other features.
- Malignancies related to systemic disease include non-Hodgkin lymphoma (NHL) and Kaposi sarcoma. Non-Hodgkin lymphoma often presents as a mass or area of destructive ulceration of the pharynx, palate, or gingivae. Kaposi sarcoma presents with multiple cutaneous and mucosal vascular nodules.
- There exists a clear relationship between deficient oral hygiene resulting in periodontal disease and cardiovascular disease and metabolic syndrome.

Table 3.15 Aetiological classification of oral manifestations of systemic diseases

Cardiovascular diseases
- Anticoagulation – purpura, ecchymosis, petechiae, spontaneous gingival haemorrhage (see *Chapter 4*)
Rheumatological conditions (see *Chapter 7*)
- Behçet disease – aphthous ulcers - Systemic lupus erythematosus - Sjögren syndrome
Gastrointestinal disorders (see *Chapter 9*)
- Coeliac disease - Inflammatory bowel disease

Endocrine disorders (see *Chapter 9*)
• Diabetes mellitus • Adrenal disease • Acromegaly • Hyperparathyroidism
Haematological diseases
• Sickle cell anaemia (see *Chapter 9*) • Graft-versus-host disease – lichenoid reactions (see *Chapter 7*)
Oral adverse effects of systemic treatments
• Drug-induced dry mouth (salivary compromise) • Oral pigmentation (see *Chapter 8*) • Gingival hyperplasia (see *Chapter 4*) • Osteonecrosis (see *Chapter 9*)

CHAPTER 4

REACTIONS OF THE ORAL MUCOSA TO LOCAL OR EXOGENOUS FACTORS

See also:
- *Section 6.4.1: Angular cheilitis; Section 6.1.1: Denture-related stomatitis*
- *Section 7.1: Aphthous ulcers; Section 7.2.4: Graft-versus-host disease*
- *Section 9.3: Angioedema due to anaphylaxis; Section 9.7: Aphthous ulcers due to coeliac disease; Section 9.8.1: Aphthous ulcers due to inflammatory bowel disease; Section 9.16: Drug-induced osteonecrosis of the jaw*
- *Section 10.3.1: Actinic keratosis of the lip; Section 10.3.4: Reverse smoker's palate*

Specific oral mucosal diseases can be due to local debris, trauma (including sharp teeth or dentures, and burns), and the effects of toxins associated with tobacco and areca nut.

4.1 Dental and oral hygiene

Dental and oral hygiene aims to care for the oral mucosa, tongue, teeth, lips, gums, and dentures. The goal is to remove or prevent the build-up of plaque and tartar, to prevent dental caries and periodontal disease, and to decrease the incidence of halitosis.

4.1.1 Adults

- Patients should see their dentist and dental hygienist once or twice a year.
- Brush teeth for 2–3 minutes twice daily using a manual or electric soft-bristle toothbrush and fluoride toothpaste. An electric toothbrush requires less effort. Remove plaque and remnants of food and drink from teeth and gums by vertical or horizontal scrubbing, rolling, or using the Bass technique.
- Use a tongue scraper to clean the tongue's surface.
- Avoid brushing your teeth straight after consuming acidic drinks and foods, to reduce the chance of dental enamel erosion.
- Replace your toothbrush every 3–4 months.
- Remove biofilm and debris between the teeth once a day using floss or an interdental brush to prevent gum disease and tooth decay.
- As bacteria, fungi, plaque, and tartar can become deposited on removable dentures, these must be taken out after every meal and cleared of food remnants under running water. They should be cleaned using a denture brush without toothpaste at least once daily.

- Oral rinses with anti-plaque, anti-cavity, anti-tartar and anti-bacterial agents reduce oral discomfort, provide moisture, and help with bad breath.

4.1.2 Children

- Children should be introduced to tooth brushing at 2 years of age with a pea-sized amount of low-fluoride toothpaste. A parent or caregiver should help with the brushing until the child is at least 3 years old. After the age of 6 years, children can safely use regular fluoridated toothpaste.
- Flossing in toddlers should be commenced as soon as primary teeth establish proximal contact.
- Mouthwashes are not recommended for children under 6 years because of the risk of swallowing.

4.1.3 Patients with oral mucositis due to radiotherapy or chemotherapy

- When pain prevents using an ordinary toothbrush, use a gauze pad, a swab stick, or a foam toothbrush (dental swab).
- To avoid mucosal irritation, select a toothpaste without menthol, cinnamon, peppermint oil, and sodium lauryl sulphate.
- Patients with a bleeding tendency should avoid interdental cleaning with dental floss.
- Use antibacterial mouthwash to prevent gingivitis and periodontitis.
- For dry mouth, choose a mouth rinse with mucin, carboxymethylcellulose and hydroxymethyl cellulose, xanthan, linseed oil and polyethylene oxide to improve viscosity and wettability.
- Patients with mucositis should avoid mouthwashes containing alcohol and chlorhexidine. Replace with salt-and-soda solution or rinse with 0.5% lignocaine.
- Using sugar-free chewing gum after eating can accelerate the clearance of dietary substances and microorganisms, promote buffers to neutralize plaque acids, and provide antibacterial substances.
- Patients with ulceration or neutropenia must not wear dentures during and after radiotherapy or chemotherapy except while eating.

4.2 Debris

4.2.1 Hairy tongue

A hairy tongue has a white, brown, or blue-black mid-dorsal surface in front of the circumvallate papillae.

- A hairy tongue affects around 13% of the general population.
- It affects about 8% of children and young adults and 57% of imprisoned drug addicts.

Causes

A hairy tongue is characterized by hypertrophy and elongation of filiform papillae, which fail to desquamate because of a lack of mechanical stimulation and debridement. Associations include the following factors:

- Edentulism
- Heavy smoking and excessive coffee drinking
- Poor oral hygiene
- A soft diet that prevents the shedding of the papillae
- Dehydration due to fasting or a febrile disease
- Dry mouth due to medication or radiotherapy
- A prolonged course of an antibiotic
- Mouthwash containing oxidizing agents
- Sometimes, *Candida albicans* or bacterial infection.

Clinical features

A hairy tongue has varying colours (see *Figs. 4.1a* and *b*) due to retained pigment from tobacco smoking, food, beverages, and candies or pigment-producing bacteria. The hairy area cannot be wiped off with gauze.
- Some patients complain of glossodynia (a burning sensation without signs), taste aberration, halitosis, gagging, and nausea.
- Cytologic smears and swabs for culture for candida are usually negative.

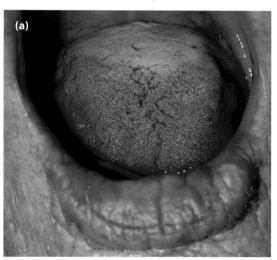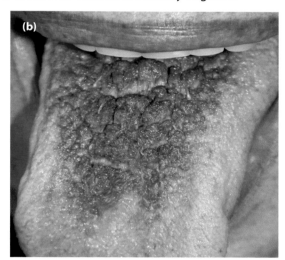

Figure 4.1 (a and b). Hairy tongue. The brown colour in image (b) was due to heavy smoking.

(a) Reproduced from Health NZ – Waikato (www.waikatodhb.health.nz) with permission.

Treatment

When treatment of hairy tongue is considered necessary, options include the following:
- Eliminate causative/predisposing factors such as anticholinergic medications or broad-spectrum antibiotics.
- Maintain oral hygiene by tooth brushing daily and scraping the tongue.
- Attempt to increase saliva production if the patient has xerostomia.
- Topical 30% urea solution and trichloroacetic acid are reported effective for severely elongated papillae.

- Treat candida-associated glossodynia with an antifungal agent.
- Clip or remove the papillae by electrodesiccation or carbon dioxide laser.

4.2.2   Materia alba

Materia alba is a soft non-mineralized whitish deposit on the tooth surface around the gingival margins.

- It is an accumulation of food debris, microorganisms, and dead cells.
- It may be associated with gingival inflammation.
- It is common among those with poor oral hygiene.

Treatment

- Remove debris by water irrigation or gentle scaling.
- Prevent recurrence by brushing the teeth daily.

4.3   Acute injury

4.3.1   Traumatic ulceration

Localized trauma results in acute ulceration (see *Fig. 4.2*).

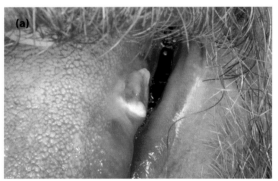

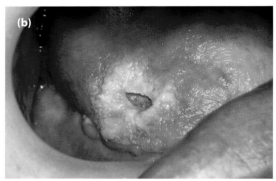

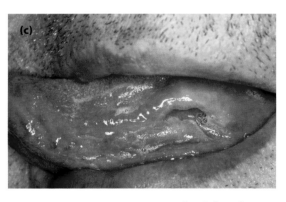

Figure 4.2 (a–c). Traumatic ulcers on the left lateral tongue.

All images reproduced from Health NZ – Waikato (www.waikatodhb.health.nz) with permission.

4.3.2   Extravascular blood

Extravascular blood results from trauma or a surgical procedure, particularly if the patient has a blood disorder, is prescribed an anticoagulant/antiplatelet drug, or has an infection such as meningococcal disease, SARS-CoV-2 infection, and others. Tissue bleeding or purpura does not blanch on pressure.

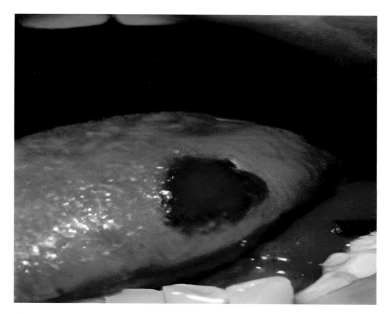

Figure 4.3. Ecchymosis of the dorsolateral tongue.

Reproduced from *Dental Research and Oral Health*, 2019;2: 047-052 under a CC-BY 4.0 licence, and included here after enhancement by AIPDerm (www.aipderm.com).

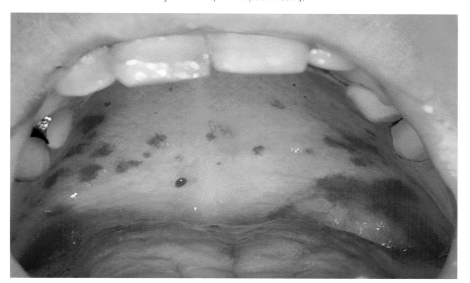

Figure 4.4. Petechiae of the marginal gingiva in a patient with severe thrombocytopenia secondary to acute leukaemia.

Reproduced with permission from *Pocket Dentistry* (Chapter 9, Bleeding disorders; www.pocketdentistry.com), and included here after enhancement by AIPDerm (www.aipderm.com).

- Ecchymosis is a flat, red, purple, or blue discolouration >1 cm due to bleeding under the skin (see *Fig. 4.3*).
- Petechiae are pinpoint 1–2mm haemorrhages (see *Fig. 4.4*).
- Spontaneous gingival haemorrhage presents as a slow ooze of blood flow.

No treatment is necessary. Tissue bleeding will resolve spontaneously in several weeks.

4.3.3   Traumatic haemorrhagic bulla

A haemorrhagic bulla is an oral blood-filled blister known as angina bullosa haemorrhagica. Traumatic haemorrhagic bulla is usually observed in adults aged 50–70.

Causes

Traumatic haemorrhagic bulla is due to masticatory trauma, especially chewing hard and crispy food. Diabetes, hypertension, and long-term steroid inhaler use may be contributory factors.

Clinical features

Traumatic haemorrhagic bulla presents as a blood-filled, red or purple subepithelial blister of the oral cavity that quickly expands and ruptures spontaneously within 24–48 hours.
- The blisters are usually observed on the soft palate (see *Fig. 4.5*). Occasionally, they may arise on the buccal mucosa, the lateral border of the tongue, or the lip.
- Although usually painless, the ruptured blister forms an ulcer, which may be painful. It heals without scarring.

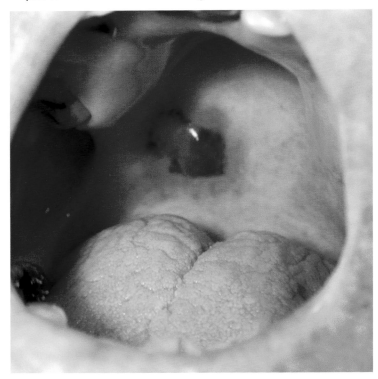

Figure 4.5. Traumatic blood-filled bulla right soft palate.

Reproduced from Health NZ – Waikato (www.waikatodhb.health.nz) with permission.

Treatment

No treatment is required for traumatic haemorrhagic bulla, which resolves spontaneously.

4.3.4 Mucosal burn

A mucosal burn may be due to heat (thermal burn), cold (frostbite or cryotherapy burn) (see *Fig. 4.6a*), chemicals, or radiation.

See also *Section 10.3.4* on reverse smoker's palate.
* The affected site may blister initially and then develop into an ulcer.
* The blister is short-lived, usually only lasting a few hours before rupturing and ulcerating.

Thermal burn

A thermal burn is a painful lesion caused by intense heat. Examples include the following:
* Scorching hot and sticky foods such as cheese or pizza.
* The burning end of the smoking device (chutta, a homemade cigar) in a reverse smoker.
* An injury during a dental procedure from an overheated impression compound.

Mucosal thermal burns are especially common in children.

Clinical features

The burn is initially red and may form a short-lasting, fluid-filled bulla. A severe burn presents as a white necrotic plaque overlying an ulcer. Frequent sites for thermal burns include the palate (see *Fig. 4. 6b*) and tip of the tongue.

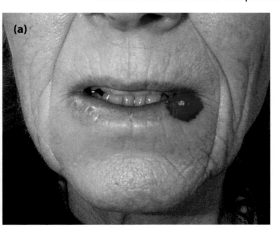 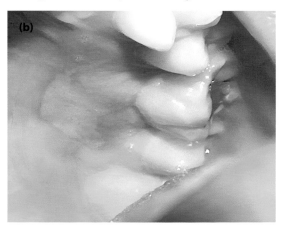

Figure 4.6 (a and b). (a) Cryotherapy burn on the left lower lip manifesting as a blood-filled blister. (b) Thermal burn of the palatal mucosa caused by microwave-heated cheese pie.

(b) Reproduced from *Cases Journal,* 2008;1:191 (https://doi.org/10.1186/1757-1626-1-191) under a CC-BY 2.0 licence, and included here after enhancement by AIPDerm (www.aipderm.com).

Treatment

Treatment of a mucosal thermal burn is symptomatic.
- Apply or spray topical lignocaine and benzydamine.
- Avoid contact with irritants and food.

The healing time depends on the size and depth of the burn.

Chemical burn

A chemical burn is a painful lesion caused by a noxious chemical agent in direct contact with the mucosa. Examples include the following:
- Aspirin that has been applied to the vestibule adjacent to a painful decayed tooth.
- A mouthwash containing chlorhexidine, alcohol, or acetone.
- Dental treatment solution containing sodium hypochlorite, formalin; an endodontic paste containing arsenic; or improper use of silver nitrate or hydrogen peroxide.

Other causative agents include acids, alkalis, urea, and organic substances.
- Acids act by coagulation necrosis through protein denaturation.
- Alkalis act by liquefaction necrosis and cause more damage than acids.

Clinical features

A chemical burn is initially erythematous, then presents as a painful, irregular ulcer covered by a white pseudomembrane (see *Fig. 4.7*). A shallow lesion has a whitish and wrinkled appearance, and a deeper one is necrotic.

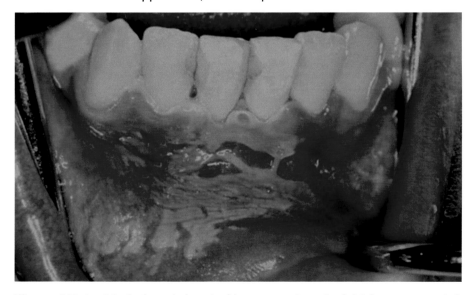

Figure 4.7. Aspirin-induced chemical burn noted on the labial mucosa and the gingiva showing white pseudomembrane.

Reproduced from *Color Atlas of Oral and Maxillofacial Diseases*, 2019; B.W. Neville, D.D. Damm, C.M. Allen & A.C. Chi, with permission from Elsevier, and included here after enhancement by AIPDerm (www.aipderm.com).

Treatment

Treatment of a mucosal chemical burn is symptomatic.
- Apply or spray topical lignocaine or benzydamine.
- A severely necrotic lesion may be treated by topical/intralesional corticosteroid injection.

Most mucosal chemical burns heal within 7–14 days.

Chemotherapy-induced oral mucositis

Chemotherapy-induced oral mucositis affects 40–60% of cancer patients undergoing chemotherapy.

Causes and risk factors

Chemotherapy-induced oral mucositis results from a complex interaction of local tissue damage, the specific drug or drugs, the level of myelosuppression, and the patient's predisposition.
- Patients with haematological malignancies have an increased rate of oral mucositis compared with those with solid tumours.
- The occurrence and severity of mucositis depend on the intensity and duration of the chemotherapy regimen.
- The most stomatotoxic agents include the antimetabolites 5-fluorouracil, methotrexate, and cytarabine.
- Concomitant radiation therapy to the head and neck increases the risk of oral mucositis, as does hyposalivation or dry mouth from any cause.
- Younger age is associated with more severe oral mucositis.
- Chronic irritation from ill-fitting prostheses or faulty restorations predisposes patients to develop oral mucositis.

Clinical features

Mucositis occurs 7–10 days after chemotherapy, commencing with erythema that progresses towards erosion and ulceration (see *Fig. 4.8*).

Chemotherapy-induced mucositis is painful, restricts oral intake, and promotes local or systemic infection. It resolves slowly 2–3 weeks after cessation of treatment.

Diagnosis

The diagnosis of chemotherapy-induced oral mucositis is based on a history of chemotherapy for cancer, the clinical findings, and the chronology of the development of lesions.

A biopsy is not routinely necessary for diagnosis, and histopathological features may be non-specific.

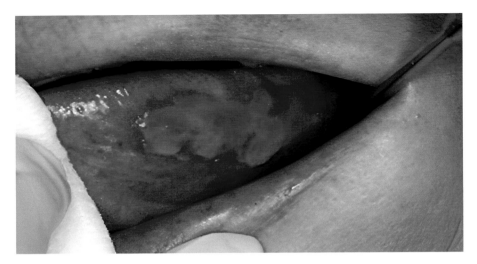

Figure 4.8. Chemotherapy-induced mucositis. Widespread mucositis of the non-keratinized mucosa of the lateroventral side of the tongue induced by chemotherapy.

Reproduced from *Handbook of Oral Pathology and Oral Medicine*, 2022; S.R. Prabhu, with permission from Wiley-Blackwell, and included here after enhancement by AIPDerm (www.aipderm.com).

Treatment

Management of oral mucositis may include:
- Oral debridement (e.g. brushing, flossing) and mucolytic agents to help dislodge dried secretions
- An antimicrobial mouthwash
- Topical and systemic pain relief
- Sucking ice chips or sipping cold water during infusions of chemotherapy.

Where available, palifermin (endogenous keratinocyte growth factor) may reduce the incidence, duration, and severity of mucositis.

Radiation mucositis

Radiation mucositis is an expected tissue injury induced by ionizing radiation, and it affects up to 90% of head and neck cancer patients treated with radiotherapy. It is also called radiation-induced oral mucositis.

Risk factors and causes

Patient-related risk factors include concomitant chemotherapy, poor oral hygiene, poor nutritional status, periodontal disease, hyposalivation, smoking, alcohol abuse, low body mass index (BMI <18.5), and immunosuppression due to co-morbidities such as diabetes mellitus, old age, and female gender.

Treatment-related risk factors include radiation source, total dose, daily fractionation, previous radiotherapy, chemotherapy (dependent on dosage, type of drug and timing), and medications designed to target cancer cells without affecting normal cells (targeted therapy).

The pathogenesis of radiation mucositis consists of four phases:
1. Initial inflammatory/vascular phase
2. Epithelial phase
3. Pseudomembranous ulcerative/bacteriological phase
4. Healing phase.

Clinical features

Radiation mucositis causes pain, odynophagia, and reduced oral intake.

Four phases follow oral radiotherapy:
1. Grade I mucositis during the second week — erythema, intolerance to spices, and burning pain
2. Grade II mucositis during the third week — erosions and desquamation
3. Grade III mucositis in the fourth and fifth weeks — ulceration covered by pseudomembrane composed of cell debris, keratin, and fibrin (see *Fig. 4.9*)
4. Grade IV mucositis in the fifth and sixth weeks — ulceration, necrosis, and sometimes bleeding.

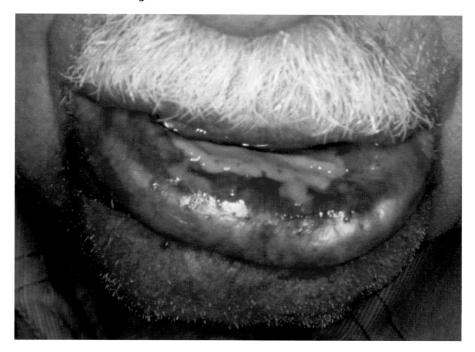

Figure 4.9. Radiation mucositis shows ulceration covered by pseudomembrane.

Reproduced from Health NZ – Waikato (www.waikatodhb.health.nz) with permission.

Treatment

Pre-treatment preparation:
- Dental assessment of the oral cavity
- The patient should use a soft-bristle toothbrush to maintain oral hygiene
- Avoid hot and spicy food, alcohol, and smoking

- Rinse mouth with normal saline, alkali (soda bicarbonate), benzydamine, or aloe vera
- Apply sucralfate or granulocyte–macrophage colony-stimulating factor to treated areas.

Pain management:
- Liquid/semi-solid high-calorie and high-protein food
- Application of honey (not suitable for people with diabetes)
- Apply local anaesthetic (2% lignocaine gel) before food
- Topical rinse with aspirin, doxepin, or benzydamine
- Analgesics, including opioids, if necessary
- Treatment of bacterial or candida infection.

4.3.5   Traumatic neuroma

Traumatic neuroma, also known as amputation neuroma, is a localized proliferation of neural tissue.

Causes

Traumatic neuroma follows an injury. The nerve bundle degenerates distal to the severed or damaged nerve. As the proximal end of the nerve regrows along the old nerve pathway, it may be blocked by scar tissue. The continued growth of the nerve then produces a nodule.

Clinical features

A traumatic neuroma of the oral mucosa is a smooth-surfaced nodule.
- Symptoms may include altered nerve sensation (numbness, tingling) or pain, which can be spontaneous or triggered by manipulation of the lesion.
- The most common intraoral site is the mental foramen due to traumatic tooth extraction.
- They may also arise on the tongue and lower lip.

Treatment

A traumatic neuroma and a small portion of the proximal nerve bundle can be surgically excised. Recurrence is uncommon.

4.3.6   Pyogenic granuloma / vascular epulis

Pyogenic granuloma is a reactive inflammatory lesion that may arise on the skin, lips, or oral mucosa. A gingival pyogenic granuloma is also known as a vascular epulis or angiogranuloma.

Causes

Oral pyogenic granuloma is more common in females than males.
- A history of minor trauma is commonly elicited.
- Irritation from calculus or an overhanging restoration may cause gingival pyogenic granuloma.
- Pregnancy predisposes to pyogenic granuloma on the gingiva, when the lesion is called a pregnancy tumour or epulis (see *Fig. 4.10a*).

Clinical features

- A pyogenic granuloma can occur anywhere in the oral cavity, but most commonly occurs on the maxillary anterior facial surfaces of the gingiva.
- It is a smooth or lobulated soft red–purple papule that may be pedunculated or sessile (see *Fig. 4.10b*). It bleeds on slight trauma.
- The lesion's surface may be smooth, ulcerated, or lobulated and often covered with a yellowish fibrinous membrane.
- During pregnancy, pyogenic granuloma usually starts in the first trimester and peaks in the third trimester. It may resolve postpartum.
- Dermoscopy shows red–purple structures separated by white strands.
- Histopathology reveals proliferating vascular channels, immature fibroblastic oedematous connective tissue, and scattered inflammatory cells.

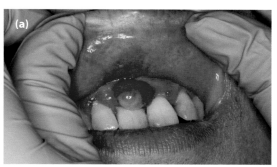

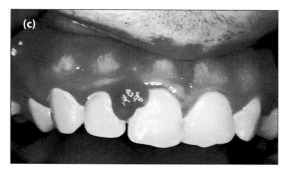

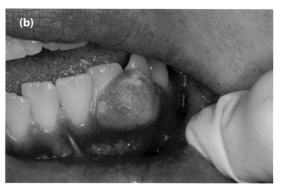

Figure 4.10 (a–c). (a) Pregnancy tumour; (b) and (c) pyogenic granuloma of the gingiva in a non-pregnant woman. Histologically both lesions show similar features.

(b) Reproduced with permission from Professor Nagamani Narayana, University of Nebraska Medical Centre, NE, USA. (c) Reproduced with permission from *Pocket Dentistry* (Chapter 9; www.pocketdentistry.com), and included here after enhancement by AIPDerm (www.aipderm.com).

Treatment

Pyogenic granuloma is treated by conservative surgical excision. Gingival lesions should be excised down to the periosteum with scaling of adjacent teeth to remove any calculus and plaque.

The prognosis is excellent, and recurrence is uncommon.

4.4 Chronic repetitive injury

Irritation within the mouth can cause a hyperplastic response, with the specific name relating to its location or appearance.

4.4.1   Fibroepithelial polyp and fibrous epulis

A fibroepithelial or fibrous polyp is a common finding on the buccal mucosa, along the occlusal line, lip, or the tip of the tongue (see *Fig. 4.11*).

A gingival fibroepithelial polyp is also known as a fibrous epulis. They are most often diagnosed in children and young adults.

Causes

Fibroepithelial polyp arises as a reaction to habitual biting or irritation.

Clinical features

Fibroepithelial polyps are painless, firm, pink, dome-shaped pedunculated or sessile papules ranging from a few millimetres to a centimetre or more.
- Usually painless, they may ulcerate following trauma.
- Histopathology shows dense, hypovascular and hyperplastic fibrous tissue.

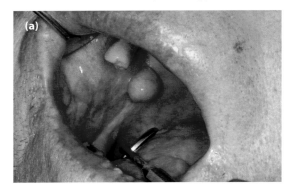
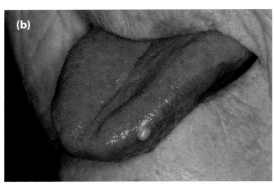
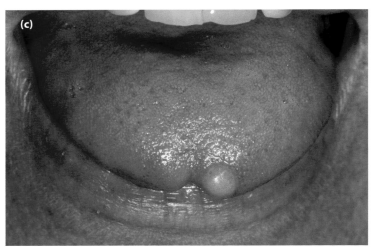

Figure 4.11 (a–c). Fibroepithelial polyp on (a) buccal mucosa, (b) left lateral tongue, and (c) tip of the tongue.

All images reproduced from Health NZ – Waikato (www.waikatodhb.health.nz) with permission.

Treatment

Fibroepithelial polyps can be surgically removed. Recurrence is uncommon.

4.4.2 Giant cell epulis

Giant cell epulis is also known as peripheral giant cell granuloma. It occurs on the gingiva and alveolar mucosa, usually interdentally. It most often affects women aged 30–60.

Causes

Giant cell epulis is due to chronic low-grade local irritation or trauma to the periodontal ligament or periosteal tissues.

Clinical features

A giant cell epulis is more prominent and darker red than a fibrous epulis.
- It is a circumscribed soft, painless, dark-red or purple nodule and is sessile or pedunculated.
- It is usually located anterior to the permanent molars (see *Fig. 4.12*).
- It may grow up to 2cm in diameter.
- It can push teeth aside or erode alveolar bone.
- Histopathology shows inflammatory cells, foreign body giant cells, haemorrhage, and fibroangiomatous stroma.

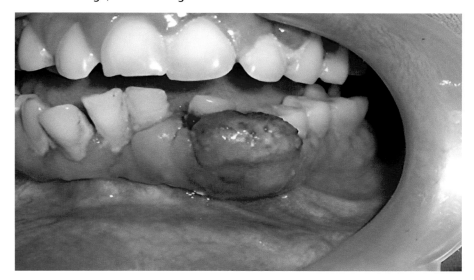

Figure 4.12. Peripheral giant cell epulis anterior to the lower premolars.

Reproduced from *Handbook of Oral Pathology and Oral Medicine*, 2022; S.R. Prabhu, with permission from Wiley-Blackwell, and included here after enhancement by AIPDerm (www.aipderm.com).

Treatment

The treatment of giant cell epulis is surgical excision. Curettage of the underlying bone may be required to prevent a recurrence.

4.4.3   Denture-induced hyperplasia

Denture-induced mucosal hyperplasia is also known as inflammatory fibroepithelial hyperplasia of the oral mucous membrane caused by a denture, denture granuloma, and epulis fissuratum.

Causes

Chronic trauma from the flange of ill-fitting dentures results in exuberant fibrous tissue.

Clinical features

Denture-wearing may induce pink, broad-based, firm, lobulated and leaf-like hyperplastic tissue on the buccal mucosa, gingiva, or labial sulcus (see *Fig. 4.13*).
* Single or multiple sites may be affected.
* The posterior edge of the upper denture may irritate the palate, causing a 'leaf fibroma'.
* Fissuring may occur, but ulceration is uncommon.
* Histopathology shows fibrous hyperplasia with a mild inflammatory cell infiltrate.

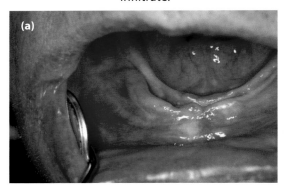 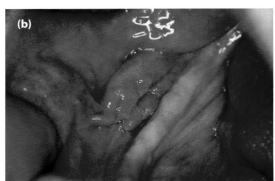

Figure 4.13 (a and b). Denture-induced hyperplasia (epulis fissuratum). Note leaf-like hyperplastic tissue in the buccal mucosa.

Both images reproduced from Health NZ – Waikato (www.waikatodhb.health.nz) with permission.

Treatment

The hyperplastic tissue can be removed surgically or by laser ablation. Ill-fitting dentures must be corrected or replaced.

4.4.4   Papillary hyperplasia

Dentures can also cause papillary hyperplasia on palatal mucosa covered by a denture.
* Papillary hyperplasia is also known as denture stomatitis or denture sore mouth.
* It occurs in 50–60% of denture wearers.
* Non-denture-bearing mucosal surfaces may rarely develop similar pathology.

Causes

Papillary hyperplasia of the palate in complete denture wearers is attributed to chronic infection by *Candida albicans* and mechanical irritation.

Clinical features

Oral papillary hyperplasia presents as asymptomatic diffuse erythema, oedema, and multiple pinpoint papules on the palate (see *Fig. 4.14*).
- Occasional white spots or petechiae may be observed.
- Lesions should be differentiated from leukokeratosis nicotina palati.

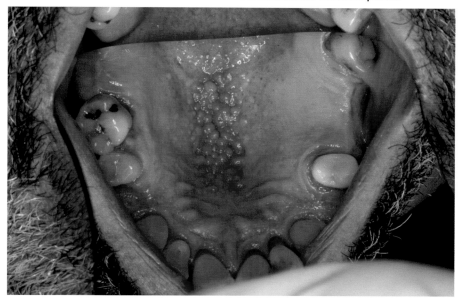

Figure 4.14. Oral papillary hyperplasia of the palate.

Treatment

Denture hygiene: soft brush twice daily, using toothpaste free of sodium lauryl sulphate.

Oral papillary hyperplasia may respond to topical antifungal therapy.

4.4.5 Peripheral ossifying fibroma of the gingiva

Peripheral ossifying fibroma, also known as cementifying or calcifying fibroma, is reactive gingival hyperplasia containing mineralized tissues, bone, cementum-like material, or dystrophic calcification. Peripheral ossifying fibroma is more common in females than in males, with a peak in the second decade of life.

Causes

Peripheral ossifying fibroma is thought to be due to irritating local agents such as dental calculus, plaque, orthodontic appliances, and ill-fitting restorations. The growth arises from the periodontal ligament.

Clinical features

Peripheral ossifying fibroma is a solitary, slow-growing nodule with an ulcerated or smooth surface (see *Fig. 4.15*).
- A peripheral ossifying fibroma is usually <1.5 cm in size.
- It may be pedunculated or sessile.
- The most common site is the anterior maxilla.
- Histopathology shows areas of dystrophic calcification within a cellular fibrous connective tissue covered by stratified squamous epithelium. An inflammatory infiltrate is usually present.

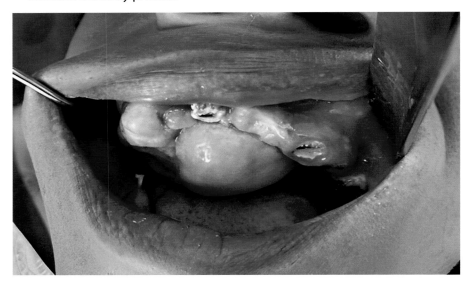

Figure 4.15. Peripheral ossifying fibroma.

Reproduced with permission from Dr Fadi Titinchi, University of Western Cape South Africa, and included here after enhancement by AIPDerm (www.aipderm.com).

Treatment

Peripheral ossifying fibroma is removed surgically down to the bone, with the adjacent periosteum and the periodontal ligament.

Recurrence rates after surgery range from 8% to 45%.

4.4.6   Frictional keratoses

Frictional keratoses are a group of hyperkeratotic white patches or plaques on the buccal mucosa. The surface of frictional keratoses can be rough, warty, wrinkled, or corrugated. Frictional keratoses are asymptomatic, and they may be unilateral or bilateral.

They are classified by their site and cause. Some examples include the following:
- Chronic cheek biting. A white plaque inside the cheeks may be due to chronic cheek biting (morsicatio buccarum) (see *Fig. 4.16*).

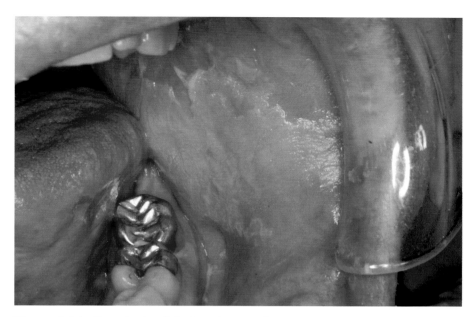

Figure 4.16. Chronic cheek biting showing keratotic white lesion on the buccal mucosa.

Reproduced with permission from Professor Nagamani Narayana, University of Nebraska Medical Centre, NE, USA.

- Alveolar ridge keratosis. This affects the retromolar trigone (60%) or the edentulous alveolar ridge (40%) and is caused by chewing without natural teeth or a dental prosthesis (see *Fig. 4.17*).
- Linea alba. This is a white keratotic line on the buccal mucosa at the occlusal plane (see *Fig. 4.18a*) or on the lateral border of the tongue and is due to contact with teeth (see *Fig. 4.18b*).
- Excessive tooth brushing. White plaques on the attached gingiva, especially the maxillary arch, may be due to excessive and inappropriate tooth brushing.

Alveolar ridge keratosis tends to affect edentulous middle-aged males at a mean age of 50–55 years. It is less common in females, with a reported ratio of 3.7:1. Other forms of oral frictional keratoses affect males and females of all ages. Prevalence has been reported to range between 2.7% and 11.5%.

Causes

Frictional keratosis is due to chronic repetitive trauma, which stimulates epithelial acanthosis, a granular layer, and the production of excessive keratin, i.e. a white plaque.

The trauma may be due to the following:
- Habitual cheek/lip/tongue biting
- Broken appliances or teeth
- Improper tooth brushing
- Teeth grinding (bruxism).

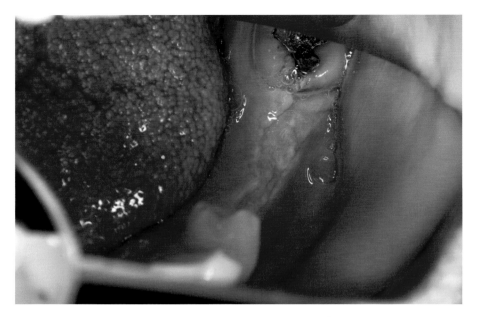

Figure 4.17. Alveolar ridge keratosis showing a white lesion with a corrugated surface on the retromolar trigone.

Reproduced from Health NZ – Waikato (www.waikatodhb.health.nz) with permission.

Diagnosis

Frictional keratoses are usually diagnosed clinically.
- A biopsy is recommended if there are atypical features, the lesion fails to resolve when friction is eliminated, or there is ulceration.
- Histopathology of frictional keratosis shows orthokeratosis, parakeratosis, hypergranulosis, and acanthosis of the surface epithelium. A patchy chronic inflammatory infiltrate may occur in the dense, fibrous connective tissue.

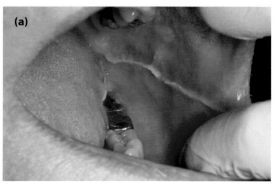
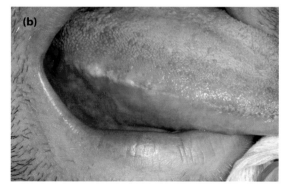

Figure 4.18 (a and b). Linea alba. Note keratotic linear line on the buccal mucosa at the level of occlusal line (a) and the lateral border of the tongue.

Images reproduced with permission from Professor Nagamani Narayana, University of Nebraska Medical Centre, NE, USA.

Treatment

- Remove any frictional irritants where possible. Repair fractured or rough tooth surfaces or irregularly fitting dentures or other appliances.
- Encourage the patient to discontinue biting, sucking, or chewing; a psychological evaluation may be appropriate.

If causative factors are eliminated, frictional keratoses resolve in 1–3 weeks. Avoidance of further friction will prevent a recurrence.

4.4.7 Verruciform xanthoma

Verruciform xanthoma is an uncommon benign reactive lesion. It is also known as verrucous xanthoma.

- It can occur at any age, most often in the fifth to seventh decades, with equal sex incidence.
- It has been reported in the oral cavity of about 300 individuals.
- A smaller number of similar lesions have been reported in anogenital sites.

Causes

Verruciform xanthoma is an immune response to local trauma or inflammation.

Clinical features

Oral verruciform xanthoma usually presents as an asymptomatic solitary, sessile or pedunculated, red or white papule 2–15 mm in size.

- Oral verruciform xanthoma commonly involves the gingiva, alveolar mucosa, and palate.
- The lesion surface can be rough or pebbly.

Diagnosis

Histopathological examination is essential to make a definitive diagnosis of oral verruciform xanthoma.

It is histologically characterized by epithelial parakeratosis and lipid-laden macrophages (foam cells) in the connective tissue papillae.

Treatment

The treatment of verruciform xanthoma is surgical excision. Recurrence is rare.

4.4.8 Contact stomatitis

Contact stomatitis is inflammation of the oral mucosa caused by external substances.

- Irritant contact stomatitis is usually due to acidic or sharp food. It can complicate other inflammatory disorders, such as lichen planus.
- Allergic contact stomatitis is a T-cell-mediated delayed hypersensitivity reaction to a specific allergen. It is much less common than allergic contact dermatitis.
- Lichenoid contact reaction to mercury in an amalgam filling.

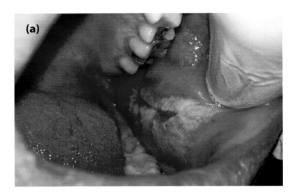
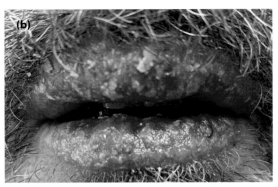
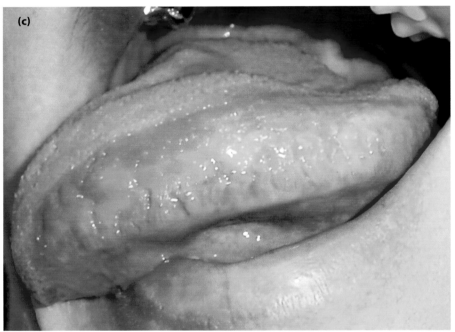

Figure 4.19 (a–c). (a) Lichenoid contact stomatitis of the buccal mucosa due to amalgam; (b) contact allergic cheilitis caused by propolis; (c) contact reaction on tongue caused by cinnamon.

(a) Reproduced with permission from Professor Yeshwant Rawal, University of Milwaukee School of Dentistry, Milwaukee, WI, USA; (b) reproduced from Health NZ – Waikato (www.waikatodhb.health.nz) with permission; (c) reproduced from *Diagnosis and Management of Oral Lesions and Conditions: A resource handbook for the clinician*; Eds: CA Migliorati and FS Panagakos (http://dx.doi.org/10.5772/57597) under CC BY 3.0 licence. © 2014 InTech.

Causes of allergic contact stomatitis

Contact allergy to oral flavourings, preservatives, metals, rubber compounds, propylene glycol, and many other substances may cause stomatitis.
- Allergens are found in oral hygiene products, foods, dental restorations, and topical medications.
- Oral fragrances include balsam of Peru, cinnamon, cinnamic aldehyde, menthol, and peppermint.

- Preservatives such as parabens are found in various foods, including salad dressing, spicy sauces, mustard, jellies, jams, fruit juices, syrups, and candies. They are also used in lipsticks, toothpaste, and dental hygiene products.
- Allergens in dental prostheses include metals (e.g. nickel, palladium, gold, mercury, and zinc), formaldehyde, acrylate monomer, resins, rubber accelerants, and colophonium.
- Propylene glycol is found in tobacco formulations, food colours, and flavouring agents.

Clinical features

Contact stomatitis presents with pain, burning sensation, or itchiness. A contact allergy should be suspected when oral examination reveals erythematous plaques, vesiculation, and ulceration (see *Fig. 4.19*). A lichenoid reaction presents as a white plaque adjacent to the amalgam.

Diagnosis

Contact stomatitis may be suspected based on history and examination. Investigations include the following:
- Patch testing to identify a contact allergen
- A mucosal biopsy to exclude other causes of stomatitis.

Treatment

Contact irritants and any identified or potential allergens should be identified and avoided.

Contact stomatitis is treated with topical corticosteroids. Severe and extensive stomatitis may require short-term systemic corticosteroids. Oral antihistamines are ineffective.

4.5 Toxins

4.5.1 Areca nut

Oral submucous fibrosis

Oral submucous fibrosis is a chronic debilitating disorder characterized by inflammation and progressive fibrosis of the submucosal tissues. It is potentially malignant.

The incidence of oral submucous fibrosis differs with diet, habits, and culture.
- In India, the incidence ranges from 0.2–2.3% in males and 1.2–4.6% in females, with an age range of 11–60 years.
- Sporadic cases of South Asians have also been reported in South Africa, the UK, and Europe.

Causes

The main cause of oral submucous fibrosis is areca nut chewing.
- 'Paan' (in India) is a betel leaf filled with chopped areca nut and slaked lime (calcium hydroxide).

- Areca nut is a confirmed carcinogen, genotoxin, and mutagen.
- Areca nut contains alkaloids (arecoline, arecaidine, guvacine, and guvacoline), flavonoids, and copper. These alkaloids stimulate fibroblasts to produce collagen.
- Oral submucous fibrosis results from increased biosynthesis and reduced clearance of collagen.

Other associated factors include the following:
- Chewing smokeless tobacco
- Autoimmunity
- Vitamin B, vitamin C, and iron deficiencies
- Consumption of spicy foods
- HPV infection.

Clinical features

The initial symptoms of oral submucous fibrosis include xerostomia, mucosal burning sensation, and the formation of vesicles.

With continued exposure to areca nut:
- mouth opening becomes progressively limited (the normal range is 40–74mm in males and 35–70mm in females)
- palpable fibrous bands arise in the buccal mucosa, retromolar areas, and around the mouth
- the tongue appears smooth as the papillae on the tongue involute
- tongue protrusion is impaired
- the mucosa appears marble white (see *Fig. 4.20*).

Diagnosis

The diagnosis of submucous fibrosis depends on a history of habitual chewing of areca nut, the clinical findings, and biopsy features.
- Histopathology of submucous fibrosis reveals an atrophic epithelium, chronic inflammation, excessive collagen, local inflammation in the lamina propria and deep connective tissues, and degenerative changes in the underlying muscles.
- Occasionally, oral submucous fibrosis may show epithelial dysplasia.

Treatment

Cessation of the use of betel quid (paan) and areca nut chewing is essential. Iron and vitamin B complex deficiencies should be corrected.

In patients with moderate oral submucous fibrosis, treatment may include:
- topical steroids and weekly submucosal intralesional steroid injections
- topical hyaluronidase
- submucosal administration of aqueous human placental extract (unapproved).

Surgical treatment (simple excision of fibrous bands) is indicated in patients with severe trismus or biopsy, revealing dysplastic or neoplastic changes. Oral submucous fibrosis is not curable.
- Monitor the patient long-term.
- Oral squamous cell carcinoma develops in 1.9–9% of patients with submucous fibrosis (see also *Section 10.4.1*).

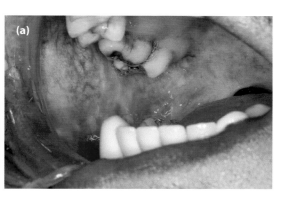

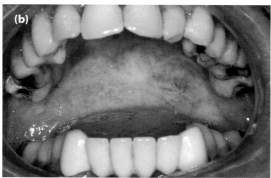

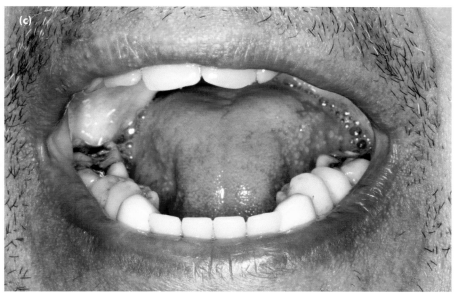

Figure 4.20 (a–c). Oral submucous fibrosis; pallor and fibrous bands on (a) the buccal mucosa and (b) the palate; (c) reduced mouth opening.

All images reproduced with permission from Professor Yeshwant Rawal, University of Milwaukee School of Dentistry, Milwaukee, WI, USA.

Oral verrucous hyperplasia

Oral verrucous hyperplasia is a histopathological diagnosis. It resembles verrucous carcinoma clinically and histologically and may evolve into frank verrucous carcinoma over time (see also *Section 10.4.1* on verrucous carcinoma).

Causes

Oral verrucous hyperplasia is strongly associated with tobacco smoking and areca nut chewing.

Clinical features

Oral verrucous hyperplasia presents as a solitary whitish or pink plaque or exophytic mass >1cm in an intraoral site (see *Fig. 4.21*).

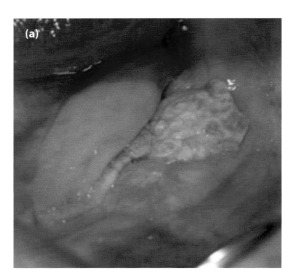
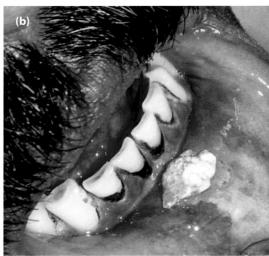

Figure 4.21 (a and b). Oral verrucous hyperplasia.

Reproduced from *Asian Pac J Cancer Prev,* 2016;17(9):4491 under a CC-BY-SA licence.

- Oral verrucous hyperplasia has a verrucous or papillary surface.
- It is classified as sharp or blunt:
  - sharp verrucous hyperplasia has long, narrow, heavily keratinized white structures
  - blunt verrucous hyperplasia has broader, flatter structures that are not heavily keratinized.
- Oral verrucous hyperplasia may co-exist with oral submucous fibrosis.

Diagnosis

Histopathology is necessary to distinguish oral verrucous hyperplasia from oral verrucous carcinoma.

- Verrucous hyperplasia is best distinguished from verrucous carcinoma in a biopsy taken at the margin of the lesion. In the former, the verrucous processes and the greater part of the hyperplastic epithelium are superficial to adjacent normal epithelium.
- Oral verrucous carcinoma has an exophytic and an endophytic growth pattern with broad, elongated rete processes resembling an elephant's feet.
- Oral verrucous hyperplasia has an exophytic growth pattern with pointed, ragged, slender, and anastomosing rete processes.

Treatment

Treatment options for verrucous hyperplasia include surgical excision and laser ablation.

4.5.2   Smokeless tobacco keratosis

Smokeless tobacco keratosis is a grey/white plaque on oral mucosa that is in frequent contact with a smokeless tobacco product such as chewing tobacco, moist snuff, or dry snuff.

It is also known as:
- tobacco pouch keratosis
- snuff dipper's keratosis.

Smokeless tobacco keratosis is common among adult smokeless tobacco users. The reported prevalence in the USA is 1.5% in smokeless tobacco users. Young men and males over 65 are affected more commonly than females.

The severity of smokeless tobacco keratosis is dependent on the following:
- Habit duration
- Brand of tobacco
- Early onset of use
- Total hours and amount of daily use
- The number of sites used for tobacco placement.

It usually takes 1–5 years to develop a smokeless tobacco keratosis.

Clinical features

Smokeless tobacco keratosis has a wrinkled or fissured corrugated surface. The most common locations are the lower labial or buccal vestibule (see *Fig. 4.22*). The plaque cannot be wiped off with gauze.

Diagnosis

Smokeless tobacco keratosis is usually diagnosed clinically.
- A biopsy is required if the lesion shows ulceration or does not resolve within 2–6 weeks of smokeless tobacco use.

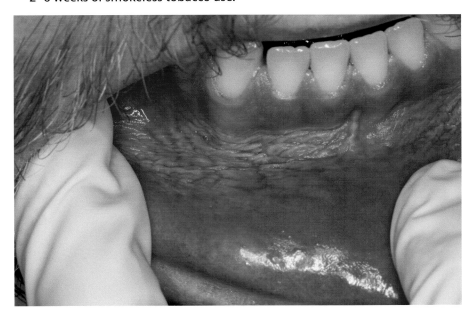

Figure 4.22. Smokeless tobacco keratosis showing a wrinkled white lesion in the labial vestibule.

Reproduced with permission from Professor Nagamani Narayana, University of Nebraska Medical Centre, NE, USA.

- Histopathology of smokeless tobacco keratosis reveals hyperkeratosis, parakeratin chevrons (V-shaped pattern), glycogen-rich clear superficial epithelial cells, and acanthosis. The connective tissue may show amorphous material, increased sub-epithelial vascularity, and vessel engorgement.

Treatment

No treatment is required.
- Encourage patients with smokeless tobacco keratosis to stop using tobacco.
- Epithelial changes resolve in 90% of lesions within 2–4 weeks of quitting smokeless tobacco use.

Verrucous carcinoma and squamous cell carcinoma have rarely been reported at the site of smokeless tobacco keratosis (see *Chapter 10* for more).

4.5.3   Tobacco smoking

Leukokeratosis nicotina palati

Leukokeratosis nicotina palati is an asymptomatic benign diffuse white lesion covering most of the hard palate.

It is also known as:
- nicotine stomatitis
- nicotinic stomatitis
- nicotine palatinus
- stomatitis palatini
- smoker's palate
- smoker's keratosis
- palatal leukokeratosis.

Leukokeratosis palati is common in smokers. A study in Saudi Arabia showed leukokeratosis nicotina palati affected 29.6% of all smokers and 60% of pipe smokers. It occurs in middle-aged and older individuals, with a male preponderance.

Causes

Leukokeratosis nicotina palati is mucosal hyperkeratosis due to the combined effects of tobacco products and heat.

It is associated with the following:
- Heavy, long-term pipe smoking
- Cigar smoking
- Hand-rolled reverse cigarette/cigar smoking.

It is less common with cigarette smoking.

Clinical features

Leukokeratosis nicotina palati presents as uniform white plaques on the palatal mucosa, sometimes with fissuring. The mid-palate inflamed mucous glands appear as umbilicated papules with red centres (see *Fig. 4.23*). Leukokeratosis nicotina palati cannot be wiped off.

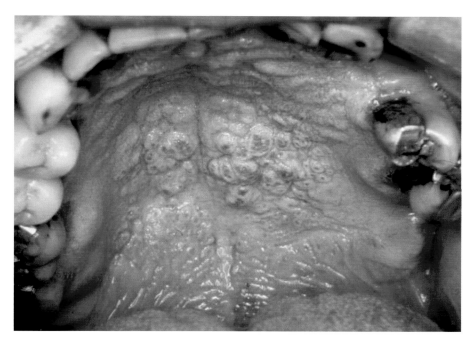

Figure 4.23. Nicotinic stomatitis (smoker's palate).

Reproduced from *Diagnosis and Management of Oral Lesions and Conditions: A resource handbook for the clinician*; Eds: CA Migliorati and FS Panagakos (http://dx.doi.org/10.5772/57597) under CC BY 3.0 licence. © 2014 InTech.

Diagnosis

Leukokeratosis nicotina palati is usually diagnosed clinically.
- A biopsy is warranted if the structure is irregular and ulcerated or if the patient places the burning end of the smoking device inside the mouth (see *Section 10.3.4* on reverse smoker's palate).
- Histopathology of leukokeratosis nicotina palati reveals acanthosis and orthokeratosis without cellular atypia or loss of polarity. Fibrosis of the lamina propria is a consequence of chronic inflammation.

Treatment

No treatment is required.
- Encourage patients with leukokeratosis nicotina palati to stop smoking.
- Leukokeratosis nicotina palati is reversible with smoking cessation.

Smoker's melanosis

Smoker's melanosis is a characteristic pigmentary change to the oral mucosal surfaces because of tobacco habits. It is due to increased melanin production by melanocytes in the basal cell layer of the epithelium and the accumulation of melanophages within the connective tissue.
- Smoker's melanosis is common among dark-skinned adult smokers.
- In females, it has been associated with birth control pills.

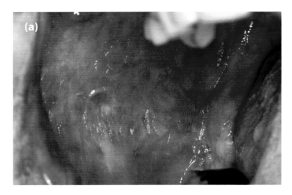

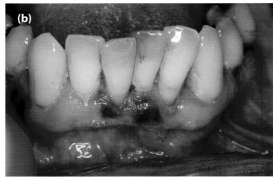

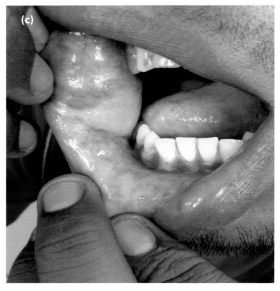

Figure 4.24 (a–c). Smoker's melanosis. Brown and black pigmentation of the oral mucosa in a heavy smoker.

(a) and (b) Reproduced from Health NZ – Waikato (www. waikatodhb.health.nz) with permission; (c) Reproduced from Wikimedia Commons (https://commons.wikimedia.org/ wiki/File:Smoker%27s_melanosis.jpg) under a CC-BY-SA 3.0 Unported licence.

- It usually presents as a diffuse hyperpigmented patch on the attached gingiva and buccal mucosa and is less common in other mucosal areas (see *Fig. 4.24*).
- Pigmentation decreases following cessation of smoking and other tobacco habits.

4.6   Adverse drug reaction

An oral mucosal adverse drug reaction to a topical or systemic medication usually presents as ulceration. Diagnosis is based on the chronology of an ulcer appearing after drug administration or dose escalation.

Causes

Adverse drug reactions are classified as Type A and Type B.
- Type A reactions are dose-dependent, based on drug pharmacology.
- Type B reactions are idiosyncratic and may be immunological (either T-cell or antibody-mediated) or non-immunological (for example, direct mucosal toxicity due to conventional and targeted anti-cancer therapy).

Pharmacogenetics influences the risk of some adverse drug reactions. For example, in Han Chinese and South-East Asian populations, the HLA-B*1502 polymorphism is associated with an increased risk of SJS/TEN with anticonvulsants.

Clinical features

Drug-induced oral mucosal ulceration may present with cheilitis (for example dryness due to isotretinoin) (see *Fig. 4.25*), aphthous-like ulcers, a lichenoid eruption, lupus-like ulcers, or trigger an immunobullous eruption. The ulcers may closely resemble an inflammatory disease that is not induced by a drug (see *Sections 7.1, 7.2,* and *7.4*).
- Ulceration may occur within days, weeks, or months of starting the responsible medication, such as methotrexate (see *Fig. 4.26*).
- Fixed drug eruptions recur at the same site with further exposure to the causative drug.

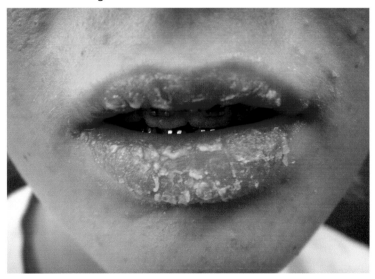

Figure 4.25. Cheilitis due to oral isotretinoin.

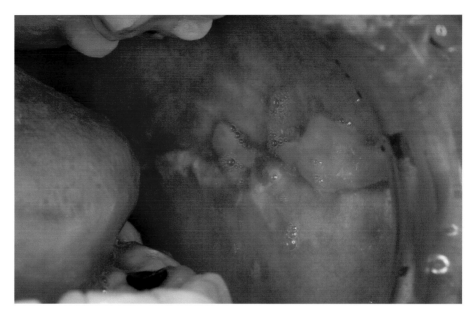

Figure 4.26. Ulceration of the left buccal mucosa due to methotrexate.

Image reproduced from Health NZ – Waikato (www.waikatodhb.health.nz) with permission.

4.6.1   Chemical burn

A chemical burn is due to direct contact of the mucosa with a causative drug, such as aspirin or cocaine.

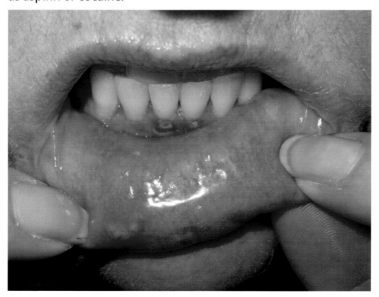

Figure 4.27. Aphthous ulceration induced by an NSAID.

Image reproduced from Health NZ – Waikato (www.waikatodhb.health.nz) with permission.

4.6.2   Aphthous-like ulceration

Aphthous or aphthous-like ulcers (see *Fig. 4.27*) can result from an oral non-steroidal anti-inflammatory drug (NSAID: naproxen, piroxicam, indomethacin), the anti-anginal nicorandil, an antihypertensive (captopril, labetalol, losartan), an antibiotic (trimethoprim-sulfamethoxazole), a bisphosphonate (alendronate, etidronate, risedronate), or an mTOR inhibitor (sirolimus, everolimus).

4.6.3   Fixed drug eruption

Oral mucosal fixed drug eruption has been reported from a single exposure or multiple exposures to a causative drug, which includes analgesics (paracetamol, naproxen, etoricoxib, piroxicam), the antihistamine levocetirizine, an antimicrobial agent, (trimethoprim-sulfamethoxazole fluconazole, clarithromycin, ornidazole, tetracycline), gabapentin, or simvastatin.

Fixed drug eruption presents as one or more acute blisters on an erythematous or purplish base resolving with hyperpigmentation. It recurs in identical sites on re-exposure to the causative drug. Fixed drug eruption can present with painful ulcers on the lips and tongue (see *Fig. 4.28*).

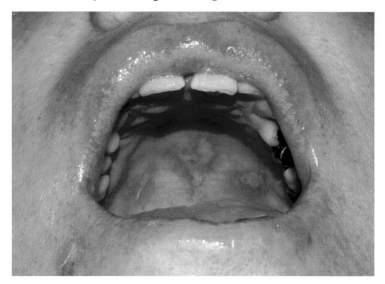

Figure 4.28. Fixed drug eruption.

Image reproduced from Health NZ – Waikato (www.waikatodhb.health.nz) with permission.

4.6.4   Lichenoid drug eruption

The wide range of drugs causing oral lichenoid reactions includes:
- analgesics – aspirin, diclofenac, ibuprofen, indomethacin, naproxen, piroxicam
- antidiabetics – glibenclamide, glipizide, metformin, tolbutamide
- antihypertensives – atenolol, captopril, enalapril, methyldopa, nifedipine, prazosin, propranolol

- antimicrobials – chloroquine, ethambutol, isoniazid, ketoconazole, rifampicin, sulfamethoxazole, tetracyclines
- antirheumatics – gold, penicillamine, sulfasalazine
- biologic agents – imatinib, sunitinib, etanercept, abatacept, adalimumab, infliximab, nivolumab, pembrolizumab
- diuretics – bendrofluazide, frusemide, hydrochlorothiazide
- other drugs – carbamazepine, allopurinol, lithium, pravastatin, simvastatin, and levothyroxine.

They present as painful lichen planus-like white streaks and ulcers, most often affecting the buccal mucosa (see *Fig. 4.29*).

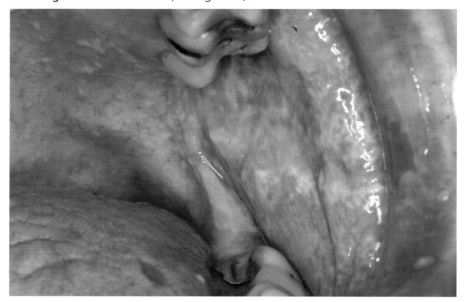

Figure 4.29. Lichenoid drug reaction associated with nivolumab. Nivolumab is used in the treatment of non-small cell lung cancer, kidney cancer, head and neck cancer, melanoma, Hodgkin disease, and liver cancer.

Image reproduced from Health NZ – Waikato (www.waikatodhb.health.nz) with permission.

4.6.5 Lupus-like reaction

Drugs that may cause oral lupus-like ulceration include antihypertensives (captopril, hydralazine), antimicrobials (minocycline, isoniazid), and others (carbamazepine, chlorpromazine, penicillamine, sulfasalazine, anti-TNF-α inhibitors, procainamide).

4.6.6 Immunobullous reaction

A bullous adverse reaction to a drug may present as an acute SCAR (a severe cutaneous adverse reaction such as SJS/TEN or bullous drug hypersensitivity syndrome (see *Fig. 4.30*). Drugs that can also induce bullous pemphigoid (e.g. vildagliptin) or pemphigus vulgaris (e.g. vancomycin) may involve the oral mucosa. Other drugs reported to cause bullous eruptions include anticonvulsants (carbamazepine, lamotrigine, phenytoin), antibiotics (amoxicillin/clavulanic acid, trimethoprim-sulfamethoxazole, rifampicin), xanthine oxidase inhibitor (allopurinol), NSAID (diclofenac), or others (chlorpromazine, frusemide, spironolactone, and penicillamine.

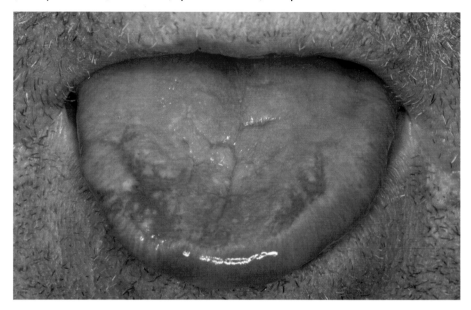

Figure 4.30. Bullous drug eruption due to sulfamethoxazole-trimethoprim, with widespread cutaneous bullae, oral blisters, and erosions seen here on the tongue.

Image reproduced from Health NZ – Waikato (www.waikatodhb.health.nz) with permission.

4.6.7   Drug-induced gingival hyperplasia

Drug-induced gingival hyperplasia is a peri-dental side-effect of certain drugs, causing swelling, bleeding, and problems with chewing, aesthetics, and pronunciation.

The drugs causing gingival hyperplasia include the following:
- Anticonvulsants, particularly phenytoin (50%)
- Immunosuppressants, particularly ciclosporin (30%)
- Calcium channel blockers, such as nifedipine (20%).

Clinical features

Drug-induced gingival hyperplasia presents as a firm, pale pink, painless, nodular enlargement of the interdental papilla, limited to the keratinized gingiva and extending to the facial and lingual gingival margins (see *Fig. 4.31*).
- Typically, it does not affect edentulous areas.
- The gingival overgrowth resolves when teeth are extracted.
- Histopathology shows an excessive accumulation of extracellular matrix-like collagen.

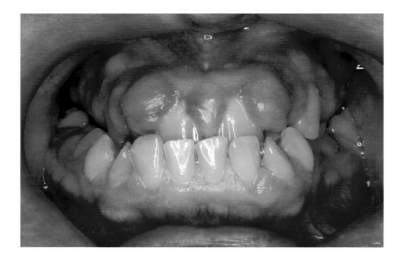

Figure 4.31. Drug-induced gingival hyperplasia (ciclosporin). Ciclosporin is an immunosuppressant medication.

Image reproduced from Health NZ – Waikato (www.waikatodhb.health.nz) with permission, and included here after enhancement by AIPDerm (www.aipderm.com).

Treatment

Options for treatment include:
- plaque control
- discontinuing or changing the inducing drug
- scalpel gingivectomy.

4.6.8   Stevens–Johnson syndrome / toxic epidermal necrolysis

Stevens–Johnson syndrome / toxic epidermal necrolysis (SJS/TEN) is a rare acute mucocutaneous emergency requiring hospitalization. The area of detached skin classifies the disease.
- SJS: skin detachment of <10% of body surface area
- Overlap SJS/TEN: detachment between 10% and 30% of body surface area
- TEN: skin detachment of >30% of body surface area.

SJS/TEN can affect children and adults. Incidence is equal in males and females, involving about 1 to 2 cases per million per year. It is more commonly experienced in people of Chinese ancestry than in Europeans.

Causes

SJS/TEN is a severe cutaneous adverse reaction, most often to a drug, such as an antibiotic (40%), an anticonvulsant, allopurinol, or targeted immunotherapy.
- In about 20% of cases, the cause is an infection or vaccination.
- There is a genetic predisposition with HLA associations for reactions to specific drugs in certain races.
- Cytotoxic lymphocytes mediate skin detachment.

Clinical features

The prodrome varies from a few days to two months, depending on the causative drug. The patient rapidly becomes extremely ill.

- Initial symptoms of SJS/TEN are high fever, sore throat, conjunctivitis, myalgia, and arthralgia.
- A tender, painful rash begins abruptly on the trunk and rapidly extends to the face and limbs over 4 days.
- It comprises erythematous macules, diffuse erythema, blisters, and targetoid lesions.
- The Nikolsky sign is positive. The skin detaches, exposing bright red, oozing dermis.
- The oral mucosal disease presents with haemorrhagic crusting of the lip, painful blisters, crusted erosions, and ulceration (see *Fig. 4.32*) causing odynophagia and dysphagia.
- The disease may affect ocular, oesophageal, anogenital mucosa, respiratory and gastrointestinal tracts, heart, liver, and kidneys.
- The acute stage of the illness lasts 1 or 2 weeks, but re-epithelialization can take weeks.

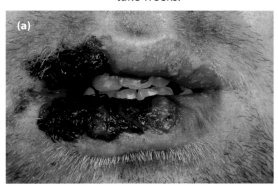 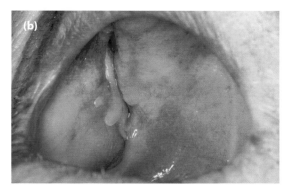

Figure 4.32 (a and b). Lip and oral mucosal crusting and ulceration in Stevens–Johnson syndrome / toxic epidermal necrolysis.

Image reproduced from Health NZ – Waikato (www.waikatodhb.health.nz) with permission.

Diagnosis

The diagnosis of SJS/TEN is clinical.

- Typical histopathological features are full-thickness epithelial necrosis and keratinocyte apoptosis. Intra-epithelial vesicles and perivascular lymphocytic infiltration are characteristic.
- Investigations are undertaken to identify and monitor systemic effects of the reaction.

Treatment

Stop the causative drug immediately; the patient should avoid it lifelong. The patient should be referred to a hospital, ideally to a burns unit.

Prognosis

The prognosis of SJS/TEN depends on the extent of epidermal detachment, patient age, and systemic co-morbidities.
- Mortality is up to 10% for SJS and >30% for TEN.
- Recovery may be accompanied by blindness and scarring of skin, nails, and mucosa.

4.7   Reaction to infection or vaccination

4.7.1   Infection-related mucositis

Erythema, oedema, and erosions can rarely arise in association with a viral infection (see *Fig. 4.33*).

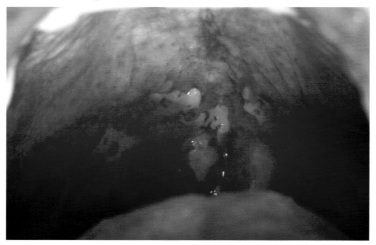

Figure 4.33. Acute mucositis associated with Covid-19 infection.

Image reproduced from Health NZ – Waikato (www.waikatodhb.health.nz) with permission.

4.7.2   Erythema multiforme

Erythema multiforme (EM) is an uncommon mucocutaneous reaction to an infection or other trigger. It usually affects young adults, with an annual incidence of about 1%.

Classification is based on the degree of mucosal involvement and the nature and distribution of skin lesions.
1. EM minor – affects only one mucosa and is associated with symmetrical target lesions on the extremities.
2. EM major – affects two or more mucous membranes with more variable skin involvement.

Causes

Erythema multiforme is often due to HSV infection (~70%).
- Other viral infectious triggers include orf and Covid-19.

- *Mycoplasma pneumoniae* causes an erythema multiforme-like distinct syndrome known as *Mycoplasma pneumoniae*-induced rash and mucositis (MIRM).
- Rare triggers of EM include vaccination, systemic illness, and medication such as an NSAID, antibiotic, or anti-epileptic.

Clinical features

Erythema multiforme is an acute reaction characterized by target lesions, oral or lip ulceration, and mild systemic symptoms.
- Lesions are present in the oral mucosa, other mucosal sites, and the skin.
- Oral lesions most frequently affect the buccal mucosa and vermilion border. They range from minor erythema to extensive and painful, deep haemorrhagic bullae, crusted erosions, and ulcers (see *Fig. 4.34*).
- EM may also affect ocular, nasal, pharyngeal, laryngeal, upper respiratory, and anogenital mucosa.
- Classic target lesions are concentric rings of central epidermal blistering/ necrosis, intermediate zone oedema, and peripheral erythema. They are pruritic and painful. Target lesions and atypical erythematous plaques start on the hands and feet and appear on the distal limbs. Target lesions may also affect the cheeks, ears, and chest. The distribution is symmetrical.
- Recurrent EM is uncommon and is nearly always triggered by herpes labialis.
- Chronic EM is rare.

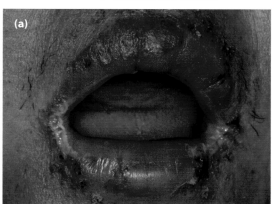
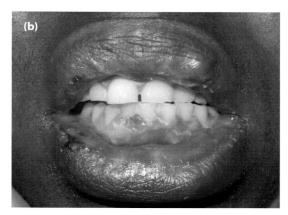

Figure 4.34 (a and b). Erythema multiforme showing (a) crusted vermilion, and (b) vesicles and erosions on gingiva and lips.

Image reproduced from Health NZ – Waikato (www.waikatodhb.health.nz) with permission.

Diagnosis

The diagnosis of EM is clinical. Typical histopathological features are dermal oedema and individual keratinocyte necrosis, but the histology is often non-specific.

Treatment

Supportive therapy includes analgesics, local anaesthetic/antiseptic mouthwash, hydration, nutritional supplementation, a topical corticosteroid, and bed rest.

Systemic steroids may be prescribed in patients with EM major, but their use is controversial.

Prognosis

In most cases, EM resolves within 3 weeks, but recovery may take up to 6 weeks for EM major.
- EM does not usually cause scarring except for rare ocular or pharyngeal involvement.
- Episodes of recurrent EM associated with HSV may be reduced by prophylactic oral aciclovir or valaciclovir.

4.8 Pigment

4.8.1 Amalgam tattoo

Amalgam tattoo, also known as focal argyrosis, is the impregnation of amalgam particles into focal areas of the oral mucosa during tooth extraction or replacement of an existing amalgam restoration.

Clinical features

Amalgam tattoos are the most common focal pigmented lesions of the oral mucosa.
- An amalgam tattoo is usually an incidental clinical finding during a routine oral examination.
- Typically, there is a solitary, blue–black, well-defined, or diffuse pigmented macule (see *Fig. 4.35*).
- Most amalgam tattoos are found on the gingivae or edentulous ridges.

Diagnosis

Clinical diagnosis is usually sufficient.
- An X-ray may reveal a large tattoo to be radiodense due to metal in the paradental tissues.

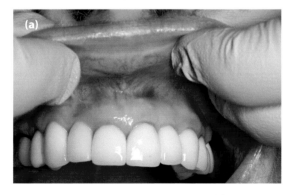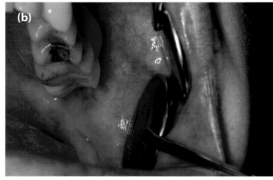

Figure 4.35 (a and b). Amalgam tattoo showing blue–black pigmentation in the missing lower premolar region.

(a) Reproduced with permission from Professor Nagamani Narayana, University of Nebraska Medical Centre, NE, USA.

- Histology shows foreign particulate material within macrophages and multinucleated giant cells or extracellularly around blood vessels in the connective tissue.

Treatment

No treatment is required for most amalgam tattoos, but they may be excised; for example, to exclude mucosal melanoma.

4.8.2   Cosmetic tattoo

Tattooing of soft tissues is popular in many countries, and it may be culturally significant in developing countries, while in developed countries, it is a social custom. While cutaneous tattooing is more common, mucosal tattooing may also be observed.

Clinical features

Tattoos should be differentiated from physiologic pigmentation and smoker's melanosis.
- The tattoo colour may vary from dark green to black.
- The gingiva, labial mucosa, and palate are the most common intraoral sites for tattooing.
- Periodontal disease increases the risk of procedure-related infection.
- The colour fades more rapidly in the mouth than when implanted in the skin.

Treatment

The pigment used for tattoos is usually harmless, and no treatment is required. Contact allergy, granulomas, and lichenoid reactions to intraoral cosmetic tattoos have been rarely described.

4.8.3   Drug-induced pigmentation

Pigmentation of the oral mucosa is reported to be induced by many medications:
- Antimalarial (chloroquine phosphate, hydroxychloroquine, quinidine, quinacrine)
- Chemotherapy (doxorubicin, busulfan, bleomycin, cyclophosphamide, clofazimine, imatinib)
- Antiretroviral agent (zidovudine, azidothymidine)
- Antibiotic (tetracycline, minocycline)
- Tranquillizer (chlorpromazine)
- Antifungal (ketoconazole)
- Laxative (phenolphthalein).

Clinical features

Drug-induced mucosal pigmentation may present as linear, diffuse, or multifocal discrete macules. Brown or grey pigmentation may affect the gingivae or other mucosal sites (see *Fig. 4.36*).

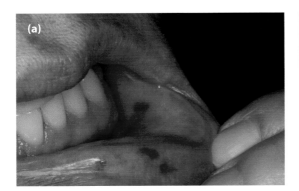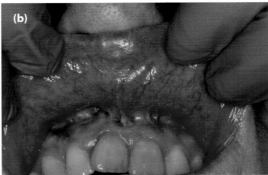

Figure 4.36 (a and b). Drug-induced pigmentation. Multifocal discrete macules (a) and patchy diffuse pigmentation (b).

- Diagnosis is usually on clinical grounds and a history of chronic drug use.
- Intraoral fixed drug eruption and lichenoid drug eruption may also result in pigmentation following an inflammatory phase.
- A biopsy may be required for confirmation.

Treatment

No treatment is required for asymptomatic drug-induced pigmentation. Patient education and reassurance are recommended.

4.8.4   Postinflammatory pigmentation

Inflammatory skin conditions such as lichen planus may result in localized hyperpigmentation as they resolve, especially in patients with skin of colour.

4.8.5   Heavy metal pigmentation

Heavy metal pigmentation is rare and is caused by excessive ingestion or exposure to bismuth, lead, mercury, and silver.

Clinical features

Pigmentation appears on the skin and oral mucosa in a patient with a metallic taste, gastrointestinal disturbance, and a history of exposure to heavy metals.
- A thin linear deposit of the gingiva is the most common sign of heavy metal pigmentation. Diffuse pigmentation may also occur.
- A biopsy reveals black particulate deposits in the lamina propria. These are the products of the oxidation of the metal within the tissues.

Treatment

Treatment involves avoiding further exposure to heavy metals and referral to a hospital facility.

4.9 Reaction to an underlying disease

4.9.1 Acanthosis nigricans

Acanthosis nigricans refers to hyperpigmented velvety plaques affecting the skin folds in the neck, groin, and axillae. Acanthosis nigricans may also affect the oral cavity.

- Acanthosis nigricans is more commonly observed in people of African and Polynesian descent than in Europeans and Asians.
- Acanthosis nigricans may become apparent at any age. When associated with malignancy, it most frequently occurs after 40 years of age.

Causes

Acanthosis nigricans is a sign of insulin resistance and is most often associated with obesity and systemic diseases such as diabetes. Elevated levels of insulin and insulin-like growth factor cause epithelial cells to proliferate.

- Acanthosis nigricans is sometimes caused by a medication (e.g. insulin, glucocorticoids, niacin, oral contraceptive, or a protease inhibitor).
- It may be inherited as an autosomal dominant trait due to mutations in fibroblast growth factor receptor 3.
- Malignant or paraneoplastic acanthosis nigricans is most often associated with gastric adenocarcinoma and less commonly with lung, ovary, and breast cancers.
- Malignant acanthosis nigricans is related to the secretion of various tumour products such as epidermal growth factor, transforming growth factor-alpha, and hormones that stimulate the growth of melanocytes, keratinocytes, and fibroblasts.

Clinical features

Acanthosis nigricans is characterized by hyperpigmentation and abnormal thickening of the sides and back of the neck, axillae, groin, and anal/genital region. Oral involvement is rare.

- Acanthosis nigricans of the oral mucosa is characterized by painless soft, papillomatous plaques on the lips, perioral region, palate, gingiva, and tongue (see *Fig. 4.37*).
- The mucosal lesions have the same colour as the surrounding mucosa.
- Oral acanthosis nigricans may be the first clinical sign of internal cancer.

Diagnosis

The diagnosis of acanthosis nigricans is based on personal and family history and clinical evaluation. Endocrine tests and imaging may follow.

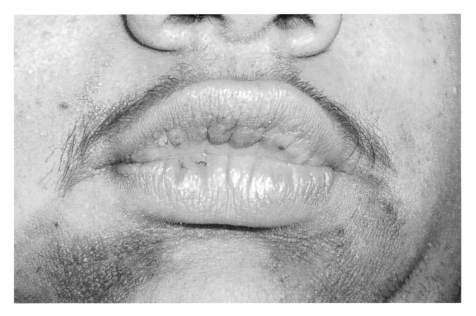

Figure 4.37. Acanthosis nigricans affecting vermilion.

Image shown here after enhancement by AIPDerm (www.aipderm.com).

Treatment

There is no specific treatment for oral acanthosis nigricans. Treatment of any underlying medical problem is helpful, such as weight loss in those with obesity.

4.9.2   Plummer–Vinson syndrome

Plummer–Vinson syndrome (also known as the Paterson–Kelly syndrome) is a triad of:
1. dysphagia
2. iron-deficiency anaemia
3. oesophageal webbing.

It is associated with an increased risk of oral squamous cell carcinoma (SCC) and SCC of the pharynx and oesophagus, with 3–15% of patients developing upper gastrointestinal tract cancer.
- Plummer–Vinson syndrome is rare, with most patients of Caucasian background, middle-aged, and female.
- Its causes are unknown.
- Dysphagia may be painless and intermittent or progressive over many years. It may limit dietary options and, in some cases, result in significant weight loss.
- Anaemia may result in weakness, pallor, and fatigue.
- Oral manifestations of long-standing anaemia include glossitis and angular cheilitis (see *Section 6.4.1*).

4.9.3 Mouth ulcers due to underlying bowel disease

Aphthous or aphthous-like ulceration is sometimes associated with underlying bowel disease, when treatment of the bowel disease can result in improvement or resolution of the mouth ulcers. See also *Section 9.7* on coeliac disease and *Section 9.8* on inflammatory bowel disease.

4.10 Reactive gingival hyperplasia

4.10.1 Localized juvenile spongiotic gingival hyperplasia

Localized juvenile spongiotic gingival hyperplasia primarily affects children and young adults. Its cause is unknown.

Clinical features

Juvenile spongiotic gingival hyperplasia results in bright red plaques on the attached gingiva.
- They have a papillary or granular surface.
- Histopathological examination shows subtle papillary epithelial hyperplasia with spongiosis, neutrophil exocytosis and engorged capillary vascular spaces in the lamina propria.

Treatment

Persistent juvenile spongiotic gingival hyperplasia can be surgically excised and does not recur if completely excised.

4.10.2 Hormone-related gingivitis

According to the US CDC, 60–75% of pregnant women have gingivitis.

Causes

Gingival disease in pregnancy is initiated by dental plaque and changes in oral microbiota due to fluctuations in oestrogen and progesterone levels. Oral contraceptive medications can provoke similar features, and hormone-related gingivitis may occur in postmenopausal women.

Clinical features

Gingivitis in pregnancy is characterized by erythematous swollen gingiva with increasing periodontal probing depths and bleeding upon probing.

Treatment

Maintenance of good oral hygiene is essential.

Consider surgical reduction of gingival hyperplasia.

CHAPTER 5

ORAL MUCOSAL DISEASES OF DEVELOPMENTAL AND GENETIC ORIGIN

See also:
- *Chapter 1: Anatomical features and variants of the oral cavity*
- *Section 8.2: Cysts*
- *Section 9.3: Hereditary angioedema; Section 9.14: Sickle cell anaemia*
- *Section 10.1.5: Infantile proliferative haemangioma*

5.1 Congenital disorders

5.1.1 Congenital macroglossia

Macroglossia is an abnormally large tongue that protrudes beyond the alveolar ridge in a resting position. It can be congenital or acquired.
- Congenital macroglossia has a prevalence of fewer than 5 per 100 000 births.
- It is twice as common in females as in males.
- It is twice as common in African Americans compared to those of European ancestry.

Causes

Congenital macroglossia may be isolated or associated with inherited or other congenital disorders.
- These include Down syndrome, Apert syndrome, Beckwith–Wiedemann syndrome, acromegaly, primary amyloidosis, and congenital hypothyroidism.
- Local abnormalities causing congenital macroglossia include vascular or lymphatic malformations, infantile haemangioma, and neurofibromatosis.
- Isolated congenital macroglossia can be genetic with autosomal dominant inheritance.

Clinical features

Macroglossia may be asymptomatic. When symptomatic, macroglossia may cause drooling, speech impairment, difficulty eating, stridor, snoring, airway obstruction, abnormal growth of the jaw and teeth, ulceration, and crenations on the lateral borders of the tongue (see acquired macroglossia in acromegaly (*Fig. 9.12*) and amyloidosis (*Fig. 9.13*)).

Diagnosis

Congenital macroglossia is usually diagnosed at birth due to the tongue's size. *In utero*, an ultrasound scan can detect macroglossia.

Treatment

Congenital macroglossia can resolve as the child grows, as the tongue and oral cavity adapt to accommodate the larger tongue.

Surgery may rarely be considered for severe persistent macroglossia.

5.1.2   White sponge naevus

White sponge naevus is a rare inherited disorder in which there are persistent white plaques in the oral mucosa and less commonly in the nasal, oesophageal, laryngeal, or anogenital mucosa. There are no associated abnormalities of skin, hair, or nails.

White sponge naevus is also known as:
- Cannon disease
- familial white folded gingivostomatitis
- hereditary leukokeratosis
- white gingivostomatitis
- exfoliative leukoedema.

White sponge naevus is rare, having a prevalence of under 1 in 200 000, without gender or racial predilection.

Causes

White sponge naevus is a developmental anomaly.
- It is inherited as an autosomal dominant trait with variable expressivity and high penetrance.
- There are defects in keratin 4 and keratin 13, expressed in the oral mucosa's spinous cell layer.
- It can occasionally be sporadic, with no history of affected family members.

Clinical features

White sponge naevus is usually present at birth or early childhood, occasionally developing during adolescence.
- White sponge naevus presents as one or more asymptomatic, diffuse, symmetrical, white, soft, corrugated, or velvety plaques.
- They are in the buccal mucosa (see *Fig. 5.1a* and *b*) or less often in the labial or gingival mucosa, the floor of the mouth, or the tongue (see *Fig. 5.1c*).
- Less often, similar plaques occur in the nasal, oesophageal, laryngeal, and anogenital mucosa.

The white colour persists when the tissue is stretched. The lesion cannot be removed by rubbing.

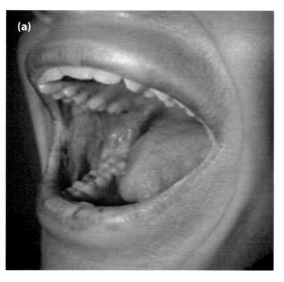

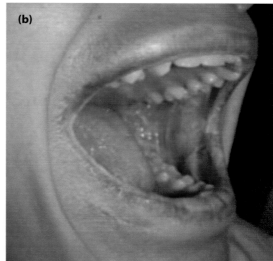

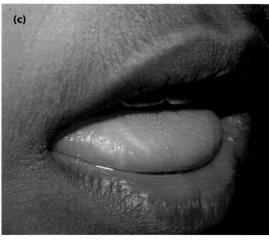

Figure 5.1 (a–c). White sponge naevus in the right (a) and left (b) buccal mucosa and on the dorsal tongue (c).

(a and b) Reproduced from *Pediatric Dermatology*, 2012;29, 1–3 with permission from John Wiley & Sons, and included here after enhancement by AIPDerm (www.aipderm.com). (c) Reproduced from Health NZ – Waikato (www.waikatodhb. health.nz) with permission.

Diagnosis

White sponge naevus is diagnosed from history and clinical examination. A biopsy is not usually required.

- Family history may or may not be present.
- The histopathology of white sponge naevus shows epithelial hyperkeratosis and acanthosis. The suprabasal cells exhibit intracellular oedema with pyknotic nuclei and compact aggregates of keratin intermediate filaments within the upper spinous layer. There may be a few mitotic figures, but there is no evidence of dysplasia.

Treatment

White sponge naevus is benign. It remains unchanged after the first few months of onset, and no treatment is necessary.

- A topical antifungal agent (nystatin oral solution) can be prescribed if symptomatic when colonized by candida.
- Rarely, if a lesion extends onto the lip vermilion border, the plaque may be removed surgically for aesthetic reasons.

5.1.3 Vascular malformation

A vascular malformation is a developmental condition affecting blood vessels, including arteries and veins, arterioles and venules, capillaries, or lymphatic vessels. Vascular malformations are primarily present at birth but can enlarge over time. They can be isolated or part of a syndrome involving several organs.

- Port wine stain (capillary malformation – see below)
- Slow-flow venous and lymphatic malformations
- Fast-flow arteriovenous malformations and arteriovenous fistulas
- Syndromes such as Klippel–Trenaunay, Parkes–Weber, Osler–Weber–Rendu, CLOVES, and blue rubber bleb naevus syndrome.

Port wine stain

Port wine stain, also known as naevus flammeus, is a cutaneous capillary vascular malformation present at birth and which persists for life.

Port wine stain affects 0.3% to 1% of the population, and females are affected twice as often as males. The occurrence is usually sporadic, but a 10% familial incidence has been reported.

Clinical features

Approximately 90% of port wine stains are located on the face, with the remainder usually found on the neck, trunk, and extremities. Most facial port wine stains are unilateral in a trigeminal dermatomal distribution (see *Fig. 5.2*).

- Port wine stain can also involve the oral mucosa and gingiva, resulting in complications such as macrocheilia and gingival bleeding.
- An initial pink patch becomes a reddish–purple plaque over time. Vascular nodules arise in 50%.
- Port wine stains are a component of the Sturge–Weber syndrome (encephalotrigeminal angiomatosis), Parkes–Weber syndrome, Klippel–Trenaunay syndrome, Proteus syndrome and some arteriovenous malformations.

Treatment

The current treatment for port wine stain is photocoagulation of the abnormal blood vessels by pulsed dye laser. Other lasers may also be effective. Surgical intervention is needed to revise any anatomical distortion of the dental and jaw tissues.

5.1.4 Lymphatic malformation

Lymphatic malformations occur mainly in infancy and early childhood and frequently affect the head and neck region. Intraoral lesions are rare.

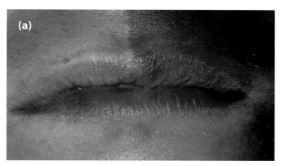
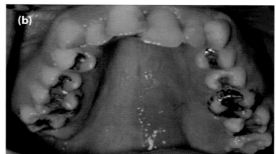
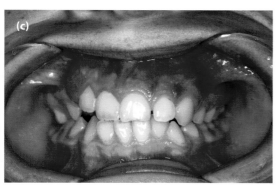

Figure 5.2 (a–c). Port wine stains showing unilateral distribution in (a) trigeminal dermatomal region of the face and (b) the palate; (c) showing V1/V2 distribution resulting in enlargement of the maxillary alveolus and gingiva.

(a and b) Reproduced with permission from *Pocket Dentistry* (https://pocketdentistry.com/sturge-weber-syndrome-case-report), and included here after enhancement by AIPDerm (www.aipderm.com). (c) Reproduced from Health NZ – Waikato (www.waikatodhb.health.nz) with permission.

Causes

A lymphatic malformation arises from a localized abnormal development of lymphatic vessels.

Clinical features

The most common form of lymphatic malformation is an asymptomatic translucent to purple, smooth or nodular plaque composed of multiple fluid-filled spaces or microcysts.
- The alternative term lymphangioma is a misnomer as the lesion is not a proliferative tumour.
- Lymphatic malformations may be stable or slowly enlarge.
- The most common intraoral site is the anterior two-thirds of the tongue, causing macroglossia.
- Lingual lymphatic malformations may be superficial, involve muscle, or extend more widely within the oral cavity.
- They are usually asymptomatic, translucent, smooth plaques, often with a pebbly surface composed of lymph-filled vesicles (see *Fig. 5.3*). These may be haemorrhagic.

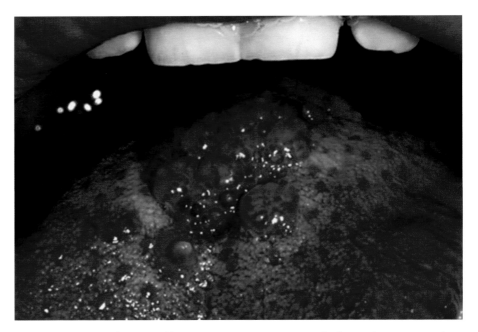

Figure 5.3. Lymphatic malformation. Mass composed of translucent papules on the dorsal tongue.

Reproduced from *Color Atlas of Oral and Maxillofacial Diseases*, 2019; B.W. Neville, D.D. Damm, C.M. Allen & A.C. Chi, with permission from Elsevier.

Complications of lingual lymphatic malformations:
- Airway obstruction
- Recurrent infection
- Dysphagia
- Orthodontic abnormalities and malocclusion
- Excessive salivation
- Speech problems.

Diagnosis

The diagnosis of lymphatic malformation is generally based on history and clinical findings.
- A biopsy may be undertaken for histopathological confirmation, but it may cause bleeding.
- MRI may be undertaken to determine the extent of the lesion.

Treatment

Minor lymphatic malformations may require no intervention but rarely regress spontaneously.
- Treatment options include surgery, laser ablation, radiofrequency ablation, and sclerotherapy.
- Management of significant lymphatic malformations is complex, requiring multidisciplinary care.

- Recurrence after treatment is common.
- Close follow-up is recommended.

5.1.5 Ectodermal dysplasia

Ectodermal dysplasia refers to the genetically determined abnormal development of ectodermal structures — the skin, sweat glands, hair, nails, teeth, and mucous membranes.

Signs may include:
- Abnormal or missing teeth (see *Fig. 5.4*)
- Abnormal nails
- Abnormal or absent sweat glands
- Sparse, thin hair.

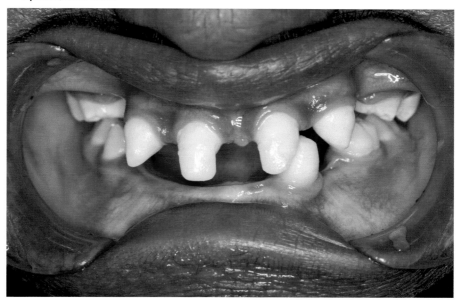

Figure 5.4. Missing and abnormal teeth in ectodermal dysplasia.

Reproduced from Health NZ – Waikato (www.waikatodhb.health.nz) with permission.

5.1.6 Focal dermal hypoplasia

Focal dermal hypoplasia is a sporadic form of congenital ectodermal and mesenchymal dysplasia characterized by patchy dermal hypoplasia. Focal dermal hypoplasia is also known as Goltz syndrome or Goltz–Gorlin syndrome.

Focal dermal hypoplasia causes deformities of teeth, hair, nails, extremities, and the central nervous system. It is usually lethal in males *in utero*, so 90% of affected living individuals are female.

Causes

Focal dermal hypoplasia is an X-linked dominant disorder caused by mutations or deletions in the porcupine *O*-acyltransferase gene (*PORCN*) located at Xp11.23. The mutation arises *de novo* in 95% and is inherited in 5%.

Clinical features

Skin lesions generally follow the lines of Blaschko, pathways of epidermal cell migration and proliferation during fetal development. Characteristics include:
- pink or red, tender, atrophic or slightly raised areas of the thin or absent dermis with herniated fat, sometimes ulcerated
- arranged with symmetrical linear, angular, or reticulated patterns
- multiple raspberry-like papillomas, apocrine naevi, and multiple hydrocystomas
- hypohidrosis and anhidrosis
- sparse and brittle scalp and body hair.

Typical facial, ocular, and auditory deformities may include:
- asymmetry of the face with hemiatrophy
- sparse eyebrows and eyelashes
- colobomata of the iris, retina, and choroid (in 30% of cases)
- asymmetry of ears and auricular appendages.

Oral and dental defects include prognathism, overbite, agenesis or dysplasia of the teeth, delayed tooth formation/eruption, microdontia, irregular spacing and malocclusion, enamel defects, and notching of the incisors or extra incisors, high-arched palate, double lingual frenulum, cleft lip, cleft palate, absence of a labial sulcus, hypertrophy of the gums, taurodontism, and papillomas of the gums, tongue, palate, and buccal mucosa.

Skeletal features are variable:
- Short stature
- Aplasia of the bones with complete or partial absence of an extremity
- Syndactyly, split hands and feet, claw hands, clinodactyly, adactyly, polydactyly, oligodactyly.

Gastrointestinal, cardiopulmonary, and genitourinary abnormalities have also been reported in patients with focal dermal dysplasia.

Diagnosis

Babies with focal dermal dysplasia are usually recognized at birth.
- Chest X-ray, eye examination, abdominal MRI, kidney ultrasound, hearing evaluation, and medical genetics consultation provide important clues to diagnosis.
- DNA testing for mutations in the *PORCN* gene confirms the diagnosis.

Treatment

Treatment for patients with focal dermal dysplasia is directed at the symptoms.
- Moisturizing creams and protective dressings relieve skin discomfort and prevent secondary infections.
- Avoidance of heat and excessive exercise.
- Dentures and hearing aids as required.
- Occupational therapy, assistive devices, or surgery for limb deformities.
- Surgical or laser therapy for dysphagia due to large fat deposits in the throat.

Most individuals with focal dermal dysplasia live to adulthood.

5.1.7   Cystic fibrosis

Cystic fibrosis is an autosomal recessive metabolic disorder affecting 1 per 2000 live births in the Caucasian population. The usual age of diagnosis is with newborn screening or before 2 years of age.

Cause

Cystic fibrosis results from one of numerous possible mutations in the *CFTR* (cystic fibrosis transmembrane conductance regulator) gene; the most common mutation is delta F508. Both parents must carry a mutation.

Clinical features

Cystic fibrosis symptoms and signs are due to thick sticky mucus (mucoviscidosis).
- Cystic fibrosis affects the lungs, pancreas, liver, intestines, sinuses, and sex organs.
- Abnormally salty sweat enables early diagnosis by a sweat test.
- Breathing difficulties, cough, recurrent pneumonia, and progressive loss of lung function.
- Digestive difficulties result in poor absorption of nutrients.

Oral manifestations of cystic fibrosis:
- Dental and skeletal maturation is delayed
- Permanent teeth develop with hypoplastic enamel
- Saliva produced by submandibular, sublingual, and minor salivary glands has increased pH and buffering capacity; this leads to a reduction in caries and periodontal disease
- The lips may be swollen, dry, and scaly due to the involvement of minor salivary glands
- Malocclusion including anterior open bite results from mouth breathing associated with chronic nasal and sinus obstruction.

Diagnosis
- Sweat chloride test
- DNA testing
- Imaging and other blood tests depend on clinical features.

Treatment

Treatment of cystic fibrosis is complex and requires a multidisciplinary approach beyond the scope of this book.

5.2   Disorders usually diagnosed in childhood

5.2.1   Darier disease

Darier disease is an autosomal dominantly inherited disorder characterized by:
- mucous membrane lesions
- scaly crusted papules in a seborrhoeic distribution
- nail abnormalities.

Darier disease is also known as keratosis follicularis.
- Darier disease occurs worldwide and shows geographic variation.
- The prevalence of Darier disease has been estimated to range from 1 in 30 000 in Scotland to 1 in 100 000 in Denmark.
- Males and females are equally affected.
- The chance of a child inheriting the abnormal gene if one parent is affected is 1 in 2 (50%).
- Not all people with abnormal genes will develop clinical features of the disease.
- Family history is absent in half of the affected individuals.

Causes

Darier disease is due to a mutation of the gene *ATP2A2* on chromosome 12q23–24.1.
- *ATP2A2* codes for the SERCA (sarco-/endoplasmic reticulum calcium-ATPase) enzyme or pump, which transports calcium within the cell.
- The cause of cell dyshesion remains unclear. However, desmosomes only assemble appropriately if there is sufficient calcium.

Clinical features

The symptoms and signs of Darier disease vary markedly between individuals and over time. The onset of skin changes is usually in adolescence.

Oral lesions

Darier disease affects the oral mucosa in up to 50% of affected patients. It may also affect pharyngeal, oesophageal, and anogenital mucosa.
- The primary lesion is a firm white papule (see *Fig. 5.5a*) with a rough sandpaper-like surface and a central depression.
- Papules may coalesce into plaques with a cobblestone pattern (see *Fig. 5.5b*).
- They may be skin-coloured, white, reddish, yellow–brown, or brown.
- They are found on the buccal mucosa and hard palate.

Intraoral mucosal lesions

These are detected in approximately 50% of patients with Darier disease. They are usually asymptomatic and discovered during a routine oral examination.
- Papules primarily affect the hard palate and alveolar mucosa and, less often, the oral mucosa, gingiva, and tongue.
- Palatal lesions may mimic papillary hyperplasia associated with dentures, smoker's palate, or intraepithelial neoplasia.

Skin lesions
- Cutaneous Darier disease presents with persistent, greasy, scaly papules coalescing into malodorous warty plaques.
- These are found on the scalp margins, forehead, ears, around the nostrils and sides of the nose, eyebrows, beard area, neck, central chest and back, axillae, groin, and the submammary zone.

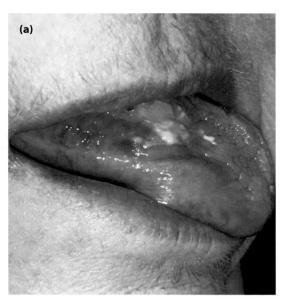
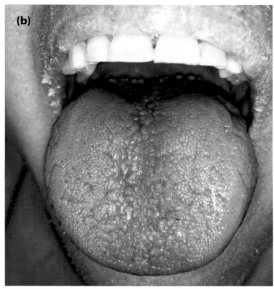

Figure 5.5 (a and b). Darier disease: (a) white hyperkeratotic plaque and (b) cobblestone appearance on the dorsal surface of the tongue.

Images reproduced from Health NZ – Waikato (www.waikatodhb.health.nz) with permission.

Nail disorders
- Longitudinal red or white stripes affect some or all fingernails.
- A V-shaped nick may be present at the free edge of the nail.

Diagnosis

Usually, Darier disease is diagnosed by its appearance and family history.

The histopathology of Darier disease includes acantholysis forming suprabasal clefts and superficial corps ronds and grains. Corps ronds in the granular cell layer show central round dyskeratotic basophilic masses surrounded by a clear halo-like zone.

Treatment

Patients with Darier disease should wear loose, covering clothing and sunscreen. Genetic counselling may be necessary.
- Flares are triggered by sun exposure, excessive sweating, and skin infection.
- Secondary bacterial infection is usually due to *Staphylococcus aureus* and may require oral antibiotics.
- Herpes simplex can be severe/extensive and is treated with high dose aciclovir or valaciclovir.

Limited or localized Darier disease may be treated with:
- a topical retinoid (isotretinoin, tazarotene, or adapalene)
- 5-fluorouracil cream
- surgical excision, dermabrasion, or carbon dioxide laser ablation of intractable plaques.

Generalized Darier disease may be treated with an oral retinoid (isotretinoin or acitretin).

Prognosis

The prognosis of Darier disease is variable. In most patients, general health remains good regardless of its severity. However, Darier disease can have a significant impact on psychosocial functioning.

5.2.2 Dyskeratosis congenita

Dyskeratosis congenita is a rare inherited bone marrow failure syndrome characterized by:
- white intraoral plaques
- reticular skin pigmentation
- abnormal nails.

In some individuals, dyskeratosis congenita is also associated with:
- congenital aplastic anaemia
- myelodysplastic syndrome
- leukaemia
- a solid tumour.

Variants include:
- autosomal dominant dyskeratosis congenita: MIM* #127550
- autosomal recessive dyskeratosis congenita: MIM #224230
- X-linked dyskeratosis congenita: MIM #305000
- sporadic forms of dyskeratosis congenita.

(*MIM is an abbreviation for Mendelian Inheritance in Man)

Dyskeratosis congenita is estimated to have an incidence of one in one million people. No racial predilection has been reported. The reported male-to-female ratio is approximately 3:1.

Causes

Mutations in fourteen genes have been identified in patients with dyskeratosis congenita.

Clinical features

Dyskeratosis congenita usually presents in childhood.

Oral lesions

White patches on the buccal mucosa, tongue (see *Fig. 5.6*) and oropharynx are found in approximately 80% of patients. The white patch may become verrucous or ulcerated.

Oral changes in dyskeratosis congenita have been reported to include:
- oral leukoplakia
- brown pigmentation
- increased dental caries

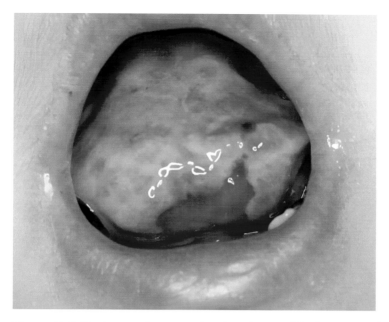

Figure 5.6. Dyskeratosis congenita showing a white lesion on the tongue.

Reproduced with permission from *Pocket Dentistry* (Chapter 25; www.pocketdentistry.com), and included here after enhancement by AIPDerm (www.aipderm.com).

- aggressive periodontitis
- hypodontia
- thin enamel
- tooth loss
- taurodontism (enlarged tooth pulp)
- blunted roots.

Any involved mucosal site may be constricted and stenosed in dyskeratosis congenita. Eye disease can also occur. Dyskeratosis congenita predisposes oral and other mucosal surfaces to squamous cell carcinoma.

Skin lesions

The main feature is hyperpigmented or hypopigmented macules and patches in a reticulated pattern on sun-exposed skin, including the upper trunk, neck, and face.

Other features
- Alopecia of the scalp, eyebrows, and eyelashes, with premature greying of the hair
- Hyperhidrosis
- Hyperkeratosis of the palms and soles
- Loss of dermatoglyphics (fingerprints).

Nail dystrophy
- Ridging of the nails and longitudinal splitting affects 90% of patients.
- The nails may become thinned, spoon-shaped, and atrophic.

- There may be pterygium formation or absent nails.
- The changes in the fingernails and toenails may worsen over time.

Systemic disease

Approximately 90% of patients have peripheral cytopenia, and about 70% of deaths relate to bleeding and opportunistic infections resulting from eventual bone marrow failure.

Diagnosis

A clinical diagnosis of dyskeratosis congenita may be confirmed by:
- dermoscopy of hyperpigmented macules showing lines of brown dots and globules arranged in a netlike pattern
- telomere length testing by multicolour flow cytometry fluorescence *in situ* hybridization (flow-FISH) showing very short telomeres compared to age-matched controls
- genetic testing, which detects a mutation in approximately 50% of cases.

Consider a diagnosis of dyskeratosis congenita in young people with:
- oral leukoplakia with no history of tobacco use
- bone marrow failure or lung fibrosis, where no other cause has been identified
- cancer.

General examination, including skin, nails, mucous membranes, chest, and neurological system, may be supplemented by:
- CBC to detect bone marrow failure
- chest X-ray and pulmonary function tests
- faecal occult blood to screen for gastrointestinal malignancy.

A skin biopsy from reticulated pigmentation typically shows non-specific mild hyperkeratosis, epidermal atrophy, superficial telangiectasia, and melanophages in the papillary dermis.

Treatment

There is no known cure for dyskeratosis congenita.

Management is multidisciplinary. Signs and symptoms develop at different ages and rates, making long-term surveillance important.

Dyskeratosis congenita carries a poor prognosis, with most deaths related to infection, bleeding, or malignancy.
- Life expectancy ranges from infancy to the 7th decade, with a mean survival of 30 years. Up to 40% of patients will have bone marrow failure before age 40.
- Genetic counselling is essential when planning future pregnancies. Antenatal diagnosis has been achieved successfully.

5.2.3   Epidermolysis bullosa

Epidermolysis bullosa (EB) is a group of genetically determined skin fragility disorders characterized by mechanical stress-induced blistering of the skin and mucous membranes. The four main types of EB are distinguished by the ultrastructural level of blister formation with at least 40 distinct clinical phenotypes.

- The overall incidence of epidermolysis bullosa is rare at fewer than 20 cases per one million live births.
- There is no gender predilection.
- The onset of epidermolysis bullosa is at birth or within the first year of life, depending on the subtype.
- Epidermolysis bullosa is broadly classified as EB simplex, junctional EB, dystrophic EB, and Kindler EB.

Causes

Epidermolysis bullosa is caused by mutations within the genes that encode at least nineteen structural proteins.

- The mode of inheritance varies depending on the type of epidermolysis bullosa.
- The site of the affected proteins within the epidermis, dermal–epidermal junction, or uppermost papillary dermis, determines the ultrastructural location of the blisters.

Clinical features

Epidermolysis bullosa is characterized by fragile skin, erosions, and in many cases, blisters (see *Fig. 5.7*).

- Epidermolysis bullosa may also involve the oral cavity, eyes, and gastrointestinal, genitourinary, and respiratory tracts.
- Oral manifestations may include mucosal fragility with blistering and scarring from previous disease activity, which may lead to microstomia. Structural defects of teeth include enamel hypoplasia.
- Blisters commonly form on the skin after minor trauma.
- Atrophic scarring can occur in any subtype.
- Some forms of epidermolysis bullosa lead to dystrophic or absent nails, milia, and scarring alopecia.

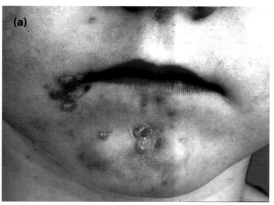
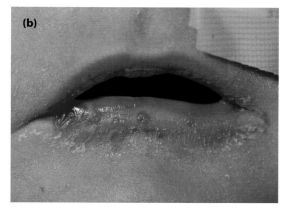

Figure 5.7 (a and b). (a) Epidermolysis bullosa simplex resulting in perioral blistering; (b) blistering on the lip in a patient with recessive dystrophic epidermolysis bullosa.

Images reproduced from Health NZ – Waikato (www.waikatodhb.health.nz) with permission.

Diagnosis

In the dominant subtypes of epidermolysis bullosa, a positive family history contributes to a clinical diagnosis. Diagnostic tests include:
- A skin biopsy of a newly induced blister for immunofluorescence antigen mapping.
- Transmission electron microscopy.
- Genetic testing.

Treatment

There are currently no specific therapies for epidermolysis bullosa.
- Management is primarily preventive and supportive, requiring a multidisciplinary approach.
- Regular dental attendance is required for preventive treatment and the management of generalized enamel hypoplasia.
- It is important to minimize trauma, particularly during dental appointments and whilst performing oral hygiene. Dental treatment may be complicated by microstomia and oral mucosal scarring.
- Lubrication of the lips and oral mucosa may reduce shear force and tissue damage.

Prognosis

The prognosis is dependent on the type of epidermolysis bullosa.
- Milder forms tend to have a reasonably good outcome, with an average life expectancy.
- Severe epidermolysis bullosa may lead to scarring, disfigurement, and failure to thrive. Very few patients with severe epidermolysis bullosa live into adulthood.

5.2.4   Fanconi anaemia

Fanconi anaemia is an autosomal and X-linked recessive disorder characterized by bone marrow failure, acute myelogenous leukaemia, solid tumours, and developmental abnormalities.

The risk of developing oral SCC in patients with Fanconi anaemia is 500–1000 times greater than in the general population.
- Cells derived from patients with Fanconi anaemia display hypersensitivity to DNA cross-linking agents, resulting in increased numbers of chromosomal abnormalities, including translocations and radial chromosomes.
- Oral SCC in Fanconi anaemia patients occurs in patients younger than the general population (15–50 years) without traditional risk factors (such as smoking and excessive alcohol consumption).
- The tumours frequently affect the gingiva and tongue.
- They behave aggressively with a high recurrence rate. Survival rates are poor.
- Haematological disorders in patients with Fanconi anaemia may be treated with an allogeneic haematopoietic stem cell transplant. However, this increases the risk of developing oral SCC.

5.2.5   Hereditary benign intraepithelial dyskeratosis

Hereditary benign intraepithelial dyskeratosis is a rare inherited disorder characterized by white epithelial plaques on the ocular and oral mucous membranes, and red eyes.

- It was first described as affecting Haleiwa Indians and their descendants (North Carolina, USA).
- It has been sporadically reported in a limited group of tri-racial families in Halifax County, North Carolina, and Europe (white, Native American, and black).

Causes

Hereditary benign intraepithelial dyskeratosis is caused by mutations (duplications) of *HBID* (hereditary benign intraepithelial dyskeratosis gene) on chromosome 4q3 (MIM #127600).

Inheritance is autosomal dominant.

Clinical features

The onset of hereditary benign intraepithelial dyskeratosis is in childhood.

Mouth
- Mouth lesions are large, superficial, soft white, spongy plaques with varying thicknesses and folds.
- They occur in the buccal mucosa, oral commissures, ventral tongue, the floor of the mouth, and less commonly on the gingiva and palate.

Eyes
- Ocular lesions are white granular to gelatinous, triangular, perilimbal, or bulbar conjunctival plaques.
- Dilated conjunctival vessels are usual.
- Lesions are typically bilateral and may encircle or extend over the cornea.
- Photophobia is common in children.

Diagnosis

The hereditary benign intraepithelial dyskeratosis diagnosis depends on positive family history, clinical findings, and the distinctive ocular and oral lesions histology.

Histopathology reveals parakeratosis, acanthosis, and many dyskeratotic 'tobacco' cells in the upper epithelium (they are called tobacco cells because of their brown colour with a Papanicolaou stain). Sometimes these dyskeratotic cells are surrounded by epithelial cells, resulting in a cell-within-a-cell appearance.

Treatment

There is no effective treatment for oral or ocular lesions. They may be excised for aesthetic reasons; however, the abnormal epithelium almost invariably recurs after excision.

5.2.6   Hereditary gingival fibromatosis

Hereditary gingival fibromatosis is rare and is characterized by slowly progressive fibrous enlargement of the gingiva. Usually, gingival enlargement starts before the age of 15 years, mostly in infancy.

Causes

There are at least five forms of autosomal dominant and recessive forms of hereditary gingival fibromatosis with known cytogenetic locations (CINGF1, GINGF2, GINGF3, GINGF4, GINGF5). Gingival fibromatosis can also occur as part of severe rare diseases and syndromes.

Clinical features

Gingival enlargement is usually generalized. Occasionally it may be localized to one or two quadrants.
- The enlarged gingiva is of normal colour, firm, and non-tender.
- The teeth are usually partly covered by the enlarged gingiva and may be malpositioned.
- Maxillary gingivae are more frequently affected than mandibular gingivae.

Treatment

Hereditary gingival fibromatosis is treated by surgical gingivectomy. Recurrence is expected but not inevitable.

5.2.7   Ligneous gingivitis

Ligneous gingivitis, also known as destructive membranous periodontal disease, is a rare disease characterized by fibrin-rich pseudomembranes. Females are affected more frequently than males (3:1 ratio).

Causes

Ligneous gingivitis is due to impaired extracellular fibrinolysis and abnormal wound healing associated with inherited type 1 plasminogen deficiency, in which there is a marked deficiency in PLG antigen due to an autosomal recessive mutation in the *PLG* gene.

Clinical features

Ligneous gingivitis often first presents in childhood. Features include:
- localized nodules or generalized gingival enlargement with ulceration
- associated ligneous conjunctivitis
- rapid loss of teeth and significant periodontal disease
- alveolar bone loss
- histologically, eosinophilic acellular material (fibrin) deposition occurs in the lamina propria
- blood tests confirm reduced plasma plasminogen activity.

Treatment

The affected gingival tissues can be removed by surgery, electrocautery, or laser ablation but recurrence of ligneous gingivitis is usual. Topical and systemic plasminogen activators have had variable success.

5.2.8 McCune–Albright syndrome

McCune–Albright syndrome is a sporadic disorder due to mutations in the gene *GNAS*. As these occur after the fertilization of the embryo, the syndrome is not inherited.

Three key features characterize McCune–Albright syndrome:
1. Polyostotic fibrous dysplasia
2. Hyperfunctioning endocrinopathies
3. Café-au-lait skin pigmentation.

Though not common, oral mucosal pigmentation has been reported in this syndrome.

5.2.9 Pachyonychia congenita

Pachyonychia congenita is a rare genetic disorder characterized by:
- white patches in mucous membranes
- thickened nails (pachyonychia)
- thickened skin of the palms and soles.

Both sexes are affected equally.

In January 2021, the International Pachyonychia Congenita Research Registry (IPCRR) reported more than 1000 individuals with genetically confirmed pachyonychia congenita.

Causes

Pachyonychia congenita is caused by a mutation in the genes encoding keratin, *K6a, K16, K17, K6b* and *K6c* (listed in decreasing frequency). By January 2021, 118 mutations had been described by the IPCRR.

Clinical features

The clinical features of pachyonychia congenita involve skin, nails, and mouth and depend on which keratin gene is involved.

Mouth
- Oral leukokeratosis on the tongue (see *Fig. 5.8*) and buccal mucosa are present at birth or develop within the first year in about 70% of patients.
- Natal or prenatal teeth are uncommon and are typically a feature of mutations in *K17*.
- Children with *K6a* mutation may experience intense pain when first eating. This is known as first-bite syndrome.
- Children may develop angular cheilitis.

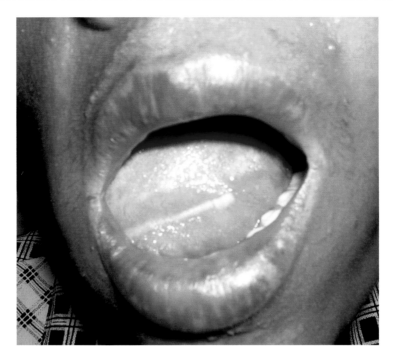

Figure 5.8. Pachyonychia congenita showing leukokeratosis of the tongue.

Image reproduced from Health NZ – Waikato (www.waikatodhb.health.nz) with permission.

Skin
- Thickened or calloused palms and soles are usual.
- Focal palmoplantar keratoderma may be the only feature of pachyonychia congenita in patients with mutations of *K6c*.
- Plantar pain affects 95% of patients with pachyonychia congenita and may have a neuropathic component. The pain may be constant and severe, particularly in patients with mutations of *K6a* and *K16*.
- Hyperhidrosis can accompany keratoderma.
- Blisters may be precipitated by friction and warm weather.
- Due to follicular hyperkeratosis, friction sites such as knees and elbows may be dry.
- Steatocystoma and pilosebaceous cysts are common.

Nails
- Nail changes are most severe with mutations of *K6a* and *K16*.
- Nail thickening is apparent early in life.
- The nails often have a brownish discolouration.
- All fingernails are commonly involved, and toenails are to a lesser extent.

Diagnosis

Pachyonychia congenita is usually diagnosed clinically.
- Skin biopsy of the affected tissues will only show non-specific changes.
- Molecular genetic studies may detect mutations in the affected keratin genes.

- Prenatal testing may be available if a pregnant woman or her partner has pachyonychia congenita.
- Pre-implantation diagnosis has been reported in embryos fertilized *in vitro*.

Treatment

There is no cure for pachyonychia congenita.

Therapy is directed towards symptoms:
- Specially constructed shoes, orthotic inserts, insoles, protective socks, and gloves
- Mechanical thinning of keratotic nails
- A systemic retinoid (isotretinoin or acitretin) reduces follicular keratoses and palmoplantar keratoderma
- Surgical excision of cysts.

Patients with pachyonychia congenita can expect an average lifespan. Genetic assessment and counselling are recommended.

5.2.10 Peutz–Jeghers syndrome

Peutz–Jeghers syndrome is a rare inherited disease characterized by gastrointestinal polyps and pigmentation of the skin and mucous membranes.

Polyps are benign hamartomas that may undergo malignant transformation. The risk of developing internal cancer is fifteen times greater for patients with Peutz–Jeghers syndrome than in the general population.

Causes

Peutz–Jeghers syndrome is due to germline mutations in the Serine Threonine Kinase tumour-suppressor gene *STK11/LKB1* found on chromosome 19p13.3.
- The gene abnormality may be inherited or arise sporadically (35%).
- Peutz–Jeghers syndrome has an autosomal dominant inheritance, so the offspring of affected individuals have a 50% chance of inheriting the disease.

Clinical features

Melanocytic macules appear in 95% of patients around the mouth and elsewhere.
- Deep brown or bluish–black 1–5mm macules appear around the mouth, lips (see *Fig. 5.9*), gingivae, buccal mucosa, eyes, hands and feet, fingers and toes, anus, and genital areas.
- Pigmentation usually appears before 5 years of age and may fade after puberty.
- Gastrointestinal polyps occur later in life and are rare in childhood. They may cause bleeding, abdominal pain, and intestinal obstruction, and risk becoming malignant.
- Approximately 50% of patients with Peutz–Jeghers syndrome develop and die from cancer by 57 years. The overall risk of cancer over adult life is 93%.
- Cancer may arise in the breast, ovary, testicle, pancreas, uterus, oesophagus, or lung.

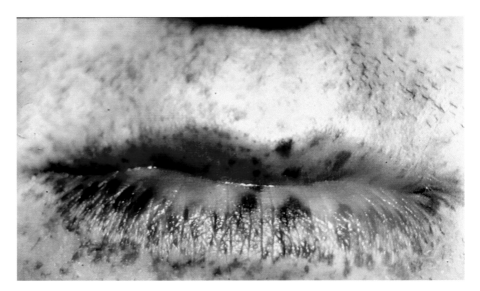

Figure 5.9. Peutz–Jeghers syndrome showing perioral pigmentation.

Reproduced with permission from Professor David Wilson, Adelaide, Australia, and included here after enhancement by AIPDerm (www.aipderm.com).

Treatment

There is no specific treatment for Peutz–Jeghers syndrome. The main goals are to manage and prevent intestinal obstruction and intussusception and to diagnose cancer early.

5.2.11   Multiple endocrine neoplasia type 2B

The multiple endocrine neoplasia syndromes are genetic diseases that result in adenomatous hyperplasia and malignant tumours of several endocrine glands.

Mucosal neuromas are a feature of multiple endocrine neoplasia type 2B (MEN 2B), also known as MEN type 3 and mucosal neuroma syndrome. It is rare, accounting for about 5% of the MEN syndromes.

Other characteristics of MEN 2B are:
- medullary thyroid carcinoma
- phaeochromocytoma
- multiple mucosal neuromas
- intestinal ganglioneuromas
- Marfanoid habitus (long limbs and digits)
- other skeletal abnormalities (such as lordosis, kyphosis, and scoliosis).

Causes

95% of MEN 2B cases are caused by a specific mutation in the *RET* gene (a protooncogene). MEN 2B is inherited as an autosomal dominant trait with a high degree of penetrance and variable expressivity. However, more than 50% are due to *de novo* mutations, and thus presentation may be sporadic rather than familial.

Clinical features

Multiple neuromas are soft papules on the lips, tongue, buccal mucosae, and eyelids that arise during childhood and are often the earliest sign of MEN 3 (see *Fig. 5.10*). See also *Section 10.1.4*.

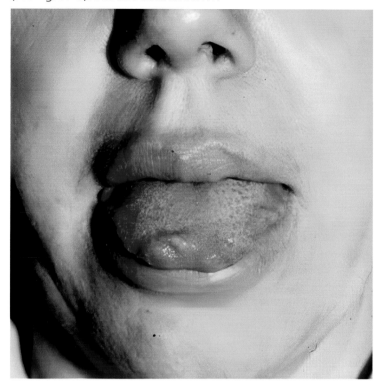

Figure 5.10. Multiple endocrine neoplasia type 2B. Facies showing prominent lips with lip and tongue neuroma.

Reproduced from *The Oncologist*, 2009;14:571, with permission from Oxford University Press, and included here after enhancement by AIPDerm (www.aipderm.com).

Diagnosis

Clinical suspicion of MEN 2B should lead to family history and confirmatory tests.
- Genetic testing of *RET* gene
- Plasma-free metanephrines and urinary catecholamines for phaeochromocytoma
- Serum calcitonin measurements for medullary thyroid carcinoma.

MRI and CT are used to search for phaeochromocytoma and medullary thyroid carcinoma.

Treatment

The standard treatment protocol for MEN 2B is the surgical excision of tumours and prophylactic thyroidectomy. Prophylactic thyroidectomy is recommended for carriers of the abnormal gene before one year of age.

5.2.12   Cowden syndrome

Cowden syndrome is a genetic disorder characterized by multiple benign hamartomas and an increased risk of developing certain cancers. It is also called multiple hamartoma syndrome and PTEN hamartoma tumour syndrome.

Cowden syndrome is estimated to affect about one in 200 000 people.

Cause

The most common mutations in Cowden syndrome affect the *PTEN*, *KLLN*, or *WWP1* genes responsible for preventing cell division. Cowden syndrome is inherited in an autosomal dominant pattern and can also arise due to a sporadic prenatal mutation.

Clinical features

Hamartomas in Cowden syndrome most commonly affect the skin, mouth, and gastrointestinal tract and may be evident in childhood or not occur until the 20s or later in life. They include:
- oral mucosal papillomatosis (see *Fig. 5.11*)
- trichilemmomas
- multiple lipomas
- palmoplantar or generalized keratoses
- papillomas
- sclerotic fibromas
- vascular malformations.

Oral mucosal papillomatosis results in a furrowed tongue, macroglossia, mucosal telangiectasia, high-arched palate, and fibromas; thyroglossal duct cysts are occasionally present.

Benign tumours may also occur in the thyroid, breast, uterus, gastrointestinal tract, and brain.

Other signs and symptoms of Cowden syndrome include:
- macrocephaly or dolichocephaly (long head shape)
- autism spectrum disorder, learning and developmental delays.

Malignancies affecting people with Cowden syndrome include melanoma and carcinoma of the breast, thyroid, endometrium, kidney, colon, and rectum.

Cowden-like syndrome may be used to describe people with some Cowden syndrome characteristics.

Diagnosis

The essential components of the diagnosis include a medical and family history and a physical examination. Laboratory tests may consist of skin biopsy and genetic testing.

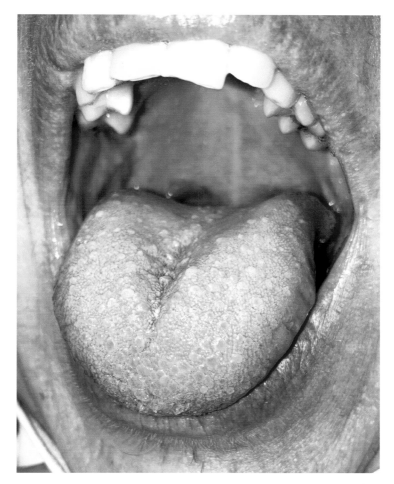

Figure 5.11. Cowden syndrome: papillomatosis affecting the dorsum of the tongue.

Image reproduced from Health NZ – Waikato (www.waikatodhb.health.nz) with permission.

Lifelong surveillance to check for internal malignancies should include:
- skin examination
- blood tests – at least CBC and thyroid function
- faecal occult blood
- urinalysis
- imaging – mammogram and breast and pelvic ultrasound examination
- colonoscopy and endoscopy.

Genetic counselling and testing of relatives are recommended.

Treatment

Benign lesions and malignancies in Cowden syndrome are treated similarly to those that occur sporadically in patients without a hereditary cancer syndrome.

5.2.13   Lipoid proteinosis

Lipoid proteinosis is a rare genetic skin disease in which an amorphous hyaline material is deposited in the skin, mucosa, and internal organs. It presents in childhood as hoarseness and papules on the skin and mucosal surfaces (see *Fig. 5.12*).

Causes

Lipoid proteinosis has an autosomal recessive inheritance. The genetic defect is the loss of function mutations in a gene encoding extracellular matrix protein 1 (*ECM1*) on band 1q21.

Clinical features

Clinical features are variable depending on the site of hyaline deposition and tend to be progressive.

Cutaneous features include:
- blisters at the site of trauma
- yellowish beaded papules on the eyelids
- waxy papules at sites of friction
- absent eyebrows and eyelashes.

Oral mucosal features include:
- cobblestone papillomatosis of the lips, tongue, and gingiva
- reduced mobility of the tongue
- swollen salivary glands
- dry mouth
- dental decay and missing teeth.

Hyaline infiltration affects the respiratory tract, central nervous system, and eye with a variety of significant symptoms.

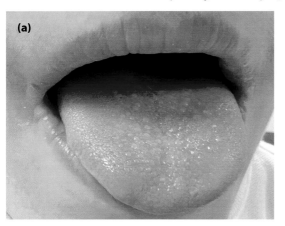
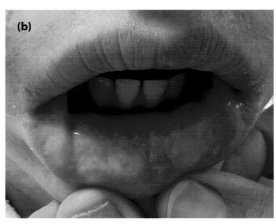

Figure 5.12 (a and b). Lipoid proteinosis: cobblestone papillomatosis affecting (a) the dorsum of the tongue and (b) lips.

Image reproduced from Health New Zealand Waitaha Canterbury (www.cdhb.health.nz) with permission.

Diagnosis

Lipoid proteinosis is confirmed by skin biopsy, imaging, and genetic testing. Genetic counselling should be provided to family members.

Treatment

There is no known treatment for lipoid proteinosis.

5.3 Disorders usually diagnosed in adult life

5.3.1 Fordyce spots

Fordyce spots or Fordyce granules are ectopic or heterotopic sebaceous glands within the oral mucosa. They are visible in 20% of children, 30% of adolescents, and up to 90% of adults.

Fordyce spots may be commonly seen in males and people with:
- greasy skin
- rheumatic disorders
- colorectal cancer
- hyperlipidaemia.

Clinical features
- Fordyce spots are clusters of 1–3mm white to yellow macules and papules on the oral mucosa. They may coalesce into plaques.
- They arise on the vermilion border of the upper lip, the buccal mucosa (see *Figs. 1.4* and *1.7*), the tongue, the gingiva, the retromolar region, and the palate.
- Fordyce spots can also occur on the glans or shaft of the penis (Tyson glands), the vulva, the vagina, or the areolae of the breasts (Montgomery glands).

Diagnosis

Fordyce spots are diagnosed clinically.
- Dermoscopy/mucoscopy shows multiple monomorphic whitish–yellow round or oval clods.
- The histopathology of Fordyce spots shows mature sebaceous lobules of rounded cells with clear granular cytoplasm.

Treatment

Fordyce spots do not require any treatment.

Electrosurgery and vaporizing laser treatment (CO_2 laser) of Fordyce spots result in scars.

5.3.2 Hereditary haemorrhagic telangiectasia

Hereditary haemorrhagic telangiectasia (HHT), or Osler–Weber–Rendu syndrome, is an autosomal dominant condition characterized by skin and mucosal telangiectasia and arteriovenous malformations.

HHT becomes apparent during adolescence or later, although it is estimated that 90% of affected people are unaware they have the disorder. It affects males and females equally.

Causes

HHT is due to a mutation in endoglin on chromosome 9 or activin receptor-like kinase-1 on chromosome 12. These genes are implicated in vascular development and repair.
- The vascular endothelial growth factor, VEGF, may modulate angiogenesis in HHT.
- Telangiectasias occur when capillaries fail to develop between arterioles and venules.

Clinical features

Telangiectasia affects the face, lips (see *Fig. 5.13*), tongue, oral mucosa, nose, gums, conjunctiva, trunk, arms, and fingers.
- 1–2mm red to purplish superficial blanchable vessels on the skin and mucous membranes.
- Dermoscopy of telangiectasia reveals red clods, serpiginous and linear vessels on a pink background.
- In many patients, epistaxis is the first sign of the disease. Oral lesions may also bleed.

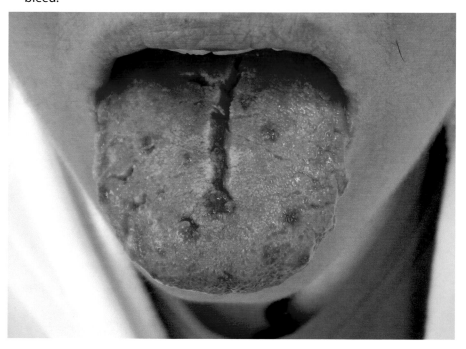

Figure 5.13. Superficial vessels on the tongue in hereditary haemorrhagic telangiectasia; the patient also has a plicated tongue.

Image reproduced from Health NZ – Waikato (www.waikatodhb.health.nz) with permission.

Diagnosis

The diagnosis of HHT is based on a detailed patient and family history and a thorough clinical examination.

Treatment

No treatment is required for asymptomatic patients. When symptomatic, the treatment of HHT is directed at specific symptoms.
- Bleeding vessels are cauterized, ligated, or treated by a vascular laser.
- Intravenous bevacizumab (an antiangiogenic drug) can be given intermittently to reduce nosebleeds and anaemia.

5.3.3 Laugier–Hunziker syndrome

Laugier–Hunziker syndrome is the combination of hyperpigmented macules on the skin, oral mucosa and nails. Often sporadic, it is thought to have a genetic origin.

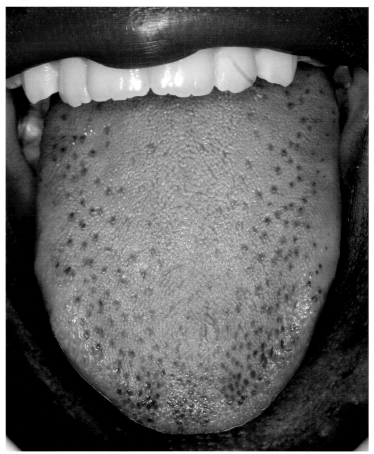

Figure 5.14. Laugier–Hunziker syndrome affecting the tongue with multiple 1–5mm pigmented macules.

Image reproduced from Health NZ – Waikato (www.waikatodhb.health.nz) with permission.

- Brown, black or slate-coloured 1–5mm macules typically appear during early to middle adulthood (see *Fig. 5.14*).
- The buccal mucosa and the lower lip are the most common sites in the mouth. Pigmentation may also affect the gingiva, tongue, soft palate, and hard palate.
- Pigmented macules may also arise on all the digits, the palms, soles, and genital mucosa.
- Dermoscopy of mucosal macules shows various patterns of regular reticular or linear pigmentation.
- Longitudinal melanonychia often affects several nails with single or multiple bands or diffuse nail pigmentation.

Treatment

Treatment may be sought for cosmetic reasons. Options include various pigment lasers and cryosurgery.

5.3.4 Leukoedema

Leukoedema describes an asymptomatic opalescent white appearance of the buccal and labial mucosa and is a normal variation (see *Fig. 1.3*).
- Leukoedema occurs in almost 90% of adults with black skin and 50% with white skin.
- The incidence of leukoedema increases up to 40–49 years and then declines.
- There is no sex predilection.

Causes

The white appearance of leukoedema is thought to be due to intracellular oedema of the superficial epithelial cells and parakeratosis.

Diagnosis

Leukoedema is diagnosed clinically. It diminishes upon stretching the mucosa, distinguishing it from frictional keratosis, lichen planus, and leukoplakia.

Treatment

No treatment is required.

5.3.5 Venous lake

A venous lake is a localized area of vascular dilatation. It is most often diagnosed on the lower lip; other sites include the earlobe, face, neck, or upper trunk.

Clinical features

A venous lake presents as a soft purple or bluish, often blanchable, macule or papule (see *Fig. 5.15a*) that disappears on compression by a glass slide or the lens of a contact dermatoscope. Dermoscopy shows uniform bluish discolouration (see *Fig. 5.15b*).

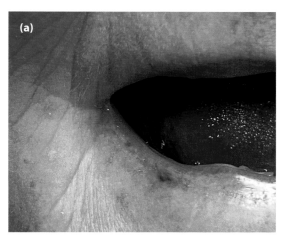 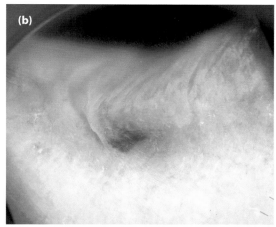

Figure 5.15 (a and b). (a) Bluish venous lake on the lower lip; (b) dermoscopy image.

Image reproduced from Health NZ – Waikato (www.waikatodhb.health.nz) with permission.

Treatment

Available aesthetic treatment options include cryotherapy, electrocautery, sclerotherapy, and vascular laser therapy.

CHAPTER 6

ORAL MUCOSAL INFECTIONS

> See also:
> - *Section 4.10.2: Hormone-related gingivitis; Section 4.1: Dental and oral hygiene*

6.1 Fungal infections

6.1.1 *Candida albicans* infections

In asymptomatic individuals:
- Candida can be detected in the mouths of 30–45% of healthy adults, 45% of neonates, and 50–65% of people who wear removable dentures.
- *C. albicans* is found in the mouths of 90% of patients with acute leukaemia undergoing chemotherapy and 95% of patients with HIV.

White plaques caused by *C. albicans* are classified as:
- acute or chronic pseudomembranous candidosis (oral thrush)
- chronic hyperplastic candidosis (a premalignant disorder)
- chronic mucocutaneous candidosis (a congenital form of immunodeficiency).

In this text we have used the term 'candidosis'; this is synonymous with 'candidiasis'.

Other types of fungal infections are rare in the mouth.

Pseudomembranous candidosis

Pseudomembranous candidosis (oral thrush) is characterized by a white pseudomembrane consisting of desquamated epithelial cells, fibrin, and fungal hyphae.

Risk factors

Pseudomembranous candidosis occurs if there are local or systemic predisposing risk factors.

Local factors include:
- wearing dentures at bedtime
- smoking
- impaired salivary gland function
- inhaled corticosteroid
- inflammatory disease (e.g. lichen planus)
- oral cancer.

Systemic factors include:
- extremes of age (5–7% of infants have oral thrush)
- diabetes mellitus
- Cushing syndrome
- nutritional deficiency (protein-energy malnutrition, iron, folate, vitamin C, or vitamin B12)
- long-term use of an antibiotic, antidepressant, antipsychotic, anticholinergic, antihypertensive, or antiadrenergic agent
- haematological malignancy (oral thrush affects up to 20% during cytotoxic chemotherapy and radiation therapy)
- immunosuppressant drugs
- immunodeficiency due to HIV infection (9–31% of patients with AIDS have thrush), severe combined immunodeficiency, DiGeorge syndrome, hereditary myeloperoxidase deficiency, or Chediak–Higashi syndrome.

Causes

Oral candidosis is caused by the proliferation or infection of the oral cavity by candida (yeast).
- C. albicans is the most frequently cultured species.
- Other less common species include C. tropicalis, C. glabrata, C. pseudotropicalis, C. guillierimondii, C. krusei, C. lusitaniae, C. parapsilosis, and C. stellatoidea.

Clinical features

The pseudomembranous form of oral candidosis classically presents as acute infection; chronic pseudomembranous candidosis denotes recurrent disease.
- Patients with pseudomembranous candidosis may complain of a slight tingling sensation or foul taste.
- Typically, white to whitish–yellow creamy confluent plaques resemble milk curds or cottage cheese (see Fig. 6.1).
- These are found on the labial and buccal mucosa, hard and soft palate, tongue, and oropharynx.
- In acquired immune deficiency syndrome (AIDS) patients, the oesophageal mucosa may also be involved. Oesophageal candidosis causes dysphagia and chest pain.
- The pseudomembrane can usually be wiped off with a swab to expose an underlying erythematous mucosa.

Diagnosis

Pseudomembranous candidosis is a common clinical diagnosis.
- Typically, routine microscopy and culture of oral swabs and scrapings are unnecessary.
- Cytology of a PAS-stained smear of the pseudomembrane shows a network of candida hyphae containing desquamated cells, microorganisms, fibrin, inflammatory cells, and debris.

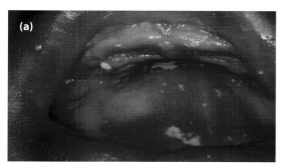

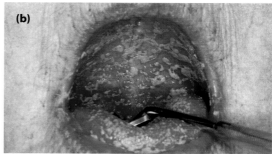

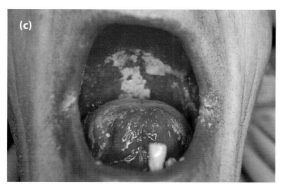

Figure 6.1 (a–c). Oral pseudomembranous candidosis; (a) in a newborn; (b) in an adult; (c) in an elderly individual. Note curd-like white deposits.

(a and c) Reproduced with permission from Professor Yeshwant Rawal, School of Dentistry, Milwaukee University, WI, USA; (b) Reproduced with permission from Professor Nagamani Narayana, University of Nebraska Medical Centre, NE, USA.

Treatment

Topical antifungal treatment is effective against candidosis in immunocompetent individuals, providing adequate contact time with the infected site. The recommended treatment regimens are shown below.

- Predisposing factors should be treated or eliminated where feasible.
- Maintain optimum oral hygiene.

The recommended treatment regimens for oral pseudomembranous candidosis:

Adults and children 2 years and older

Options are any of the following:

- Amphotericin B 10mg lozenge sucked (then swallowed) four times daily after food for 7–14 days; continue treatment for 2–3 days after symptoms resolve
- Miconazole 2% gel 2.5ml topically (then swallowed) four times daily after food for 7–14 days; continue treatment for at least 7 days after symptoms resolve
- Nystatin liquid 100 000 units/ml 1ml topically (then swallowed) four times daily after food for 7–14 days; continue treatment for 2–3 days after symptoms resolve.

Neonates and children younger than 2 years

Treat oral candidosis in neonates and children younger than 2 years with a topical antifungal. In infants, apply the dose in the front of the mouth to reduce the risk of choking. Options are:

- Miconazole 2% gel 1.25ml topically (then swallowed), four times daily after feeding for 7–14 days; continue treatment for at least 7 days after symptoms resolve*
- Nystatin liquid 100 000 units/ml 1ml topically (then swallowed) four times daily after feeding for 7–14 days; continue treatment for 2–3 days after symptoms resolve.

The three topical antifungals have similar efficacy**.
- Amphotericin B lozenges may not be suitable for a patient with a dry mouth.
- Miconazole may be systemically absorbed, so drug interactions are possible, e.g. with warfarin, whereas topical nystatin and amphotericin B have negligible systemic absorption.
- Nystatin liquid contains a high sucrose concentration, promoting plaque accumulation on the teeth and dental caries.

Oral erythematous candidosis

Oral erythematous candidosis is a localized acute or chronic infection with *Candida albicans*.

Clinical features

Oral erythematous candidosis is common among individuals infected by HIV and those undergoing prolonged broad-spectrum antibiotic or corticosteroid therapy.
- Oral erythematous candidosis is an acute or chronic, painful erythematous patch.
- Erythematous candidosis may involve the tongue in the form of rhomboid glossitis and the palate in contact with the tongue (a kissing lesion) (see *Fig. 6.2*).

Treatment

Oral erythematous candidosis is treated with a topical antifungal agent. Options include nystatin oral suspension or pastilles, amphotericin lozenges or suspension, or miconazole gel.

Underlying predisposing factors should be identified and eliminated.

Denture-related stomatitis

Denture-related stomatitis (denture sore mouth; chronic atrophic candidosis) consists of mild inflammation and erythema of the mucosa beneath a dental appliance, usually a complete or partial upper denture.

---

*   The data sheet states that miconazole gel is contraindicated in children younger than 6 months; if used in this age group, take appropriate precautions to reduce the risk of choking – use a clean finger or cotton bud to apply a small amount of gel to the inside cheeks and over the tongue. Do not use the spoon provided with the product to administer the gel.

**   Source: Therapeutic Guidelines, Oral and Dental: Version 3. Melbourne. Therapeutic Guidelines Limited (2019)

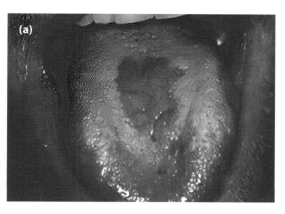
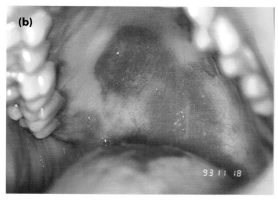

Figure 6.2 (a and b). Erythematous candidosis on (a) the dorsum of the tongue and (b) the palate in HIV-infected individuals.

Reproduced from *Handbook of Oral Diseases for Medical Practice,* 2016; Eds: L Samaranayake, HMHN Bandara and SR Prabhu, with permission from Oxford University Press, and included here after enhancement by AIPDerm (www.aipderm.com).

Cause

Fungi, such as *Candida*, are isolated in up to 90% of individuals with denture-related stomatitis, and when *Candida* species are involved in denture-related stomatitis, the more common terms 'Candida-associated denture stomatitis', 'denture-induced candidosis', or 'chronic atrophic candidosis' are used.

Clinical features

Chronic erythema and oedema of the mucosa that contacts the fitting surface of the denture, usually a complete upper denture (the denture-bearing area); the mucosa below lower dentures are rarely involved (see *Fig. 6.3*).

Treatment

Dentures should be removed and cleaned at least once daily. Cleaning options include the following:

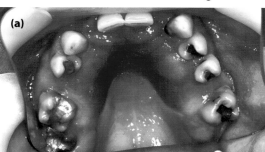
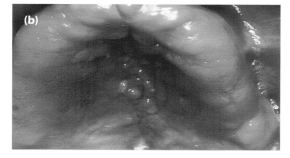

Figure 6.3 (a and b). Denture-related stomatitis. Erythematous mucosal patch of the partial denture-bearing area (a) and diffuse palatal erythema with papillary hyperplasia in a complete denture wearer (b).

Reproduced from *Handbook of Oral Pathology and Oral Medicine,* 2022; SR Prabhu, with permission from Wiley-Blackwell, and included here after enhancement by AIPDerm (www.aipderm.com).

- Mechanical cleaning by brushing with neutral soap or dentifrice
- Chemical cleaning includes soaking in sodium perborate, and sodium hypochlorite (6% bleach diluted by mixing 10 parts water and one part bleach for 10 minutes)
- For established denture stomatitis, topical antifungal applications to the denture-fitting surface and oral mucosa
- Consultation with a dentist is essential.

Chronic hyperplastic candidosis

Chronic hyperplastic candidosis is a persistent, white, keratotic plaque colonized by *C. albicans*. This lesion is also called candida leukoplakia.

- Chronic hyperplastic candidosis is no longer classified as a potentially malignant disorder.
- Chronic hyperplastic candidosis is uncommon in healthy individuals.
- The global prevalence is 0.2–11%, diagnosed in people with local and systemic predisposing conditions.
- Males are affected more frequently than females.

Causes

Chronic hyperplastic candidosis is due to chronic *C. albicans* in its hyphal form.

Local predisposing factors:
- Tobacco smoking
- Friction associated with dentures or dental trauma
- Poor denture hygiene
- Loss of vertical dimension of occlusion.

Systemic factors include haematinic deficiency, particularly iron deficiency.

Clinical features

Chronic hyperplastic candidosis is characterized by one or more asymptomatic, persistent, well-circumscribed, white lesions.

- On the buccal mucosa and labial commissures, the white plaque typically has a triangular shape tapering posteriorly, sometimes with an erythematous component (see *Fig. 6.4*).
- It can also affect the lateral border of the tongue and palate.
- On palpation, chronic hyperplastic candidosis is non-tender, rough, and occasionally nodular.
- The white plaques cannot be wiped off.

Diagnosis

Clinical suspicion of chronic hyperplastic candidosis follows a careful history and examination.

- A swab or smear is sometimes necessary to confirm the diagnosis.
- A biopsy is indicated to exclude intraepithelial neoplasia.

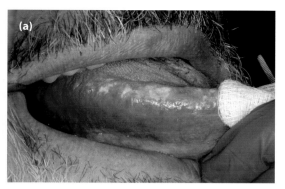

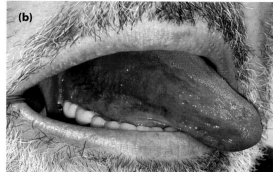

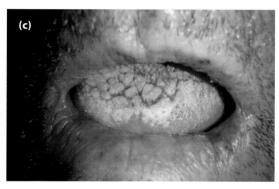

Figure 6.4 (a–c). Hyperplastic candidosis (candidal leukoplakia) of (a) lateral tongue, (b) same tongue after antifungal treatment, (c) dorsal tongue.

(c) Reproduced from Health NZ – Waikato (www.waikatodhb.health.nz) with permission.

- Histopathology of chronic hyperplastic candidosis shows parakeratosis, broad bulbous epithelial ridges, and neutrophilic microabscesses. Candida hyphae are seen within the parakeratotic stratum corneum in PAS-stained sections. The connective tissue shows mild chronic inflammatory cell infiltrate.
- Full-thickness epithelial dysplasia indicates carcinoma *in situ*.

Treatment

Topical treatment of chronic hyperplastic candidosis is applied sparingly after meals and at bedtime for 14 days. Identify and treat candidosis in other sites (e.g. angular cheilitis). Options:
- Miconazole 2% gel
- Nystatin 1:100 000 oral solution.

A systemic antifungal agent is recommended if chronic hyperplastic candidosis is resistant to topical therapy.
- Start with a 14-day course of fluconazole 100mg, two tablets on the first day and then once daily.
- If chronic hyperplastic candidosis persists, treatment may be continued for 2–3 months.
- Local and systemic predisposing factors should be treated or eliminated where feasible.
- Smoking cessation and regular dental assessments are essential.

- If there is microscopic evidence of carcinoma *in situ*, the lesion should be excised to reduce the risk of invasive squamous cell carcinoma.
- A patient with chronic hyperplastic candidosis should be followed up periodically due to its potential for malignant transformation.

Chronic mucocutaneous candidosis

Chronic mucocutaneous candidosis is a rare disorder in which recurrent or persistent superficial skin, mucous membrane, and nail infection with candida are associated with a defect in cell-mediated immunity.

- Chronic mucocutaneous candidosis may be sporadic or familial with autosomal dominant and recessive inheritance.
- The prevalence of chronic mucocutaneous candidosis is about 1 in 100 000 individuals.
- No racial or ethnic predilection has been reported.

Causes

Candida species, particularly *C. albicans*, cause chronic mucocutaneous candidosis.

Chronic mucocutaneous candidosis is associated with a defect in cell-mediated immunity limited to candida antigens or with a broader immune deficiency.

Clinical features

Chronic mucocutaneous candidosis manifests in 60–80% of cases in infancy or early childhood, with a mean age of onset of 3 years. Delayed or adult onset of chronic mucocutaneous candidosis is less frequent.

Chronic mucocutaneous candidosis presents with recurrent or persistent:
- superficial oral candidosis (thrush) and angular cheilitis
- rarely, oesophageal candidosis
- intertriginous or periorificial candidosis
- candida napkin (diaper) dermatitis
- vulvovaginal candidosis
- acral hyperkeratotic erythematous plaques, often serpiginous
- thickened dystrophic nails and erythematous, oedematous periungual tissues
- erythematous peeling skin.

Chronic mucocutaneous candidosis may occur in association with an endocrine or autoimmune disease in adolescence or adulthood, including:
- hypoparathyroidism
- thyroid disease
- autoimmune polyendocrinopathy, candidosis, and ectodermal dysplasia syndrome.

Recurrent and severe non-candida infections associated with chronic mucocutaneous candidosis include:
- septicaemia
- bacterial pneumonia

- opportunistic infections such as cryptococcal meningitis or disseminated histoplasmosis.

Other disorders associated with chronic mucocutaneous candidosis include:
- dental enamel dysplasia
- interstitial keratitis
- vitiligo
- alopecia areata.

An adult form of chronic mucocutaneous candidosis typically presents after the third decade of life. This may be associated with:
- thymoma
- myasthenia gravis
- hypogammaglobulinaemia
- abnormalities of the bone marrow.

Diagnosis

The diagnosis of chronic mucocutaneous candidosis depends on confirmation of candida infection and endocrine/immune dysfunction.
- Standard microbiology swabs for culture in a suitable medium (Sabouraud agar with chloramphenicol and cycloheximide).
- Scrapings suspended in 10–20% potassium hydroxide solution for microscopy.
- Blood glucose or glycosylated haemoglobin, thyroid function, liver function, serum electrolytes, corticotropin and serum cortisol, complete blood cell count, and HIV serology.

A skin biopsy may be helpful.
- Histopathology of chronic mucocutaneous candidosis may reveal subcorneal pustules. Granulomatous lesions of chronic mucocutaneous candidosis show hyperkeratosis and parakeratosis, with a dense mixed dermal infiltrate containing lymphocytes and plasma cells.
- PAS or silver stains can help identify yeasts.

Treatment

Chronic mucocutaneous candidosis requires multidisciplinary consultation, antifungal drugs, and immunological therapies.

General measures include the maintenance of good oral hygiene and avoiding smoking and alcohol.

Antifungal drugs:
- Topical antifungal agents for oral or vaginal candidosis are ineffective for nail disease.
- First-line oral antifungals for chronic mucocutaneous candidosis include fluconazole, itraconazole, and posaconazole.
- Second-line antifungal therapy includes voriconazole, echinocandins, terbinafine, and liposomal amphotericin B.
- Side-effects, drug interactions, and risk-to-benefit ratio must be considered.

Immunological therapies:
- Transfer factor is a cell-free protein extracted from the T lymphocytes of candida-immune donors.
- Systemic immunologic treatments include intravenous immunoglobulin G (IgG), granulocyte-macrophage colony-stimulating factor (GM-CSF) infusions, and interferon-alfa.

The prognosis of chronic mucocutaneous candidosis is variable. If the disease flares, urgent consultation may be necessary, particularly after a course of antifungals has been discontinued.

Median rhomboid glossitis

Median rhomboid glossitis describes an erythematous area around the midline of the dorsum of the tongue.

Causes

Median rhomboid glossitis is thought to be caused by *Candida albicans*.

Clinical features

Median rhomboid glossitis is a well-demarcated, symmetrical, smooth, lobulated and depapillated erythematous patch anterior to the circumvallate papillae (see *Fig. 6.5*).
- Occasionally, erythema may also be present on the adjacent palate.
- Median rhomboid glossitis is usually asymptomatic. Some patients may complain of mild soreness, irritation, or pruritus.

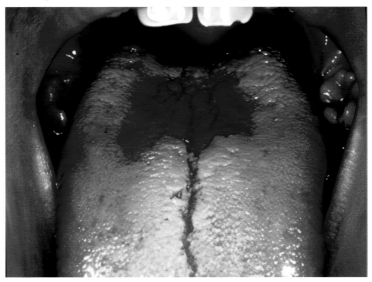

Figure 6.5. Median rhomboid glossitis: an erythematous patch anterior to the circumvallate papillae.

Reproduced from *Handbook of Oral Diseases for Medical Practice,* 2016; Ed: SR Prabhu, with permission from Oxford University Press, and included here after enhancement by AIPDerm (www.aipderm.com).

Treatment

Usually, no treatment is necessary for asymptomatic median rhomboid glossitis. Symptomatic patients may be treated with topical antifungal medication. If the lesion does not respond, a biopsy is recommended.

6.1.2   Deep mycoses

Deep mycoses are serious opportunistic fungal infections caused by aspergillus species, mucormycetes, *Histoplasma capsulatum*, *Cryptococcus neoformans*, *Blastomyces dermatitidis*, and *Paracoccidioides brasiliensis*. Treatment may require the reduction or cessation of immunosuppressive medication, surgical excision, and second-line antifungal therapy.

Aspergillosis

Aspergillus is a widespread mould that can cause allergy symptoms or, in immunocompromised individuals, chronic bronchopulmonary or sinus infections.
- Aspergillosis causes fistulae, abscesses, and aspergillomas (fungus balls).
- Oral mucosal ulceration and underlying osteomyelitis are rare.
- It has a mortality rate of approximately 30%.

Mucormycosis

Mucormycetes are a group of moulds whose spores in the air, soil, and decaying organic material cause infection via a breach in the mucocutaneous surface.
- Mucormycosis primarily affects the paranasal sinuses but may spread to the palate, orbit, lungs, skin, and brain. Arterial invasion leads to thrombosis and necrosis.
- Oral lesions present as palatal ulceration.
- The infection has a poor prognosis, with a mortality rate of 30–70%.

Histoplasmosis

Histoplasma capsulatum is found in bird and bat faeces, and infection is endemic in parts of the USA, India, Latin America, and Australia.
- Immunocompetent patients may clear the infection naturally.
- Oral mucosal lesions present as fungating ulcers and nodules and may invade bone.
- Mild histoplasmosis has a good prognosis with antifungal treatment, but untreated disseminated infection is associated with a mortality rate of 80%.

Cryptococcosis

Cryptococcus neoformans most often affects patients with untreated HIV infection; the incidence has decreased due to antiretroviral therapies.
- Cryptococcosis is spread via the bloodstream and primarily affects the lungs.
- Oral lesions may present as mucosal ulcers, nodules, and granules.
- Mild cryptococcosis has a good prognosis with antifungal treatment, but mortality is up to 40% in patients with cryptococcal meningitis.

Blastomycosis

Blastomyces dermatitidis is found in soil in the USA, India, Latin America, and Australia.
- Blastomycosis primarily affects the lungs.
- Oral mucosal lesions are rare and present as soft tissue masses or ulcers.
- The overall mortality rate is 6% but is up to 37% in immunocompromised patients.

Paracoccidioidomycosis

Paracoccidioides brasiliensis occurs in Central and South America and most often infects men who work outdoors in rural areas.
- Paracoccidioidomycosis can be asymptomatic or affect the lungs, mouth, and throat.
- Oral mucosal lesions are ulcerated erythematous or granulomatous plaques that bleed easily.
- The prognosis is good in treated immunocompetent patients, but the mortality is 50% in immunocompromised patients.

6.2 Viral infections

6.2.1 Herpes simplex

Infection with herpes simplex virus (HSV) may present in several forms in the orofacial region:
1. Primary herpetic gingivostomatitis
2. Recurrent herpes labialis
3. Recurrent intraoral herpes.

Primary herpetic gingivostomatitis

Primary herpetic gingivostomatitis occurs in 15–30% of initial HSV infections in children and is rare in adults. The peak incidence is 2–3 years of age.

Causes

Primary herpetic gingivostomatitis is due to HSV type 1 (human herpesvirus-1) in 90–95% and HSV type 2 (human herpesvirus-2) in 5–10%. Transmission is through contact with contaminated oral secretions.

Clinical features

Primary herpetic gingivostomatitis is a common febrile childhood illness characterized by crops of vesicles on the lips and mouth.
- The incubation period for primary herpetic gingivostomatitis is 3–6 days.
- Asymptomatic or subclinical infection is common.
- Some patients develop sudden-onset fever, malaise, headache, and cervical lymphadenopathy.
- Initially, oral lesions appear as swollen erythematous gingiva, followed by pin-head vesicles that rupture, forming crusted ulcers on the lips, gingiva, and tongue (see *Fig. 6.6*).

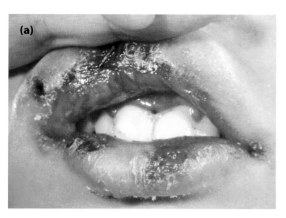

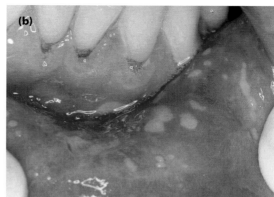

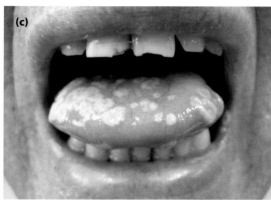

Figure 6.6 (a–c). Primary herpetic gingivostomatitis.

All images reproduced from Health NZ – Waikato (www.waikatodhb.health.nz) with permission.

- Other oral mucosal and adjacent cutaneous sites may also be involved.
- In most cases, the acute stage lasts 5–7 days, with symptoms resolving within 2 weeks.

Diagnosis

The diagnosis of primary herpetic gingivostomatitis is usually clinical. Investigations include:

- Tzanck smear – HSV can be confirmed by cytology from an oral smear showing multinucleated virus-infected giant epithelial cells (Tzanck cells)
- viral swab for culture or PCR; viral shedding continues for about 3 weeks
- tissue biopsy, which shows intraepithelial vesicles and early cytopathic changes.

HSV serology is not informative.

Treatment

Supportive therapy may include analgesics, hydration, nutritional supplementation, and rest.

- Topical anaesthetic gel (lignocaine) may ease the pain when applied before eating.
- Systemic aciclovir or valaciclovir may be effective if commenced within the first 48 hours of symptoms.

Prognosis

Most cases of primary herpetic gingivostomatitis settle within 10 days.
- Complications of primary herpetic gingivostomatitis include eczema herpeticum and secondary bacterial infection.
- Severe complications may rarely include keratoconjunctivitis, pneumonitis, meningitis, and encephalitis.
- Lifelong viral latency occurs in the ganglia of the nerves supplying the infected area.

Herpes labialis

Herpes labialis (a cold sore) is a secondary HSV infection. Herpes labialis affects 15–45% of the general population.

Causes

Herpes labialis is also due to HSV type 1 in 90–95% and type 2 in 5–10%.
- It is due to the reactivation of the latent virus that travels along the nerve from the sensory nerve ganglion to the lip.
- Trauma, stress, cold, exposure to ultraviolet radiation, viral infection, or immunosuppression can trigger reactivation.

Clinical features

Herpes labialis is a common recurring condition characterized by blisters on or around the lips.
- Many people experience prodromal tingling, paraesthesia, burning or discomfort at the site of recurrence.
- Early erythema is followed by clusters of vesicles, most often on the vermilion border of the lips (see *Fig. 6.7a*).
- The vesicles rupture within an hour of their appearance.
- They crust over in 2–3 days (see *Fig. 6.7b*) and then heal within about 10 days without scarring.
- Herpes labialis commonly recurs at the same site.

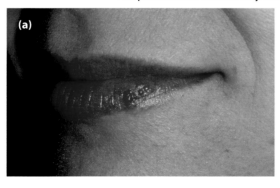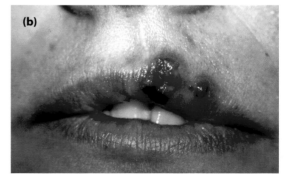

Figure 6.7 (a and b). Recurrent herpes labialis showing vesicles and crust on the vermilion border of the lower lip (a) and on the upper lip (b).

(a) Reproduced with permission from Professor Nagamani Narayana, University of Nebraska Medical Centre, NE, USA. (b) Reproduced from Health NZ – Waikato (www.waikatodhb.health.nz) with permission.

Diagnosis

The diagnosis of herpes labialis is clinical. Laboratory diagnosis is not usually required, but atypical cases may warrant viral culture, cytology of a smear, or PCR testing of vesicular fluid.

Treatment

Most people with recurrent herpes labialis do not seek treatment.
- Aciclovir 5% cream reduces symptoms when applied to the area 4-hourly for 4 days, commencing as soon as symptoms occur.
- Prophylactic application of sunscreen lip balm may reduce the reactivation of herpes simplex by sun exposure.
- Prophylactic oral aciclovir or valaciclovir may reduce the number and severity of recurrences.

Prognosis

Herpes labialis may trigger erythema multiforme in some patients.

Recurrent oral mucosal herpes

Recurrent intraoral mucosal herpes is much less common than herpes labialis.

Causes

A traumatic dental procedure such as a local anaesthetic injection or tooth extraction in an immunocompetent patient may trigger intraoral herpes. It is more common in immunocompromised patients.

Clinical features

Recurrent intraoral mucosal herpes tends to be more symptomatic than herpes labialis.
- Prodromal symptoms are not always present.
- Intraoral herpes typically affects the keratinized tissues of the hard palate and attached gingiva, although all mucosal sites may be affected.
- Fragile vesicles often develop unilaterally without crossing the midline in the mandibular and maxillary molar and premolar regions.
- Vesicles quickly rupture to form multiple, small, tender erosions. These may merge into irregular, superficial ulcerations.
- Lesions resolve within 2 weeks.

Diagnosis

The diagnosis of intraoral herpes is clinical. Laboratory diagnosis is not usually required, but atypical cases may include viral culture, cytology of a smear, or PCR testing of vesicular fluid.

Treatment

Supportive therapy includes analgesics, hydration, nutritional supplementation, and bed rest.

- Topical anaesthetic gel (lignocaine) can be applied before eating.
- Systemic antiviral agents are most effective if started within the first 48 hours.
- Systemic antiviral therapy may be indicated for immunocompromised patients, even if it commenced after 48 hours of the onset of symptoms.

Prognosis

Prophylactic antiviral therapy may be indicated in immunocompromised patients. In some patients, intraoral herpes simplex may trigger erythema multiforme. The underlying HSV infection is not always symptomatic.

6.2.2   Varicella-zoster infection

Varicella-zoster virus (VZV or HHV-3) gives rise to a primary infection, varicella, and a secondary infection, herpes zoster. The disease is transmitted via droplets or close contact with lesions.

Varicella

Varicella, or chickenpox, is a highly contagious vaccine-preventable infection typically affecting young children.

Causes

Varicella is the primary disseminated form of VZV infection. Transmission is by droplets or direct contact with an infected lesion.

Clinical features

Varicella was a common childhood febrile illness characterized by itchy, crusted vesicles primarily on the scalp, face, and trunk. It is now uncommon in many countries due to widespread vaccination.
- The incubation period for varicella is 7–14 days.
- Intraoral white–opaque vesicles on the buccal mucosa and palate may precede cutaneous involvement. The blisters rapidly rupture and ulcerate.
- Itchy papules on the scalp, face, and trunk quickly evolve into vesicles and later pustules, which dry up and crust after 3–4 days.
- Fever, malaise, anorexia, and headache are common.
- Symptoms usually last 2–3 weeks.

Diagnosis

The diagnosis of varicella is clinical.
- Viral swabs can confirm VZV infection by culture or PCR.
- Previous varicella can be confirmed by serology, for example, in a patient considering VZV vaccination before starting immunosuppressive therapy.

Treatment

Supportive therapy may include analgesics, hydration, nutritional supplementation, and bed rest. Antiviral treatment may reduce the duration of symptoms but may not be necessary.

Prognosis

Varicella is usually a self-limiting condition with a good prognosis.
- Rare but serious complications are more common in adults than children. They include encephalitis, cerebellar ataxia, septicaemia, pneumonia, and secondary bacterial infection.
- VZV establishes latency in the sensory nerve ganglia and may reactivate to cause herpes zoster.

Herpes zoster

Herpes zoster or shingles is a painful dermatomal blistering eruption typically affecting older people or the immune-compromised.

Causes

Herpes zoster is the secondary localized form of VZV infection.
- It is due to the reactivation of VZV in the sensory nerve ganglia of cranial nerves or dorsal spinal roots.
- Herpes zoster is more likely to occur when cellular immunity to VZV is impaired, especially during immunosuppression or advancing age.
- Ramsay Hunt syndrome is a herpes zoster arising within the geniculate ganglion.

Clinical features

Herpes zoster is common, especially in older individuals. It is characterized by unilateral pain and blistering confined to one or a few dermatomes.
- Prodromal tingling, itching, burning, pain, or stinging can precede the rash for several days.
- Crops of vesicles erupt on normal or erythematous skin (see *Fig. 6.8a*).
- The vesicles evolve into pustules and crusted erosions, sometimes to ulceration and necrosis.
- Intraoral prodromal pain may be very severe and present as toothache.
- Very painful oral lesions are located unilaterally in the distribution of the affected branch of the trigeminal nerve (see *Figs 6.8b* and *c*).
- Ramsay Hunt syndrome results in otitis externa, unilateral lower motor neuron facial nerve palsy, and ipsilateral ulceration of the anterior two-thirds of the tongue and soft palate. The oral lesions affect the distribution of chorda tympani.
- Herpes zoster blisters resemble herpes simplex – vesicles that quickly evolve into erosions – but in severe zoster, they may coalesce to form large irregular ulcers.
- Oral ulcers may last 5–10 days without intervention in an immunocompetent patient or longer in the immunocompromised.
- Fever, malaise, and cervical lymphadenopathy are common.

Diagnosis

The diagnosis of herpes zoster is usually clinical. Confirmatory viral swabs for VZV culture or PCR are rarely needed.

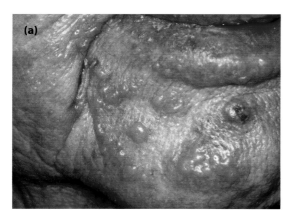

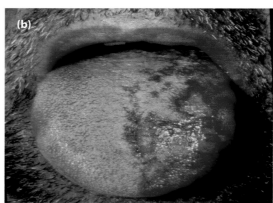

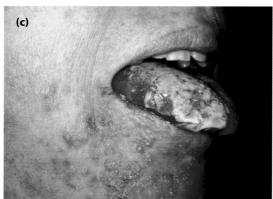

Figure 6.8 (a–c). Herpes zoster with unilateral crusted vesicles on the chin (a) and tongue (b and c) innervated by CN V3 and CN XII, branches of the trigeminal nerve.

All images reproduced from Health NZ – Waikato (www. waikatodhb.health.nz) with permission.

Treatment

Supportive therapy for herpes zoster includes wet compresses, analgesics, hydration, nutritional supplementation, and bed rest.
- Systemic antiviral therapy (aciclovir or valaciclovir) is most effective if prescribed within 48–72 hours of onset.
- Seek an ophthalmic review for any ocular or eyelid symptoms or signs.

Prognosis

Herpes zoster has a good prognosis. Postherpetic neuralgia and hyperaesthesia of the affected dermatome may affect up to 14% of patients; this is aching or burning pain that persists for 3 or more months after blisters have healed.

6.2.3   Infectious mononucleosis

Infectious mononucleosis, also known as glandular fever, is due to a primary infection with Epstein–Barr virus (EBV or HHV-4). Symptomatic infectious mononucleosis is most common between 15 and 24 years of age.

Causes

EBV is commonly transmitted via kissing (the 'kissing disease') or, less commonly, through sexual contact or by sharing utensils.

- Initially, EBV replicates within oropharyngeal epithelial cells and B cells in the oropharyngeal lymphoid tissues.
- EBV disseminates throughout the lymph system, where it may incubate for 30–50 days before becoming symptomatic.

Clinical features

Young children infected with EBV are asymptomatic. Oral signs are uvular oedema, petechiae on the soft palate, and tonsillar inflammation.
- Other symptoms include pharyngitis, moderate–high fever, headache, myalgia, and enlarged inguinal, axillary, posterior auricular, and cervical nodes.
- Hepatosplenomegaly is present in 10–50% of patients.
- Fatigue can be prominent and persistent.
- An exanthematous rash affects up to 10% of patients and may be scarlatiniform, morbilliform, urticarial, or erythema multiforme-like.

Diagnosis

Diagnostic laboratory tests support a clinical diagnosis of infectious mononucleosis.
- Lymphocytes usually comprise >50% white cells with an absolute lymphocyte count of $>4.5 \times 10^9$/L.
- A positive heterophile antibody test is present in 80–90% of cases (IgM).
- Basophilic reactive atypical lymphocytes are observed on a peripheral blood smear.

IgG antibodies against EVB persist lifelong. Viral reactivation is not associated with clinically significant symptoms except in immunocompromised people.

Treatment

Infectious mononucleosis is self-limiting, although full recovery may take 6 months. Symptomatic treatment and bed rest are adequate for most cases.

Hepatitis, especially in older adults, and swelling or rupture of the spleen are rare complications of infectious mononucleosis.

6.2.4 Cytomegalovirus

Cytomegalovirus (CMV or HHV-5) infection often results in asymptomatic latent infection, but primary infection or reactivation may be life-threatening in immunocompromised patients.
- Congenital CMV may cause significant morbidity and death.
- CMV infects 40–70% of adults in developed countries and almost 100% of the population in developing nations.

Clinical features

CMV infection is asymptomatic in approximately 90% of cases.

- Some patients will develop symptoms of acute viral infection like infectious mononucleosis (fever, chills, headache, myalgia, sore throat, fatigue, lymphadenopathy, and splenomegaly).
- Immunocompromised patients may also develop anaemia, pneumonia, retinitis, encephalitis, colitis, and hepatitis.
- Solitary mucosal ulcers may occur, more commonly in immunocompromised patients.
- Neonatal CMV infection may result in developmental tooth defects.
- The virus may develop latency and sequester the salivary glands.

Diagnosis

The diagnosis of oral CMV infection relies on CMV serology or viral PCR from a swab taken from an oral ulcer. The CMV viral load can also be measured.

Treatment

Symptomatic CMV responds to antiviral therapy, most commonly ganciclovir or valganciclovir.

6.2.5   Enterovirus

Hand, foot, and mouth disease

Hand, foot, and mouth disease is a common and highly contagious viral infection caused by various enteroviruses. It is also called enteroviral vesicular stomatitis with exanthem.

- Hand, foot, and mouth disease frequently occurs in young children under 10 years, but may also occur in adolescents and adults.
- Infection in children tends to be milder than in adults.

Causes

Hand, foot, and mouth disease is most often caused by coxsackievirus A10 or A16.

Transmission is via the faecal–oral route, droplet infection (secretions from the mouth or respiratory system by sneezing and coughing), or direct contact with blister fluid.

Clinical features

Hand, foot, and mouth disease is a mild childhood illness resulting in stomatitis and flaccid blisters on the hands and feet and, sometimes, elsewhere (see *Fig. 6.9a*).

- The incubation period for hand, foot, and mouth disease is 3–5 days.
- Symptoms include fever, sore throat, loss of appetite, and lethargy.
- Oral lesions initially appear as small red dots (see *Fig. 6.9b*), which form vesicles and subsequently develop into ulcers.
- Any oral mucosal site may be affected, particularly the buccal mucosa, gingiva, and lateral tongue.
- A vesicular rash affects perioral skin, the palms of the hands, the soles of the feet, the buttocks, and sometimes elsewhere (especially in adults).
- Acute illness usually lasts 10–14 days, and full recovery occurs within 3 weeks.

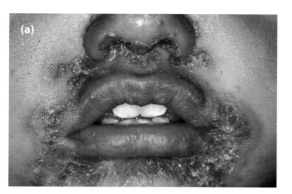
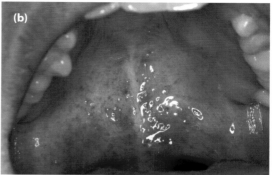

Figure 6.9 (a and b). Hand, foot, and mouth disease: (a) perioral vesicles and crusting and (b) red dots on the palate.

Images reproduced from Health NZ – Waikato (www.waikatodhb.health.nz) with permission.

Diagnosis

The diagnosis of hand, foot, and mouth disease is usually clinical. Enterovirus PCR testing of swabs taken from the throat, faeces, or a blister can confirm an atypical case. The virus can be detected in faeces for several weeks.

Treatment

Supportive therapy may include analgesics as required. Oral lesions may cause difficulty eating and drinking. Ensure adequate hydration.

Prognosis

Infection rarely recurs or persists. A minority of hand, foot, and mouth patients may develop severe complications such as persistent oral ulceration, aseptic meningitis, and rarely interstitial pneumonia, myocarditis, and pulmonary oedema.

Herpangina

Herpangina is also called enteroviral vesicular pharyngitis. It usually affects young children 3–10 years of age during summer or autumn.

Causes

Herpangina is most often due to coxsackievirus A16 or B1. Transmission is via the faecal–oral route, droplet infection, or fomites. Freshwater sources may act as a reservoir for transmission.

Clinical features

Herpangina is a mild febrile childhood illness resulting in vesicles and ulcers at the back of the mouth.
- The incubation period for herpangina is 4–14 days.
- Infection may be subclinical or asymptomatic.
- Some children experience sudden-onset pharyngitis, fever, dysphagia, malaise, cough, and lymphadenitis.

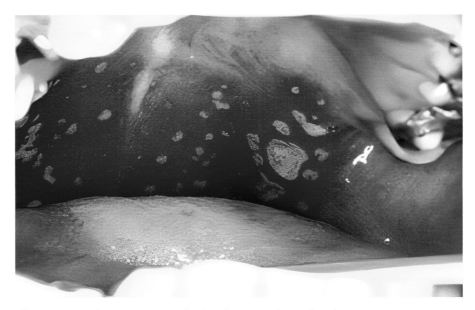

Figure 6.10. Herpangina: multiple ulcers on the soft palate.

Reproduced from *Handbook of Oral Pathology and Oral Medicine*, 2022; SR Prabhu, with permission from Wiley-Blackwell, and included here after enhancement by AIPDerm (www.aipderm.com).

- Vesicles and small ulcers follow erythema of the tonsillar region and soft palate (see *Fig. 6.10*).
- The acute illness usually lasts 4–7 days, with full recovery within 2–3 weeks.

Diagnosis

The diagnosis of herpangina is usually clinical. Enteroviral infection can be confirmed on PCR testing of an oral swab in an atypical case.

Treatment

Supportive therapy may include analgesics as required. Oral lesions may cause difficulty eating and drinking. Ensure adequate hydration.

Prognosis

Rare complications most often due to enterovirus 71 include aseptic meningitis and myocarditis.

Herpangina has rarely resulted in adverse pregnancy outcomes such as spontaneous abortion, low birth weight, or preterm delivery.

6.2.6 Measles

Measles or rubeola is an acute childhood viral respiratory infection with a rash and Koplik spots.
- Previously common, measles is now rare in many countries due to widespread childhood vaccination.
- Large outbreaks occur in unvaccinated individuals in countries where vaccination rates are low.

Causes

The measles virus is a single-stranded RNA virus (morbillivirus) of the family Paramyxoviridae.
- Measles is highly contagious.
- Transmission is via infectious droplets that can persist in the air for up to 2 hours.
- The incubation period is 14 days.

Clinical features

Measles commonly presents as a runny nose, cough, conjunctivitis, fever, and lymphadenopathy.
- The exanthem starts on the face and is 'morbilliform' (erythematous macules and papules that fade through a coppery colour) (see *Fig. 6.11a*). Buccal and labial mucosa show Koplik spots (see *Fig. 6.11b*), small white macules with surrounding erythema, usually on the buccal and labial mucosa.
- Oral lesions are followed by an erythematous maculopapular rash on the face, spreading to the trunk and limbs.
- Complications from measles include otitis media, pneumonia, bronchitis, diarrhoea, encephalitis, and death in 1–3 in 1000 infected children. Subacute sclerosing panencephalitis is a potential degenerative neurological complication of measles arising up to 10 years after infection.

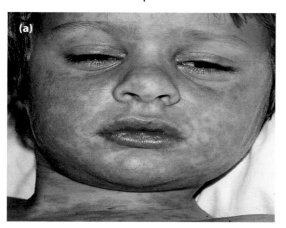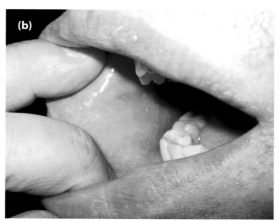

Figure 6.11 (a and b). Measles: (a) exanthem on the face and (b) Koplik spots on the buccal mucosa on day 1.

Images reproduced from Health NZ – Waikato (www.waikatodhb.health.nz) with permission.

Diagnosis

Laboratory confirmation is essential in sporadic cases, as other viral infections and adverse drug eruptions may have similar symptoms or signs.
- Throat, nasopharyngeal swab, or urine for measles PCR.
- Serology for measles-specific IgM.
- Genotyping.
- Evidence of immunity can be confirmed by IgG serology in those born after 1957.

Treatment

The management of measles is supportive.
- Isolation for 4 days
- Airborne precautions (N95 mask, personal protective clothing)
- Adequate hydration
- Appropriate analgesia
- Vitamin A in hospitalized or severe cases.

Measles is prevented by two doses of MMR (mumps, measles, rubella) or MMRV (varicella) vaccine. Typically, vaccination programmes start at 12 months of age.

6.2.7   Mumps

Mumps is an acute childhood viral infection causing painful facial swelling.

Causes

Mumps is caused by a paramyxovirus of the Rubulavirus family.
- Mumps is transmitted via droplets most often due to sharing water bottles or cups, kissing, or close contact.
- The average incubation period is 16–18 days.

Clinical features

The prodromal symptoms of mumps are a low-grade fever, myalgia, malaise, headache, and loss of appetite.
- This is soon followed by unilateral or bilateral parotid pain, tenderness, and swelling.
- Swelling peaks in 1–3 days and then subsides within 10 days.
- Classically, the swelling displaces the angle of the ear up and out.
- Less frequently, the submandibular and sublingual glands may also be affected.

Diagnosis

Mumps is usually confirmed by laboratory testing.
- Detection of viral RNA by reverse-transcriptase PCR in a buccal swab taken as soon as mumps is suspected.
- Serology for mumps IgM for current infection and IgG for earlier infection.

Treatment

Management is supportive, including adequate hydration and appropriate analgesia.

The infection is self-limiting. Second episodes are occasionally diagnosed.

Mumps is prevented by two doses of MMR (mumps, measles, rubella) or MMRV (varicella) vaccine. Typically, vaccination programmes start at 12 months of age.

6.2.8   Human immunodeficiency virus

Hairy leukoplakia

Hairy leukoplakia is a white plaque with hair-like papillae usually located on the lateral surfaces of the tongue in patients with immunocompromised status.
- Hairy leukoplakia is common in HIV-infected individuals, with a point prevalence in the USA of 25–53%.
- No racial predilection has been reported.
- When associated with HIV infection, hairy leukoplakia is more common in Europe and the USA than in Africa and Asia.

In HIV-positive patients, hairy leukoplakia is commonly observed in:
- patients with low CD4 lymphocyte count: the risk of developing hairy leukoplakia doubles with every 300-unit decrease in the CD4 count
- men who have sex with men (MSM)
- smokers.

Hairy leukoplakia also affects other immune-suppressed or unwell patients, including:
- those on chemotherapy or corticosteroids
- organ transplant recipients
- people with leukaemia, Behçet syndrome, or ulcerative colitis.

Causes

Hairy leukoplakia is caused by the Epstein–Barr virus (EBV, HHV-4).
- EBV may replicate in saliva, circulating B lymphocytes, monocytes, or within the epithelium of the tongue; when anti-EBV cell-mediated immunity is suppressed, and local antigen-presenting Langerhans cells are absent.
- EBV initiates keratinocyte hyperplasia.

Clinical features

Hairy leukoplakia usually presents as an asymptomatic white plaque along the lateral border of the tongue.
- Smooth, flat macules or irregular 'hairy' or 'feathery' corrugated plaques may occur (see *Fig. 6.12*).
- Unilateral or bilateral non-tender white lesions can also arise on the dorsal or ventral surfaces of the tongue, the buccal mucosa, or the gingiva.
- The lesions are flat and smooth on the ventral tongue, buccal mucosa, or gingiva.
- Symptoms may include mild pain, dysaesthesia, and alteration of taste.
- There is no associated erythema or oedema of the surrounding tissue.
- The white plaques are adherent and cannot be removed by scraping.

Diagnosis

Hairy leukoplakia is clinically distinct in the typical immune-suppressed patient.

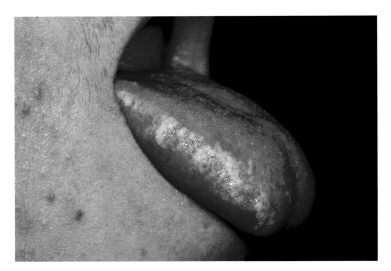

Figure 6.12. Oral hairy leukoplakia; a white hyperkeratotic plaque on the side on the tongue.

Reproduced from Health NZ – Waikato (www.waikatodhb.health.nz) with permission.

A definitive diagnosis requires histopathology and the demonstration of EBV within the epithelial cells of the lesion by immunohistochemistry or *in situ* hybridization. Five major features characterize the histopathology of hairy leukoplakia:

1. Hyperkeratosis of the upper epithelial layer ± superficial infection with bacteria or candida.
2. Parakeratosis.
3. Acanthosis with ballooning koilocyte-like cells.
4. Minimal or no inflammation in the epithelial and subepithelial tissues.
5. Normal basal epithelial layer.

Treatment

Oral hairy leukoplakia is treated with systemic antiviral medication. Topical treatment with antivirals is not necessary or effective.

- High dose aciclovir (800mg 5 times per day) usually results in the resolution of hairy leukoplakia within 1–2 weeks. Valaciclovir is an alternative.
- Tretinoin gel and cryotherapy have also been reported to be successful.
- Hairy leukoplakia usually decreases with highly active antiretroviral therapy (HAART) therapy in HIV patients but can return when HAART is reduced.
- Therapy is not curative. Antiviral drugs inhibit productive EBV replication but do not eliminate a latent infection. Recurrence following discontinuation of treatment is usual.

Linear gingival erythema

Linear gingival erythema is an intense narrow zone of erythema affecting the free gingiva on the margin of the anterior teeth. It is typically associated with HIV infection.

Causes

Subgingival colonization of candida and human herpesviruses have been proposed as triggers or cofactors. Linear gingival erythema is not related to bacterial plaque.

Clinical features

Linear gingival erythema on the free gingiva is demarcated from the normal-appearing attached gingiva. The erythema may be diffuse or petechial, and the width may vary from 1mm to several millimetres (see *Fig. 6.13*). Gingival bleeding is uncommon.

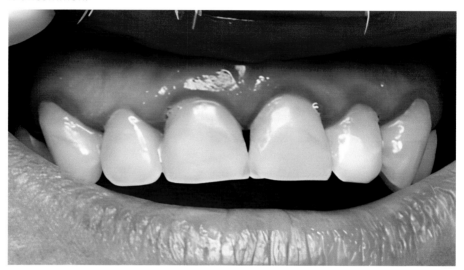

Figure 6.13. Linear gingival erythema in a patient with HIV infection.

Reproduced from *Handbook of Oral Pathology and Oral Medicine*, 2022; SR Prabhu, with permission from Wiley-Blackwell, and included here after enhancement by AIPDerm (www.aipderm.com).

Treatment

Treatment requires a combination of oral hygiene and antimicrobial agents. Options include:
- topical antifungal agent
- antiseptic mouthwash (e.g. 0.2% chlorhexidine)
- systemic antifungal agent; be aware of the interaction of azoles with antiretroviral drugs.

HIV-associated oral melanotic hyperpigmentation

HIV-associated oral hyperpigmentation can affect any part of the oral mucosa.
- Typically, there are asymptomatic, single or multiple, well-defined or irregular, light to deep brown macules of variable size and shape.
- Common sites are the gingiva and buccal mucosa (see *Fig. 6.14*).
- The cause of pigmentation may be HIV-induced cytokine dysregulation, a drug, or adrenocortical dysfunction associated with low CD4$^+$ T cell counts.

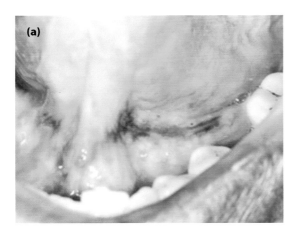
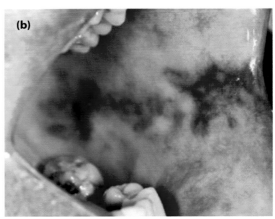

Figure 6.14. HIV-associated oral mucosal melanin hyperpigmentation (HIV-OMH). (a) Melanin hyperpigmentation of the floor of the mouth of a female 42-year-old non-smoker who was HIV-seropositive with a CD4⁺ T-cell count of 25 cells/mm³. HAART was started immediately after the diagnosis, and the hyperpigmentation appeared sometime later. (b) Irregular, non-homogeneous pigmented patch on the buccal mucosa of a 69-year-old HIV-seropositive male with a CD4⁺ T-cell count of 88 cells/mm³. HAART was started after 2 years, and the hyperpigmentation appeared 4 years later.

Reproduced from *AIDS Res Treat*. 2016;2016:8389214 (© Chandran *et al.*) under a CC-BY-SA licence.

6.2.9   Human papillomavirus

Viral warts

Oral warts are benign verrucous or papillary lesions of the oral mucosa. They are classified as verruca vulgaris, squamous papilloma, and condyloma acuminatum.
- Oral warts are common, affecting 7–8% of children and many adults. They affect males and females equally.
- Warts are frequently observed in patients with HIV infection or immune suppression.
- Verruca vulgaris, or the common wart, is most often diagnosed in children.
- Squamous cell papilloma accounts for 7–8% of all growths in children and 3–4% of all biopsied oral soft tissue lesions. In adults, it is usually diagnosed between 30 and 50 years of age.
- Condyloma acuminatum is usually diagnosed in teenagers and young adults.

Causes

Viral warts are caused by human papillomavirus (HPV) of low-risk types, often by autoinoculation from cutaneous viral warts.
- Verruca vulgaris is induced by HPV types 2, 4, and 40.
- Squamous cell papilloma is induced by HPV types 6 and 11.
- Condyloma acuminatum is also induced by HPV types 6 and 11 but is sexually transmitted.

- The incubation period ranges from 3 weeks to an undetermined period.
- Verruca vulgaris and squamous cell papilloma are usually transmitted by autoinoculation from cutaneous warts.
- There is a 50% chance of transmission of condyloma acuminatum during oral sex with an infected individual. In children, they are an indicator of possible sexual abuse.

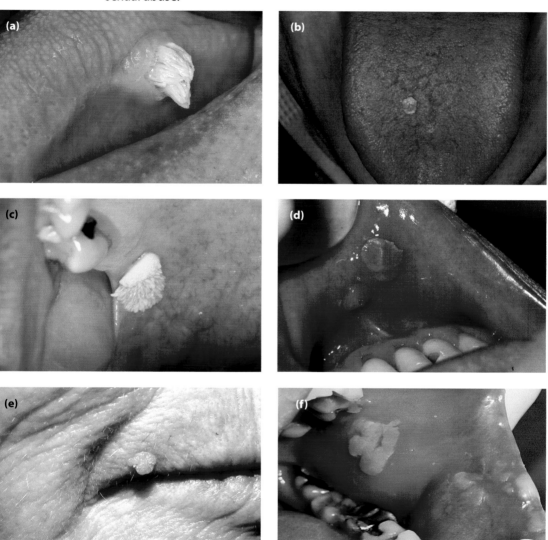

Figure 6.15 (a–f). (a) squamous papilloma left lateral tongue; (b) squamous papilloma right dorsal tongue; (c) squamous papilloma right soft palate; (d) squamous papilloma lower labial mucosa; (e) verruca vulgaris right upper lip; (f) condyloma acuminatum left buccal mucosa.

(a, c, d and e) Reproduced from Health NZ – Waikato (www.waikatodhb.health.nz) with permission; (f) reproduced from *Handbook of Oral Pathology and Oral Medicine*, 2022; SR Prabhu, with permission from Wiley-Blackwell, and included here after enhancement by AIPDerm (www.aipderm.com).

Clinical features

Oral warts may be solitary or multiple.
- Oral verruca vulgaris presents as an exophytic, sessile or pedunculated, painless, soft, white cauliflower-like lesion on the lip commissures, vermilion border, attached gingiva, or the tongue (see *Fig. 6.15a*). The average size is <5mm. They may rapidly enlarge and then remain stable for several years.
- Squamous cell papilloma forms a soft, painless, pinkish, pedunculated exophytic mass up to 1cm in diameter, with finger-like projections on the soft and hard palate, tongue (see *Fig. 6.15b*), buccal mucosa (see *Fig. 6.15c and d*), and lip (see *Fig. 6.15e*). Papillomas can also arise in the oesophagus, respiratory tract, and conjunctiva. Extraoral sites include the pharynx, larynx, oesophagus, cervix, vagina, or anal canal.
- Condyloma acuminatum presents as pinkish or whitish papules or sessile cauliflower-like blunt projections on the tongue, lips, palate, and floor of the mouth (see *Fig. 6.15e*).

Diagnosis

In most cases, oral warts are recognized clinically. Dermoscopy shows multiple whitish structures around central vessels.
- If the diagnosis is uncertain, perform a biopsy.
- Histopathology of squamous cell papilloma reveals exophytic finger-like projections of the keratinized squamous epithelium and fibrovascular connective tissue. The keratinocytes typically show (non-specific) cytopathic effects of viral infection.
- Histopathology of verruca vulgaris reveals acanthotic epidermis, hyperkeratosis, and parakeratosis with elongated rete ridges often curving towards the centre of the lesion.

Treatment

Verruca vulgaris disappears spontaneously after a year or two, and squamous cell papilloma spontaneously resolves in 20–30% of patients. On the other hand, relapses occur in 20–30% of patients who have undergone treatment.

If treatment is required, surgical excision is often the treatment of choice. Other options include:
- electrocautery
- cryotherapy
- local hyperthermia
- CO_2 laser
- topical keratolytic agents (containing salicylic acid and lactic acid)
- topical trichloroacetic acid, podophyllotoxin, or 5-fluorouracil
- intralesional infiltration of α-interferon or imiquimod.

Childhood vaccination with the nine-valent HPV vaccine markedly reduces the incidence of oral warts associated with the relevant HPV types.

Multifocal epithelial hyperplasia

Multifocal epithelial hyperplasia of the oral mucous membranes, also known as Heck disease, is characterized by painless papules and nodules with a sessile base.
- Multifocal epithelial hyperplasia affects children and adolescents between 3 and 18 years of age, with a female predilection.
- It is most often diagnosed in specific populations in the USA and Greenland. Sporadic cases involving Caucasians from other regions have been reported.

Causes

Several immune-cytochemical and *in situ* hybridization studies have identified the presence of HPV (subtypes 1, 6, 11,13, 32, and 55) as the possible causative agent of multifocal epithelial hyperplasia. Contributing factors include immune suppression, genetic predisposition, and malnutrition.

Clinical features

Multiple epithelial hyperplasia presents clinically as circumscribed papules and nodules ranging in diameter from 1–10mm (see *Fig. 6.16*). Lesions frequently coalesce into plaques.
- Painless red, grey, or whitish lesions are found on the buccal mucosa, labial mucosa, labial commissures, tongue, hard palate, and gingiva.
- Lesions may spontaneously regress or persist for years.

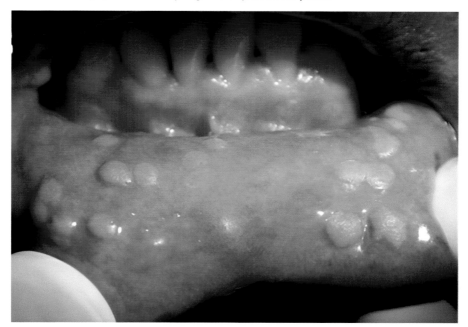

Figure 6.16. Multiple epithelial hyperplasia (Heck disease); multiple papules on the lower labial mucosa.

Reproduced from *Trends in Infectious Diseases*, 2013 (http://dx.doi.org/10.5772/57597) under CC BY 3.0 licence. © 2014 InTech, and included here after enhancement by AIPDerm (www.aipderm.com).

Treatment

Treatment options for multifocal epithelial hyperplasia include:
- surgical removal
- cryotherapy
- electrocautery
- laser ablation
- topical agents such as imiquimod, retinoic acid, or trichloroacetic acid.

6.2.10   Molluscum contagiosum

Molluscum contagiosum is a common childhood keratinocyte infection that sometimes affects adults, especially when immune-compromised (such as HIV infection).

Causes

Molluscum contagiosum is an intraepidermal infection caused by the molluscum contagiosum virus.

It is transmitted by skin-to-skin contact in wet conditions such as bathing or swimming.

Clinical features

Molluscum contagiosum is characterized by crops of umbilicated round whitish papules.
- They occur in moist body locations such as the groin and limb creases.
- Facial lesions can occur (see *Fig. 6.17*), and clusters of papules may arise on the lips, tongue, and buccal mucosa.

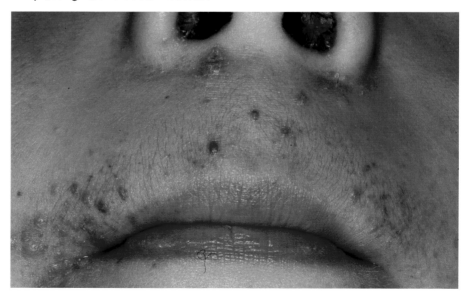

Figure 6.17. Molluscum contagiosum lesions on the face and upper lip vermilion.

Reproduced from Health NZ – Waikato (www.waikatodhb.health.nz) with permission.

- Secondary dermatitis may surround the papules.
- The dermoscopy of a papule shows a characteristic white centre with polarized white structures and peripheral crown vessels.

Treatment

White molluscum bodies can be expressed from the centre of the papules, resulting in the resolution of the individual lesions. Physically destructive treatments can be used.

Treatment is unnecessary, as lesions will resolve spontaneously within a few months, usually without scarring. Pitted scars may occur occasionally.

A mild topical steroid can be used to control dermatitis.

6.3   Bacterial infections

6.3.1   Staphylococcal infections

Staphylococcal infections commonly affect the perioral skin, particularly in children.
- Impetigo (a common localized superficial skin disease often co-infected with group A streptococcus)
- Staphylococcal scalded skin syndrome (an uncommon localized or widespread blistering skin disease affecting infants).

Impetigo

Risk factors

Staphylococcal infections can occur at all ages but are most common in children aged 2 to 5 years.
- Colonization with staphylococci may lead to bullous or non-bullous impetigo if epidermal barrier function is compromised.
- Impetigo is common in crowded conditions (e.g. day-care centres and schools) and hot or humid environments.
- It is more prevalent and severe in patients with diabetes, cancer, or who are immune-compromised.
- It can complicate surgical wounds, traumatic wounds, and skin diseases (particularly eczema).
- Intraoral impetigo is rare.
- The risk is reduced by good hand hygiene (regular soap and water or sanitizer use).

Causes
- Impetigo is caused by *Staphylococcus aureus* and *Streptococcus pyogenes*.
- These bacteria are commonly found in asymptomatic individuals in the nose (30%) and mouth (24%).
- Infection is spread by direct and indirect contact.

Clinical features

- The incubation period is about 10 days.
- Perioral impetigo presents with localized erythema, itching, and oozing patches which evolve into honey-crusted erosions (see *Fig. 6.18*). Healing occurs without scarring.
- Intraoral impetigo presents with erythema, oedema, pain, or burning discomfort affecting the gingivae.
- Intraoral impetigo is usually accompanied by angular cheilitis.
- Bullous impetigo does not affect the mucosa.

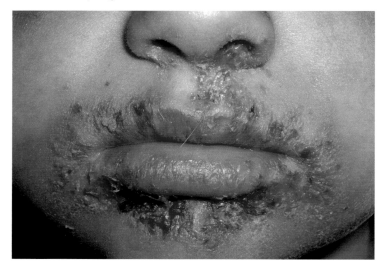

Figure 6.18. Honey-coloured crusted perioral erosions due to impetigo.

Provided by the late Dr Anthony Yung, Dermatologist, Hamilton, New Zealand.

Diagnosis

- In most cases, the diagnosis is clinical.
- Swabs can reveal methicillin-resistant *Staphylococcus aureus* or another cause of infection.

Treatment

- Topical antiseptic or antibiotic for limited disease; otherwise, oral antibiotics.
- Mild intraoral disease can be managed with chlorhexidine rinses.
- Patients should stay at home and cover their lesions until they are on antibiotics and the lesions have dried.
- Do not share, and wash clothing, linen, and towels daily.
- Good hand hygiene (wash hands frequently with soap and water or use sanitizer) and oral hygiene (brush and floss teeth and gums).

Prognosis

Complications of impetigo may include:
- dental abscess (see below)
- bacteraemia and sepsis
- toxic shock syndrome.

Staphylococcal scalded skin syndrome

Risk factors

Staphylococcal scalded skin syndrome (SSSS) most often affects neonates and children under 6 years; most are under 2 years.

- The immature renal function fails to clear the bacterial exotoxin.
- Individual susceptibility may relate to the quantity of the epidermal desmosomal protein desmoglein-1.
- SSSS sometimes occurs in adults who have renal or immunological dysfunction.

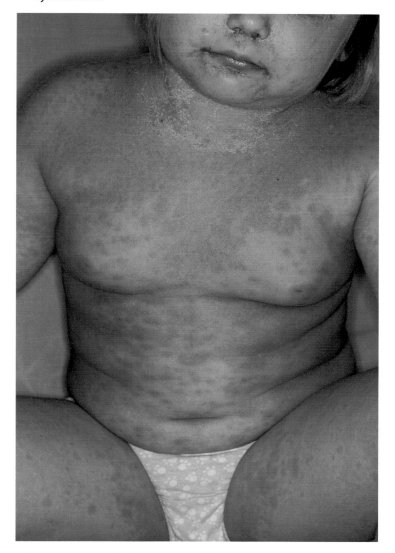

Figure 6.19. Staphylococcal scalded skin syndrome. Crusted perioral erosions and widespread erythema with erosions and desquamation.

Reproduced from Health NZ – Waikato (www.waikatodhb.health.nz) with permission.

Causes

SSSS is caused by *Staphylococcus aureus* with exfoliative toxin-producing strains. The toxin is a serine protease targeting desmoglein-1, resulting in superficial intraepidermal lysis.

Clinical features
- The rash starts as localized impetigo, often causing perioral crusting (see *Fig. 6.19*).
- The infant then develops diffuse or patchy cutaneous erythema, facial oedema, tenderness, and fever. Bullae are flaccid and break easily.
- Unlike toxic epidermal necrolysis, SSSS does not affect mucosa (*see Section 4.6.8*).
- Nikolsky sign is positive in the acute phase (stroking the involved skin results in separation of the superficial epidermis).
- Desquamation occurs within a day or so and healing within 10–14 days.

Diagnosis
- In most cases, the diagnosis is clinical.
- Swabs from the primary site may reveal *Staphylococcus aureus* but are negative from blisters in distant sites.
- Biopsy, if performed, shows cleavage below the granular cell layer.

Treatment
- Systemic antistaphylococcal antibiotics
- Supportive care.

Prognosis

Mortality is more likely if there is sepsis or a severe medical condition. It is less than 4% in infants but higher in adults.

6.3.2   Streptococcal infections

Group A streptococcal infections may cause invasive or non-invasive disease of the oral mucosa.
- Pharyngitis
- Scarlet fever (see *Section 6.3.5*)
- Impetigo (see *Section 6.3.1*).

Risk factors

Group A streptococcal infections can occur at all ages but are most common in children aged 5 to 15 years.
- They are more common in crowded conditions (e.g. day-care centres and schools).
- The risk is reduced by good hand hygiene (regular soap and water or sanitizer use) and respiratory etiquette (covering cough or sneeze).

Causes

Group A streptococcal infections are caused by certain strains of *Streptococcus pyogenes* (beta-haemolytic streptococci). They are transmitted directly from person to person through respiratory droplets or secretions.

Streptococcal pharyngitis

Clinical features

Streptococcal pharyngitis presents with a sudden onset of a sore throat, pain with swallowing and fever.
- The incubation period is 2–5 days.
- Other symptoms may include headache, abdominal pain, nausea, and vomiting.
- Examination findings are pharyngeal erythema, tonsillar hypertrophy (see *Fig. 6.20*) and possible exudate, palatal petechiae, and anterior cervical lymphadenopathy.

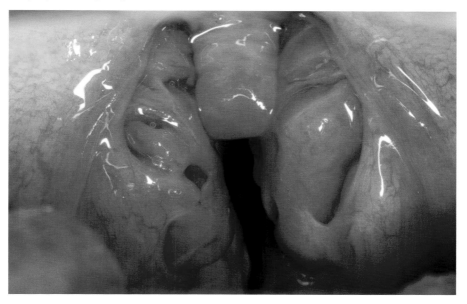

Figure 6.20. Tonsillar hypertrophy due to multiple episodes of streptococcal tonsillitis.

Reproduced from Health NZ – Waikato (www.waikatodhb.health.nz) with permission.

Diagnosis

Viral infections are more common causes of pharyngitis than group A streptococci, especially in preschool children.
- Cough, rhinorrhoea, conjunctivitis, or mouth ulcers usually accompany viral pharyngitis, but are absent in streptococcal pharyngitis.
- A throat swab rapid antigen detection test or culture confirms group A streptococcal pharyngitis.
- Consider also diphtheria, gonorrhoea, chlamydia, and *Mycoplasma pneumoniae*.

Treatment

Group A streptococcal infections are treated with oral antibiotics to reduce symptoms, transmission, and complications.

- In patients without penicillin allergy: penicillin V
- In patients with penicillin allergy: cephalexin, roxithromycin, clarithromycin (see local guidelines).
- Patients should stay home until the fever has gone and they have taken antibiotics for at least 12–24 hours.

Prognosis

Complications of streptococcal pharyngitis may include:
- peritonsillar abscess (quinsy), cervical lymphadenitis, and mastoiditis
- acute rheumatic fever or post-streptococcal glomerulonephritis.

6.3.3   Dental plaque (biofilm)

Dental plaque or biofilm is an adherent whitish substance that arises on teeth and gums within a few days of neglecting oral hygiene.
- Plaque may be supragingival or extend apical to the gingival margin (subgingival).
- Mineralized plaque is called dental calculus.
- Dental plaque and calculus lead to dental caries, gingivitis, periodontitis, and bone destruction around the teeth.

Risk factors

Dietary sugars.

Causes

Dental plaque comprises bacterial cells, soluble and insoluble salivary carbohydrates, and bacterial extracellular products.
- About 1000 commensal and pathogenic bacterial species have been found in dental plaque, including *Streptococcus mutans*, lactobacilli, and other anaerobes.
- These bacteria rapidly metabolize dietary sugars resulting in an acidic, low pH, demineralizing tooth enamel and causing dental caries.
- The periodontal pathogens *Porphyromonas gingivalis*, *P. endodontalis*, *Prevotella intermedia*, and *Parvimonas micra* form microcolonies within the biofilm, whereas spirochaetes dominate outside the biofilm.
- Bacterial virulence factors include bacterial lipopolysaccharides, which stimulate immune cells.

Treatment

Bacterial plaque, caries, and periodontal disease are prevented by daily brushing, flossing and professional tooth cleaning.

Gingivitis and periodontitis

Gingivitis and periodontitis are collectively known as periodontal diseases.
- The periodontium comprises the soft tissue and bone surrounding the tooth (gingival tissue, the periodontal ligament, alveolar bone, and cementum).
- Plaque-induced gingivitis results in localized or generalized redness, swelling and bleeding on probing (see *Fig. 6.21*).

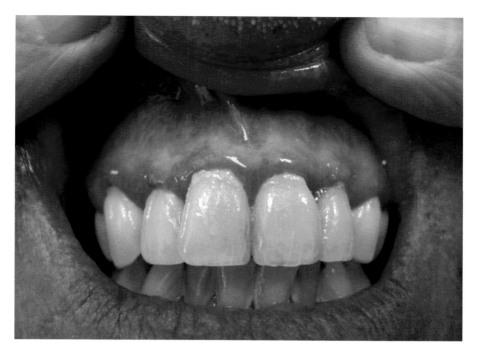

Figure 6.21. Gingivitis showing generalized redness and swelling of the marginal gingiva.

Reproduced from Health NZ – Waikato (www.waikatodhb.health.nz) with permission.

- Gingivitis alone is reversible – the inflammation spares the connective tissue attachment and alveolar bone.
- Progressive disease leading to periodontitis is irreversible – the inflammation destroys alveolar bone, leading to tooth mobility and loss.

The American Academy of Periodontology (AAP) has classified periodontitis into:
- aggressive periodontitis
- chronic periodontitis
- periodontitis as a manifestation of systemic diseases.

Causes

The most important risk factor for aggressive and chronic periodontitis is the dental plaque at and below the gingival margin associated with a destructive host-inflammatory immune response.

Risk factors for periodontitis
- A shift from a Gram-positive bacterial population associated with periodontal health to a Gram-negative population
- Lower socioeconomic status, heavy smoking, alcohol, and substance abuse
- Diabetes; periodontitis is a recognized complication of poorly controlled diabetes, due to reduced neutrophil function, especially in smokers – it can be prevented by good oral hygiene
- Leukaemia; periodontitis is due to impaired immune function

- Genetic predisposition; three genes have convincing evidence for association with chronic periodontitis: vitamin D receptor (*VDR*), Fc gamma receptor IIA (*Fc-γRIIA*) and interleukin 10 (*IL10*).

Clinical features

Severe periodontitis causes tooth loss, negatively impacting speech, nutrition, quality of life, and self-esteem.
- Bacteraemia and systemic dissemination of inflammatory mediators produced in the periodontal tissues may result in systemic inflammation and endothelial dysfunction, contributing to cardiovascular disease, atheroma, respiratory disease, and diabetes mellitus.
- Periodontitis/bacteraemia is associated with adverse pregnancy outcomes (preterm birth, low birth weight, and pre-eclampsia).

Necrotizing periodontal diseases

Necrotizing periodontal diseases include necrotizing gingivitis, necrotizing periodontitis, necrotizing stomatitis, and noma.
- Necrotizing gingivitis is limited to the interdental papilla; it has a punched-out appearance (see *Fig. 6.22a*) and results in bleeding and halitosis.
- Necrotizing periodontitis is diagnosed when there is rapid alveolar bone loss (see *Fig. 6.22b*), a pseudomembrane, lymphadenopathy, and pyrexia.
- Necrotizing stomatitis progresses to osteonecrosis and bony sequestration of the alveolar bone.
- Noma (cancrum oris) is a fast-spreading non-contagious orofacial gangrene. Noma leads to extensive soft tissue and bony destruction and may eventually be fatal.

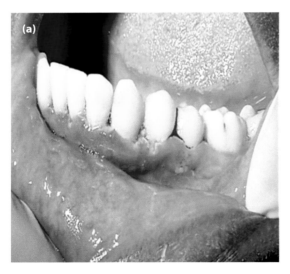 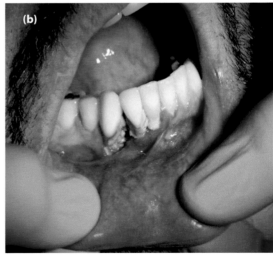

Figure 6.22 (a and b). (a) Necrotizing ulcerative gingivitis (NUG) showing characteristic ulcers of the interdental papillae; (b) necrotizing ulcerative periodontitis (NUP) with destruction of periodontal tissues.

Reproduced with permission from Professor Jeff Hill, School of Dentistry, University of Alabama, in Birmingham, AL, USA.

Causes

Necrotizing periodontal diseases are due to opportunistic infection with fusiform and spirochaete bacteria: Treponema, Selenomonas, Fusobacterium and *Prevotella intermedia.*
- Necrotizing periodontal diseases are usually diagnosed in undeveloped countries in malnourished children 3–10 years old.
- Predisposing factors include poor oral hygiene, smoking, stress, immunosuppression, malnutrition, uncontrolled diabetes, and cancer.
- Necrotizing gingivitis and necrotizing periodontitis are also common in patients with immunodeficiency, such as HIV.

Diagnosis

Diagnosis of a necrotizing periodontal disease is primarily based on clinical findings and medical history and the exclusion of recurrent gingivitis, generalized periodontitis, vesiculobullous diseases, and diseases with periodontal manifestations such as leukaemia or scurvy.

Treatment

Dentists treat necrotizing gingivitis and necrotizing periodontitis with:
- NSAIDs to alleviate pain
- antibiotics: metronidazole or amoxicillin.

Gingival and periodontal abscess

Gum abscesses can be classified into gingival and periodontal abscesses.
- A gingival abscess (also known as parulis) affects the marginal gingiva.
- A periodontal abscess (lateral periodontal abscess) affects periodontal tissues. It may destroy the periodontal ligament and alveolar bone.

Causes

A gingival abscess is usually caused by trauma such as penetration by a toothpick.
- Most periodontal abscesses are due to obstruction of a periodontal pocket.
- Local factors that increase the risk of a periodontal abscess include invaginated tooth, root grooves, a cracked tooth, and external root resorption.
- Gram-negative anaerobic bacteria dominate the microbiology.
- Diabetes mellitus can increase the incidence and progression of periodontal disease, including periodontal abscess.

Clinical features

Patients with a gingival or periodontal abscess complain of pain of varying intensity and soft red gingival swelling (see *Fig. 6.23a*). Signs of a periodontal abscess include:
- increased periodontal probing depths (usually >6mm)
- suppuration
- tooth mobility
- furcation involvement (bone loss at the branching point of the roots)

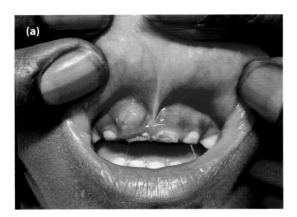
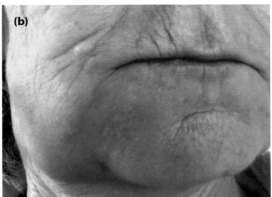

Figure 6.23 (a and b). (a) Gingival abscess (parulis); (b) facial swelling due to dental abscess.

(a) Reproduced with permission from Dr Kirsten Due, Australia.

- tenderness to palpation and lateral percussion
- facial swelling (see *Fig. 6.23b*).

Diagnosis

Diagnosis is based on the history, clinical findings, and periapical radiography of the tooth involved.

Treatment

The abscess should be incised and drained. Antibiotics may be necessary if symptoms are severe, or the patient is immunocompromised.

Drainage of pus from a periodontal abscess is followed by removing debris and calculus using mechanical scaling. Tooth repair may be required.

6.3.4   Gonococcal stomatitis

Gonococcal stomatitis is a rare manifestation of sexually transmitted infection with *Neisseria gonorrhoeae*.

Causes

N. gonorrhoeae in adults is transmitted through vaginal, oral, or anal sex. Neonatal infection can follow vaginal birth if the mother has untreated genitourinary gonorrhoea.

Clinical features

Gonococcal stomatitis presents as erythematous and eroded buccal mucosa, tongue, and gingiva.
- A yellow or white pseudomembrane may cover affected areas.
- Symptoms include sore throat and mucosal burning.
- Submandibular and cervical lymph node enlargement may occur.

Diagnosis

Diagnosis of gonococcal stomatitis is based on clinical history, presenting features and the isolation of *N. gonorrhoeae*, e.g. by PCR.

Treatment

Refer to the US Centers for Disease Control (CDC) for treatment recommendations, currently intramuscular ceftriaxone (December 2023). *N. gonorrhoeae* is prone to antibiotic resistance.

6.3.5 Strawberry tongue

Strawberry tongue describes glossitis with hyperplastic fungiform papillae associated with a febrile infection.

Causes

Strawberry tongue occurs in scarlet fever (caused by group A β-haemolytic streptococci, which produce erythrogenic toxins), some cases of toxic shock syndrome (*Staphylococcus aureus*) and other severe infections, and the non-infectious disorders Kawasaki disease and multisystem inflammatory syndrome in children (a complication of Covid-19).

Clinical features

A strawberry tongue may be white or red.
- White strawberry tongue presents as a white coating of the dorsum of the tongue through which the hyperplastic fungiform papillae protrude.
- The red strawberry tongue is revealed when the white coating is lost.
- Large red papillae are sometimes described as a raspberry tongue.
- Fever, sore throat, erythematous rash, and other symptoms and signs of infection are present.

Treatment

Patients with strawberry tongue are unwell and may require hospitalization. The systemic symptoms and signs should be carefully evaluated, and investigations should be undertaken to determine the underlying cause.

Antibiotics are prescribed for a confirmed streptococcal or staphylococcal infection.

6.3.6 Syphilis

Syphilis is a bacterial infection caused by the anaerobic spirochaete *Treponema pallidum*.
- Infection is usually sexually transmitted.
- Syphilis may also be transmitted by skin contact with an infectious lesion.
- It has a worldwide incidence of approximately 6 million cases per year.

Clinical features

There are four disease stages (primary, secondary, latent, and tertiary syphilis).
- Primary syphilis presents as a painless chancre (ulcer) (see *Fig. 6.24a*) at the inoculation site. Up to 12% of chancres occur in the oral cavity, commonly located on the tongue, palate, lip, or gingiva.
- The incubation period ranges from 10–90 days; the chancre appears and then heals up to 8 weeks later.
- 25% of untreated patients develop disseminated secondary syphilis.
- Secondary syphilis results in scaly macules and papules on the trunk and limbs, characteristically affecting the palms and soles. It can also cause hepatitis or uveitis.
- Oral lesions characterized by ulcers ('snail track' ulcers) (see *Fig. 6.24b*) develop in up to 30% of cases of secondary syphilis, resolving in 12 weeks.
- There are no visible signs of infection in latent syphilis, which can persist for many years.
- Oral tertiary syphilis is rare. It presents as an ulcerated nodule (gumma) on the tongue, palate, or lip or an irregular white hyperkeratotic plaque (syphilitic leukoplakia) on the tongue.

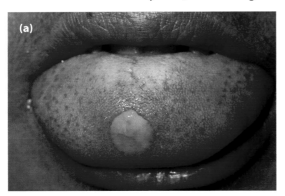 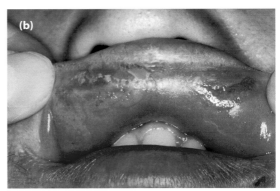

Figure 6.24 (a and b). (a) Primary syphilitic chancre on the tongue. (b) Ulcers due to secondary syphilis on the labial mucosa.

(a) Reproduced from Health NZ – Waikato (www.waikatodhb.health.nz) with permission; (b) Reproduced from *Handbook of Oral Diseases for Medical Practice*, 2016; Ed: SR Prabhu, with permission from Oxford University Press, and included here after enhancement by AIPDerm (www.aipderm.com).

Diagnosis

Darkfield microscopy of exudate from a chancre may reveal spirochaetes. Confirmation of the diagnosis of syphilis at any stage relies on serological findings, which can be hard to interpret.

Inexpensive non-specific serological tests used for screening and monitoring disease activity include:
- rapid plasma reagin (RPR) test – the titre indicates the degree of disease activity
- venereal disease research laboratory (VDRL) test.

Specific tests for active, latent, or treated syphilis include:

- enzyme immunoassay (EIA)
- chemiluminescent microplate immunoassay (CMEIA)
- treponemal pallidum particle agglutination (TPPA)
- fluorescent treponemal antibody absorption (FTA-ABS).

Warthin–Starry silver staining or specific treponemal immunohistochemistry can be applied to biopsy tissue.

Treatment

Patients with syphilis should be referred urgently to a sexual health or infectious disease physician for assessment, sexual partner notification, and treatment with benzathine penicillin or an alternative antibiotic.

Syphilitic leukoplakia

Syphilitic leukoplakia is an irregular white hyperkeratotic plaque on the dorsum of the tongue associated with tertiary syphilis. The plaque cannot be removed by gentle scraping, and it persists after treatment of the bacterial infection.
- Syphilitic leukoplakia is potentially malignant and should undergo biopsy.
- Fissuring, nodules, or erosions may be signs of malignant transformation.
- Histopathology of syphilitic leukoplakia shows hyperkeratosis, dysplasia, and a late-syphilitic chronic inflammatory cell infiltrate with plasma cells, granulomas, and endarteritis of small arteries.

6.3.7   Tuberculosis

Tuberculosis (TB) is a chronic granulomatous mycobacterial infection. Extra-pulmonary TB affects up to 25% of patients and is increasing in incidence. Oral lesions in 5% of cases may present before pulmonary symptoms.

Cause

TB is usually caused by *Mycobacterium tuberculosis*, although *M. bovis* and atypical mycobacteria have occasionally been implicated.
- Primary oral TB is rare.
- Secondary oral TB is most often caused by inoculation of the oral mucosa with infected sputum.
- Oral TB can also be due to the haematogenous spread of pulmonary TB to the submucosa.

Clinical features

TB may affect any site in the oral mucosa.
- The appearance is non-specific, with irregular erythema, granulomatous swelling, and ulceration.
- Painful or painless ulceration with ragged, irregular margins and an indurated base (see *Fig. 6.25*).
- Deep biopsy reveals epithelioid granulomas and multinucleated giant cells, with or without caseation. Ziehl–Neelsen staining may confirm the presence of acid-fast bacilli.
- The diagnosis is confirmed by culture at low temperature.

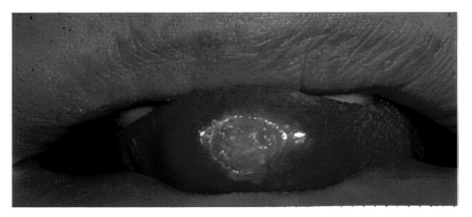

Figure. 6.25. Tuberculous ulcer of the tongue.

Reproduced from *BMC Oral Health*, 2019;19:67 (https://doi.org/10.1186/s12903-019-0764-y) under a CC BY 4.0 DEED licence, and included here after enhancement by AIPDerm (www.aipderm.com).

Treatment

The treatment of oral TB is the same as for systemic TB.
- Oral lesions usually respond well to a standardized drug regimen.
- Multiresistant TB requires alternative drugs.

6.4   Mixed infections

6.4.1   Angular cheilitis

Angular cheilitis, also known as perlèche or angular stomatitis, is a common inflammatory condition of the corners of the mouth.

Causes

Angular cheilitis is multifactorial. It is a form of intertrigo due to pooled saliva and microbial overgrowth.
- *Candida albicans*, *Staphylococcus aureus* and *Streptococcus pyogenes* may be found on culture.
- Predisposing factors include a decreased vertical dimension of occlusion in a denture wearer, downturned lips, and deep furrows due to ageing.
- It can also follow exposure to wintry weather or wind, which dry the lips resulting in fissuring.
- Angular cheilitis often complicates an acute illness, mouth breathing, or drooling.
- It can also signify an underlying systemic disease such as diabetes, HIV infection, nutritional deficiency, haematological malignancy, or solid organ tumour.
- Drugs predisposing to angular cheilitis include retinoids (acitretin, isotretinoin).

Clinical features

Angular cheilitis can be acute, relapsing, or chronic, depending on the predisposing factors.

- Most patients complain of discomfort, burning, irritation, pruritus, or pain at one or both angles of the mouth.
- The signs include red and scaly or moist, fissured plaques at the angles of the mouth (see *Figs. 6.26a, b,* and *c*).
- Occasionally, intraoral fungal infection may be present.

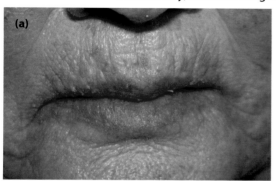

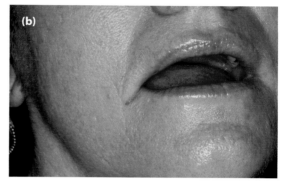

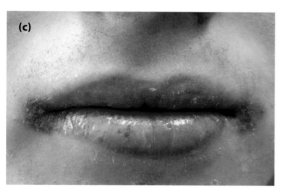

Figure 6.26 (a–c). Angular cheilitis associated with (a and b) candida and (c) *Staphylococcus aureus.*

All images reproduced from Health NZ – Waikato (www. waikatodhb.health.nz) with permission.

Treatment

Initial evaluation of local predisposing factors includes reviewing oral hygiene and the vertical dimension of any prostheses. Consider the patient's medical and drug history.

- A cream or ointment containing a combination of topical antifungal and antibacterial (e.g. nystatin and mupirocin) or antifungal, antibacterial, and steroid (e.g. nystatin, neomycin, gramicidin, and triamcinolone) is applied to the angles of the mouth two or three times daily for 1–2 weeks.
- Persistent *Candida albicans* may be treated with oral fluconazole.
- Dry lips are managed by frequently applying lip balm or plain petroleum jelly.
- Angular cheilitis may persist due to anatomic and systemic factors.

CHAPTER 7

ORAL MUCOSAL INFLAMMATORY DISEASES AND CONDITIONS

See also:
- *Section 4.6 Adverse drug reaction*
- *Chapter 6: Oral mucosal infections.*

7.1 Recurrent aphthous ulcer

Recurrent aphthous ulcer, also known as recurrent aphthous stomatitis, is an idiopathic recurrence of oral ulcers with a classic appearance.
- It is the most common cause of mouth ulcers, affecting up to 20% of the population.
- Recurrent aphthous ulcer is classified as minor (see *Fig. 7.1a*), major (see *Fig. 7.1b*), or herpetiform.

Causes

The exact cause of aphthous ulcers is unknown. Risk factors for recurrent ulcers include:
- younger age
- female gender
- genetics (HLA-A2, HLA-B5, HLA-B12, HLAB44, HLA-B51, HLA-B52, HLA-DR2, HLA-DR7, and HLA-DQ series)
- deficiency of iron, minerals, or vitamins
- smoking cessation
- stress and anxiety.

Aphthous ulcers occur in several systemic conditions, including:
- Behçet syndrome
- coeliac disease
- MAGIC syndrome (mouth and genital ulcers with inflamed cartilage)
- Sweet syndrome (neutrophilic dermatosis) (see *Fig 7.1c*)
- PFAPA syndrome (periodic fever, aphthous ulcers, pharyngitis, and cervical adenitis)
- reactive arthritis
- cyclic neutropenia.

Aphthous or aphthous-like ulcers may also be drug-induced (see *Section 4.6*).

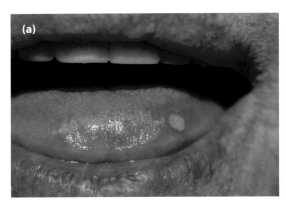

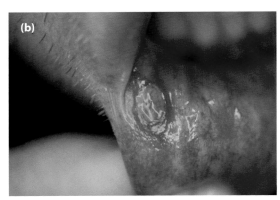

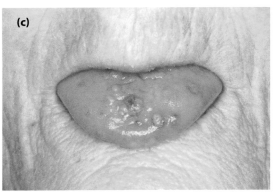

Figure 7.1 (a–c). Oral aphthous ulceration. (a) Minor aphthous ulcers, (b) major aphthous ulcer, (c) Sweet syndrome (neutrophilic dermatitis) with aphthae on the tongue.

All images reproduced from Health NZ – Waikato (www. waikatodhb.health.nz) with permission.

Clinical features

Aphthous ulcers are ovoid or round, with an erythematous halo and yellow fibrinous centre.
- The ulcers are painful and may be preceded by discomfort.
- Symptoms may be exacerbated by spicy and acidic food.

Minor aphthous ulcer (80% of cases):
- Single or multiple minor aphthous ulcers on the buccal mucosa, labial mucosa, ventral tongue, and floor of the mouth.
- Minor aphthous ulcers are <1cm in diameter (see *Fig. 7.2a*).
- Typically, they persist for up to 2 weeks.
- Minor aphthous ulcers heal without scarring.

Major aphthous ulcer (15%):
- Single or multiple major aphthous ulcers affect the labial mucosa, soft palate, and oropharynx (see *Fig. 7.2b*).
- Major aphthous ulcers are >1cm in diameter.
- They last for more than 4 weeks.
- They are painful and heal with scarring.

Herpetiform aphthous ulcer (5%):
- Herpetiform aphthous ulcers affect the ventral and lateral tongue.
- They present as crops of small ulcers (1–2mm diameter), resembling herpetic ulceration (see *Fig. 7.2c*).

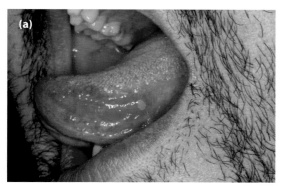

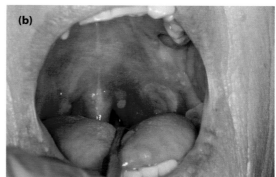

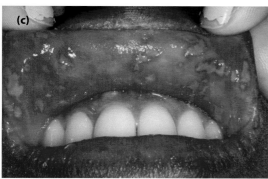

Figure 7.2 (a–c). (a) Minor aphthous ulcer on tongue; (b) major aphthous ulcer on the soft palate; (c) herpetic aphthous ulcers on the upper labial mucosa.

(c) Reproduced from *Color Atlas of Oral and Maxillofacial Diseases*, 2019; B.W. Neville, D.D. Damm, C.M. Allen & A.C. Chi, with permission from Elsevier.

- The small ulcers may coalesce to form larger ones.
- They last for 2 or 3 weeks and heal without scarring.

Diagnosis

A diagnosis of recurrent aphthous ulceration relies on history and clinical features. Investigations may include blood tests to screen for haematinic deficiencies, associated systemic disorders, and HLA typing. Histopathology is non-specific.

Treatment

Treatment of aphthous ulcer is symptomatic and may include:
- topical steroids
- anaesthetic and antiseptic mouth rinses
- short courses of systemic steroids for flares
- an immunomodulatory medication such as colchicine, dapsone, azathioprine, or thalidomide.

7.2 Lichenoid disorders

7.2.1 Oral lichen planus

Lichen planus is a chronic inflammatory mucocutaneous disease.
- Oral lichen planus (OLP) affects 1–2% of the adult population.
- It most often occurs in adults over 40, with an average age at diagnosis of 50–60 years.
- It is more common in women than men (1.4: 1).

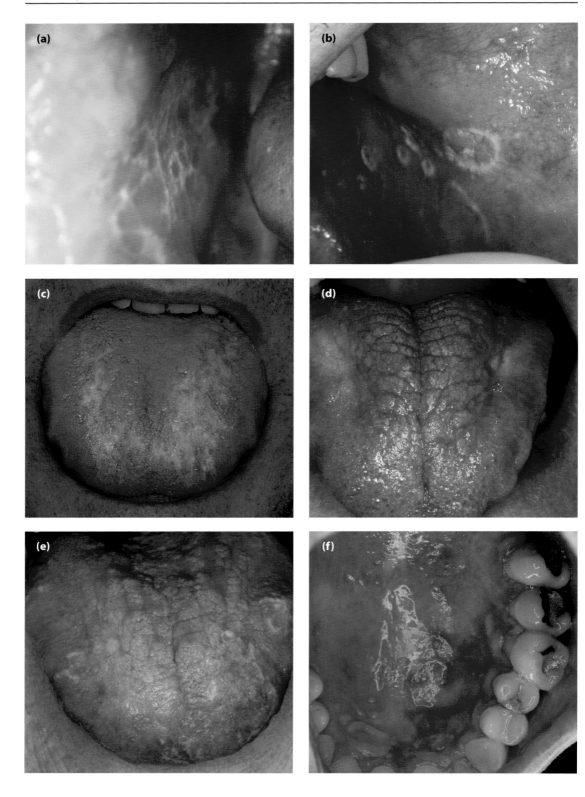

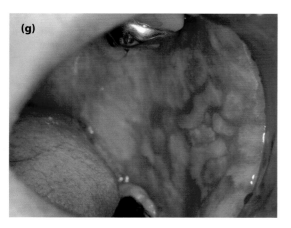

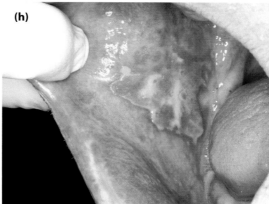

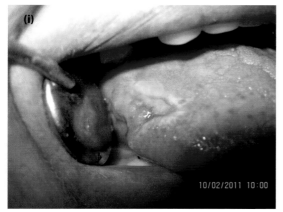

Figure 7.3 (a–i). Types of oral lichen planus. Reticular pattern on the (a) right and (b) left buccal mucosa and (c) tongue; (d) atrophic type on tongue; (e) plaque type; (f) erythema; (g) erosions and (h) ulceration on buccal mucosa, and (i) ulceration on tongue.

(a, c, f, and g) Reproduced from Health NZ – Waikato (www.waikatodhb.health.nz) with permission; (b) reproduced with permission from Professor Yeshwant Rawal, University of Milwaukee School of Dentistry, Milwaukee, WI, USA; (e and h) reproduced with permission from Professor Nagamani Narayana, University of Nebraska Medical Centre, NE, USA; (i) reproduced with permission from Professor Sandhya Tamgadge and Dr DY Patil, Dental College and Hospital, Navi Mumbai, India.

- Bullous lichen planus affects <1% of patients with OLP, i.e. 5–10 cases in a population of 100 000.
- Patients with OLP may also have cutaneous lichen planus, anogenital lichen planus, or, more rarely, lichen planus affecting other mucosal sites.
- Some patients will have a family history of lichen planus.

Causes

The precise cause of oral lichen planus has yet to be fully understood.
- It involves antigen-specific CD8[+] T lymphocytes and pro-inflammatory cytokines, which destroy the oral epithelial cells.
- Oral lichen planus is sometimes associated with chronic liver disease, hepatitis C viral infection, stress, genetic predisposition, and tobacco chewing.

Clinical features

OLP affects the buccal mucosa, the tongue, and the gingivae. It usually presents with bilateral asymptomatic or painful white lesions or erosions. These are best observed using dermoscopy/mucoscopy. Clinical variations include:
- striations (Wickham striae) with lace-like patterns (reticular OLP) (see *Figs 7.3a–c*)
- atrophic OLP (see *Fig. 7.3d*)
- patches and plaques (plaque OLP) (see *Fig. 7.3d*)
- solitary or multiple papules (papular OLP) (see *Fig. 7.3e*)
- erythema (see *Fig. 7.3f*) and erosions (erosive OLP) (see *Fig. 7.3g*); erosive lichen planus often also affects genitalia – it may result in violaceous, brown, or black postinflammatory pigmented macules, especially in darker-skinned individuals
- vesicles and bullae (bullous lichen planus). These affect the buccal mucosa and the gingiva and, less frequently, the lips. Intact bullae rupture quickly, leaving erosions and ulcers (see *Figs 7.3h* and *i*). Bullous lichen planus may also affect the skin.

Diagnosis

A history of chronic stomatitis and features on clinical examination provide clues to lichen planus. A biopsy is often performed due to its irregular clinical appearance or concern about malignant potential, as oral lichen planus may occasionally be complicated by squamous cell carcinoma.
- The histopathology of oral lichen planus is characterized by a lichenoid pattern of dense subepithelial lymphohistiocytic infiltrate, increased numbers of intraepithelial lymphocytes, and degeneration of basal keratinocytes.
- Degenerating basal keratinocytes form colloid bodies (Civatte, hyaline, cytoid bodies) which are homogenous eosinophilic globules.
- Dermoscopy of cutaneous papules may reveal characteristic white striations.

Treatment

No treatment is required for asymptomatic reticular and papular oral lichen planus.

Treatment for any symptomatic disease is with intermittent courses of topical corticosteroids twice daily after meals and bedtime until symptoms resolve.

Examples include:
- fluocinonide 0.05% gel
- betamethasone dipropionate 0.5% ointment
- fluticasone nasal solution sprayed onto the symptomatic area
- dexamethasone mouthwash (0.5mg in 5–10ml water, swish for 2 minutes and spit).

Severe oral lichen planus may require a systemic agent, such as:
- hydroxychloroquine
- prednisone or prednisolone

- methotrexate
- an immunosuppressive drug, such as azathioprine, mycophenolate, or ciclosporin.

The prognosis for oral lichen planus is uncertain.
- It can clear up within a few months or persist (with or without treatment).
- There are often periods of remission and relapse.
- About 1–4% of patients with oral lichen planus develop oral squamous cell carcinoma over 10 years, usually in the buccal mucosa or tongue.

7.2.2   Oral lichenoid reaction

An oral lichenoid reaction is a reactive lichen planus-like chronic inflammatory lesion of the oral mucosa usually induced by dental restorative materials (when it is localized) or drugs (when it may be more diffuse).

The prevalence of oral lichenoid reaction is 2–4% in the general adult population, and it is slightly more common in females than males.

Causes

An oral lichenoid reaction occurs as a response to:
- a dental material such as mercury and amalgam, epoxy resin, or composite restoration
- an NSAID, antihypertensive, antidiabetic, antimalarial, antibiotic, tricyclic antidepressant, or another medication
- a bone marrow transplant (graft-versus-host disease).

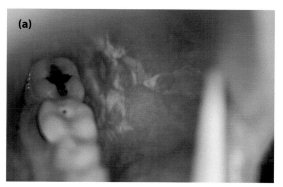

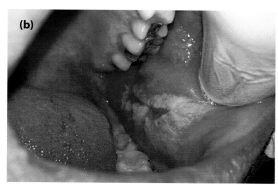

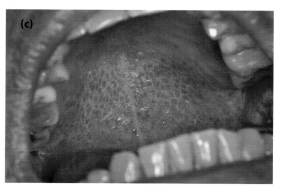

Figure 7.4 (a–c). (a and b) Localized lichenoid reaction due to hypersensitivity to amalgam; (c) diffuse drug-induced (nivolumab) lichenoid reaction on the palate.

(a) Reproduced from Health NZ – Waikato (www.waikatodhb.health.nz) with permission; (b) reproduced with permission from Professor Yeshwant Rawal, University of Milwaukee School of Dentistry, Milwaukee, WI, USA; (c) reproduced with permission from Professor Nagamani Narayana, University of Nebraska Medical Centre, NE, USA.

Clinical features

An oral lichenoid reaction (see *Fig. 7.4*) most often resembles oral lichen planus with white reticular and annular patterns. Erosions may also occur.
- White oral lichenoid papules and plaques are usually asymptomatic and unilateral.
- A reaction to a dental restoration occurs contiguously to the repair.
- Common sites are buccal mucosa and the lateral surface of the tongue and lips.

Diagnosis

An oral lichenoid reaction is suspected when clinical examination suggests oral lichen planus in a patient with a history of recent dental restoration, a new medication (see *Section 4.6*), or a bone marrow transplant.
- Skin patch testing is helpful if a dental material is suspected as the cause.
- Take a biopsy if there is any suspicion of epithelial dysplasia or carcinoma.
- Immunofluorescence may reveal linear fibrinogen at the basement membrane zone.

Treatment

Where known, remove the cause of the reaction.
- Remove and replace any dental restorative material if suspected to be responsible.
- Withdraw and replace drugs in consultation with the treating medical practitioner.
- Topical and systemic corticosteroids can be prescribed (see *Section 7.2.1* on oral lichen planus).

The prognosis is good if the cause of an oral lichenoid reaction is found and eliminated. Oral lichenoid lesions have a reported malignant transformation rate of 0.5–2%.

7.2.3   Desquamative gingivitis

Desquamative gingivitis is more common in females than in males. The most common cause of desquamative gingivitis is lichen planus. Desquamative gingivitis may also be a feature of:
- graft-versus-host disease
- lupus erythematosus
- immunobullous diseases, such as epidermolysis bullosa acquisita, mucous membrane pemphigoid, bullous pemphigoid, pemphigus vulgaris, paraneoplastic pemphigus, and linear IgA disease.

Desquamative gingivitis is rarely associated with contact allergy to oral hygiene products and other allergens.

Erythema multiforme, herpetic gingivostomatitis, and angina bullosa haemorrhagica do not cause desquamative gingivitis.

Clinical features

Desquamative gingivitis presents with vesicles, atrophy, erosion, desquamation, and diffuse erythema of the marginal and keratinized mucosa.
* Desquamation affects the anterior buccal and labial surfaces of the keratinized gingiva (see *Fig. 7.5*).
* Symptomatic patients complain of mucosal sloughing, mild–moderate gingival discomfort, soreness, bleeding, or a burning sensation especially when consuming acidic or spicy foods or beverages.

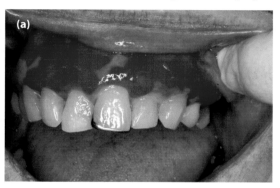
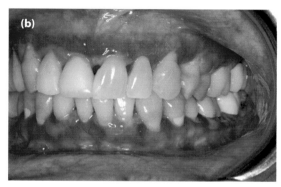
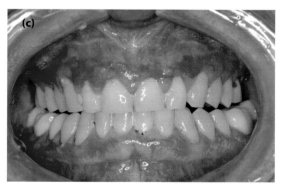

Figure 7.5 (a–c). Desquamative gingivitis due to lichen planus.

(a) Reproduced with permission from Professor Nagamani Narayana, University of Nebraska Medical Centre, NE, USA; (b) reproduced with permission from Professor Yeshwant Rawal, University of Milwaukee School of Dentistry, Milwaukee, WI, USA; (c) reproduced from Health NZ – Waikato (www. waikatodhb.health.nz) with permission.

Diagnosis

The diagnosis of desquamative gingivitis depends on a detailed medical history, clinical examination, perilesional biopsy for histopathological examination, and direct and indirect immunofluorescence tests.

Treatment

The treatment of desquamative gingivitis depends on the underlying disease.
* Local treatment of the gingivae includes oral hygiene measures and topical corticosteroids.
* Most patients also require oral corticosteroids and an immune-modulating agent such as methotrexate, azathioprine, ciclosporin, mycophenolate mofetil, dapsone, or rituximab.

7.2.4   Graft-versus-host disease

Graft-versus-host disease (GvHD) occurs after bone marrow or peripheral blood haematopoietic stem cell transplant and occasionally after solid organ transplantation. GvHD may also arise following blood transfusion, particularly if the donated blood products have not been irradiated or appropriately treated with an approved pathogen reduction system.

Indications for haematopoietic stem cell transplant include haematological and lymphoid malignancies, myelodysplastic syndrome, and non-malignant disorders such as bone marrow aplasia, severe immunodeficiency, and paroxysmal nocturnal haemoglobinuria.

The classification of GvHD was initially based on the time of onset following transplant, with acute GvHD occurring within 100 days of haematopoietic stem cell transplant and chronic GvHD occurring after 100 days. More recently, clinical and pathological features have defined consensus criteria for acute and chronic GvHD.

Causes

Three conditions are necessary for the development of GvHD:
1. Immunocompetent cells in the graft.
2. Failure of the host cells to reject the graft (immune compromise).
3. The infused cells' determination that the host is foreign (antigenic mismatch).

Immune cells in the donated tissue (the graft) recognize the recipient (the host) as foreign, mounting an immune response to reject the host's cells.

Clinical features

Acute GvHD occurs within 100 days of allogeneic haematopoietic stem cell transplantation.
- It presents with signs in the skin (erythema, maculopapular rash), liver (hepatitis, jaundice) and gastrointestinal tract (nausea, vomiting, abdominal pain, diarrhoea, anorexia).
- Oral signs in acute GvHD are uncommon and non-specific, and may include erythema with or without ulceration of the oral mucosa or lips.

Chronic oral GvHD occurs in 45–83% of patients after a haematopoietic stem cell transplant.
- Chronic oral GvHD presents as a lichenoid reaction (see *Fig. 7.6*) with mucosal atrophy, ulceration, salivary gland dysfunction, and mucocele. These features mimic oral lichen planus, Sjögren syndrome, and systemic sclerosis.
- GvHD may affect any oral mucosal site, most commonly the buccal mucosa and tongue.
- The disease is painful and may limit the intake of acidic beverages and spicy food.
- Signs include white striations and plaques, erythema, atrophy, and ulceration.
- Persistently dry mouth contributes to rampant dental caries and periodontal disease.
- Chronic inflammation of the buccal mucosa may lead to fibrosis and trismus.

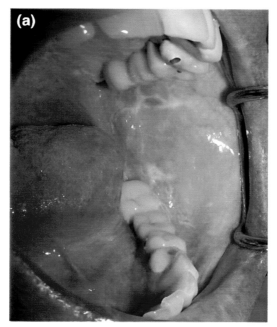
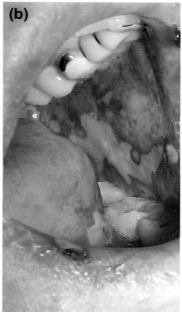

Figure 7.6 (a and b). Chronic graft-versus-host disease in the oral mucosa: (a) lichenoid lesions appear as white striations; (b) erythema, ulceration as well as subtle white striations.

Reproduced from *Int. Dental J.* 2021;71:9 (doi: 10.1111/idj.12584) with permission from Elsevier.

Diagnosis

A definitive diagnosis of GvHD requires biopsy and histopathological examination. Prolonged GvHD may lead to carcinoma *in situ* or invasive squamous cell carcinoma, especially in patients of advanced age at the time of transplant.

Treatment

Treating chronic oral GvHD is aimed at healing ulcers, minimizing mucosal pain, sensitivity, and dental sequelae, alleviating oral dryness, and improving function.

- A dry mouth can be managed with artificial saliva products, sugarless gum, and frequent sips of water. Cholinergic agonists such as pilocarpine or cevimeline hydrochloride can increase resting salivary flow rates.
- Local options for chronic oral GvHD include topical and intralesional corticosteroids, ciclosporin mouthwash, and tacrolimus ointment. In some cases, psoralens and UVA (PUVA) have also been used to treat chronic oral GvHD.
- Systemic immunosuppression for extensive multiorgan chronic GvHD may include ciclosporin, prednisone, thalidomide, and mycophenolate mofetil.
- Systemic immunosuppression may lead to opportunistic infections such as oral candidosis and herpetic infections.

7.2.5   Lupus erythematosus

Lupus erythematosus (LE) is a group of autoimmune connective tissue disorders with genetic, hormonal, and environmental influences.

Cutaneous LE is classified as acute, subacute, and chronic. Oral lesions are uncommon.
- In western countries, the estimated incidence of cutaneous LE varies between 1 and 25 per 100 000.
- Females are predominantly affected.
- The peak age at onset is 15–55 years.
- Flares may be triggered by sun exposure, stress, viral infection, or certain drugs.

Clinical features

Acute and chronic LE can affect the oral mucosa.
- Acute or systemic LE presents with fatigue, malar rash, fever, joint pain or swelling, and sun sensitivity.
- Oral lichen planus-like lesions or ulcers occur in 20% of patients.

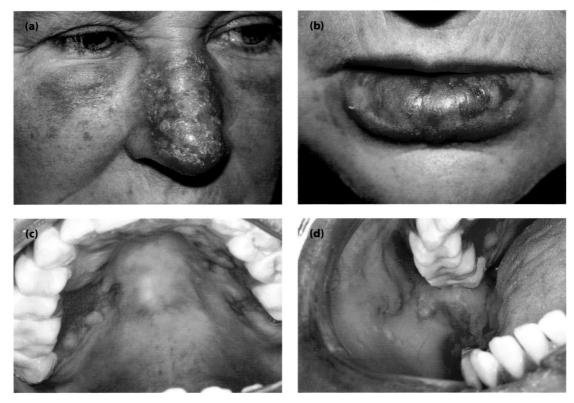

Figure 7.7 (a–d). Discoid lupus erythematosus with red, white, and eroded areas: (a) skin of the face, (b) lower lip, (c) palate, and (d) buccal mucosa.

(a and b) Reproduced from Health NZ – Waikato (www.waikatodhb.health.nz) with permission; (c and d) reproduced with permission from Professor Yeshwant Rawal, University of Milwaukee School of Dentistry, Milwaukee, WI, USA.

- Erosions and ulcers are common.
- In contrast to oral lichen planus, the palate is the most common site for oral LE.
- Chronic cutaneous LE usually presents as discoid LE. This can affect the lips and oral mucosa with unilateral, lichen planus-like reticular lesions, papules, or plaques (see *Fig. 7.7*).

Diagnosis

Oral LE should be considered if lichen planus-like oral lesions arise in a patient with a history of LE.
- Biopsy a white plaque or the edge of an ulcer to confirm LE, especially if epithelial dysplasia or carcinoma is considered.
- The histopathology features of oral LE are similar to lichen planus.
- Immunofluorescence may be positive in a new lesion (the lupus band test) but is negative in lichen planus.
- Check serology for autoantibodies such as an antinuclear antibody (ANA).
- Raised erythrocyte sedimentation rate (ESR) and C-reactive protein are supportive.

Treatment

Management of oral LE is often multidisciplinary. Treatment may include:
- withdrawal of any likely causative drug
- a topical corticosteroid (see the treatment of oral lichen planus, *Section 7.2.1*)
- an intralesional corticosteroid injection to a focal area of the disease
- an antimalarial drug (usually hydroxychloroquine).

Systemic prednisone or prednisolone and immunosuppressant drugs are helpful.

The prognosis of LE is variable. Oral LE has a very low malignant potential.

7.2.6   Chronic ulcerative stomatitis

Chronic ulcerative stomatitis is a rare erosive oral disease usually diagnosed in Caucasian females (>90% of cases), typically in their sixth and seventh decades.

The presentation is similar to oral lichen planus, but chronic ulcerative stomatitis has a distinct direct immunofluorescent pattern on histology and responds poorly to corticosteroids.

Causes

Chronic ulcerative stomatitis is classified as an autoimmune disease. Autoantibodies target the DeltaNp63alpha (ΔNp63α) antigen of a 70kD protein member of the p53 tumour suppressor gene family, which plays a role in epithelial differentiation and stratification.

Clinical features

Chronic ulcerative stomatitis presents with painful erythema and non-specific erosions in buccal and lingual mucosae.
- Like oral lichen planus, reticular striae, white papules and plaques may arise around the periphery of the ulcer.

- Desquamative gingivitis occurs in up to 50% of cases.
- 20% of patients demonstrate cutaneous lesions that resemble cutaneous lichen planus.
- Other mucous membranes, hair, and nails may be involved.

Diagnosis
- Histology shows a lichenoid inflammatory reaction with lymphocytes and plasma cells.
- Direct immunofluorescence (DIF) on perilesional tissue demonstrates a speckled IgG deposition in the keratinocyte nuclei of the basal and parabasal third of the epithelial compartment.
- The classic feature is the finding of stratified epithelium-specific antinuclear antibodies (SES-ANA) on direct and indirect immunofluorescence testing.

Treatment
Chronic ulcerative stomatitis is refractory to topical and oral steroids but is reported to respond to hydroxychloroquine.

7.3   Granulomatous disorders

7.3.1   Granulomatous gingivitis
Granulomatous gingivitis is a group of inflammatory diseases characterized by granulomas on histopathology.

Causes
Granulomatous diseases causing granulomatous gingivitis include:
- orofacial granulomatosis
- Crohn disease
- sarcoidosis
- granulomatosis with polyangiitis.

A foreign body may also induce a granulomatous reaction.

Clinical features
Granulomatous gingivitis is solitary or multiple areas of hyperplastic and erythematous inflammation involving the free and attached gingiva.
- Granulomatous gingivitis results in mild pain and discomfort.
- It is unresponsive to conventional oral hygiene treatments.
- Other clinical features may be present depending on the cause.

The diagnosis is made by finding non-caseating granulomas on histopathological examination of the affected gingiva.

Treatment
Any underlying disorder should be identified and treated.
- Gingival lesions are treated using local or systemic corticosteroids.
- Surgical intervention may be required in some cases.

7.3.2   Orofacial granulomatosis

Orofacial granulomatosis is a group of diseases characterized by non-infectious, non-caseating granulomatous inflammation in the soft tissues of the oral and maxillofacial region. Orofacial granulomatosis most often affects teenagers and young adults but can present at any age.

Causes

Orofacial granulomatosis is a delayed hypersensitivity reaction. The exact antigen inducing the response appears to vary in individual patients, and there may be a genetic predisposition.

Orofacial granulomatosis may be the oral manifestation of a systemic condition such as:
- inflammatory bowel disease (15% of patients with Crohn disease have oral signs)
- sarcoidosis
- granulomatosis with polyangiitis
- Melkersson–Rosenthal syndrome.

Some patients with orofacial granulomatosis may be hypersensitive to certain foods, additives, or flavourings.

Clinical features

Orofacial granulomatosis presents with firm, occasionally tender swelling of the lips (granulomatous cheilitis) (see *Fig. 7.8*) and oral mucosa.

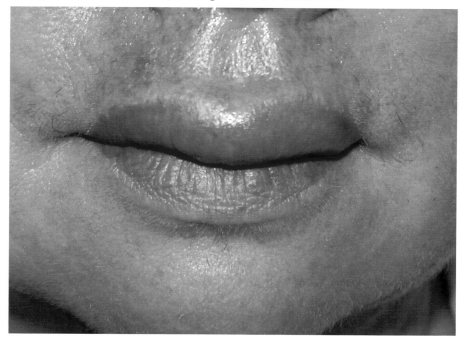

Figure 7.8. Granulomatous cheilitis affecting the upper vermilion lip.

Reproduced from Health NZ – Waikato (www.waikatodhb.health.nz) with permission.

- Melkersson–Rosenthal syndrome describes granulomatous cheilitis in combination with facial nerve palsy and a plicated (fissured) tongue.
- Signs include erythema, oedema, cobblestoning, and hyperplastic folding of the gingivae, buccal and palatal mucosae, and tongue.

Non-specific features may include:
- angular cheilitis (see *Fig. 7.9*)
- linear ulceration on the gingival and buccal sulcus
- prominent vertical fissures.

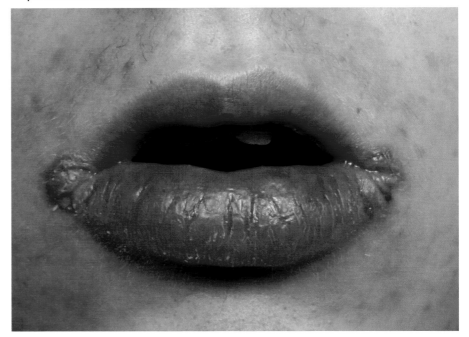

Figure 7.9. Granulomatous cheilitis affecting the lower vermilion lip and angular cheilitis in a patient with Crohn disease.

Reproduced from Health NZ – Waikato (www.waikatodhb.health.nz) with permission.

Investigations may include:
- histopathology of an oral biopsy showing non-caseating granulomatous inflammation with or without multinucleated giant cells
- identification and elimination of an inciting agent, if any
- serology for gastrointestinal malabsorption, and anti-saccharomyces cerevisiae antibodies (ASCA).

Treatment

Treatment options may include:
- intermittent clobetasol propionate ointment
- intralesional injections of triamcinolone
- systemic corticosteroids
- tetracycline (e.g. minocycline) (or a macrolide in children under 12).

Other therapies include dapsone, hydroxychloroquine, azathioprine, clofazimine, thalidomide, and TNF-α inhibitors, particularly infliximab.

7.3.3 Sarcoidosis

Sarcoidosis is a multiorgan granulomatous disease with a variable course. It mostly affects the lungs, lymph nodes, and skin. Sarcoidosis commonly affects patients under 50 years, with a female preponderance. It is more prevalent in those with African ancestry and other races with darker skin compared with white-skinned Europeans.

Causes

The cause of sarcoidosis is unknown. It is thought to develop in genetically susceptible individuals triggered by an environmental factor such as an infection.

Clinical features

Oral sarcoidosis is usually limited to lymphoid tissues and salivary glands.
- Salivary gland disease presents as persistent, painless enlargement.
- The parotid glands are most frequently involved.
- An oral submucosal mass may be noted.

Diagnosis

The diagnosis of sarcoidosis is non-specific, excludes other disorders, and is supported by finding the following features:
- Granulomatous inflammation on histopathology with Langhans giant cells (nuclei arranged peripherally), Schaumann bodies (lamellated calcifications), and asteroid bodies (stellate acidophilic inclusion bodies)
- Elevated serum angiotensin-converting enzyme levels
- Hilar lymphadenopathy on chest X-ray.

Treatment

Sarcoidosis can be difficult to treat. Organ dysfunction or extensive disease is treated with high-dose corticosteroids and immunosuppression.

7.4 Immunobullous diseases

7.4.1 Epidermolysis bullosa acquisita

Epidermolysis bullosa acquisita (EBA) is a rare chronic mucocutaneous autoimmune blistering disease.
- EBA usually presents in middle age.
- The incidence is 0.2 new cases per million population per year.
- There is no gender or racial predilection.

Clinical features

EBA has several distinct subtypes – the classical mechanobullous form, the non-classical/non-mechanobullous form, and a mucous membrane form.

- Blistering may be confined to trauma-prone sites such as elbows, knees, hands, and feet, or the disease may result in widespread pruritic, erythematous plaques.
- Oral vesicles or bullae on any mucosal site quickly rupture, forming irregular, painful ulcers and desquamative gingivitis.
- A positive Nikolsky sign may be observed.
- Oral lesions may heal with scarring, leading to microstomia.
- The disease may affect conjunctiva and nasopharyngeal, oesophageal, gastrointestinal, and anogenital mucosa.

Causes

EBA is an autoimmune bullous disease with autoantibodies directed against structural proteins of the basement membrane zone.

- It is caused by the pathogenic binding of autoantibody to the target antigen, type VII collagen (COL7), which anchors the epithelial cells and basement membrane to the underlying connective tissue.
- The functional absence of COL7 leads to the separation of the mucosa and the formation of subepithelial bullae.

Diagnosis

Diagnosis of EBA depends on history, clinical findings, histology, DIF, and serological investigations.

- Histologically, there is a subepithelial separation of the epithelium and underlying connective tissue.
- DIF demonstrates a dermal binding pattern of IgG, or less often IgA, with a U-serrated pattern.
- IgG localizes to the blister floor (the dermal side of split skin) in EBA.
- Serology (IIF) is positive in 50% of cases.
- Enzyme-linked immunosorbent assay (ELISA) to detect antibodies against type VII collagen is definitive when positive.

Treatment

Patients with EBA should minimize direct trauma to the skin and mucous membranes.

- Topical corticosteroid preparations such as dexamethasone mouth rinse may be sufficient to control mild oral disease, although more commonly, these are adjuncts to systemic therapy.
- Most patients require systemic medication, including corticosteroids, dapsone, azathioprine, and mycophenolate mofetil.
- Rituximab (anti-CD20) is reported to be effective for EBA.

Prognosis

EBA disease activity often fluctuates between partial remission and flares.

- Complications include infection of open wounds, scarring leading to dysfunction and restricted movement, conjunctival scarring resulting in impaired vision, and periodontal disease.
- Medication side-effects may add to morbidity.

7.4.2   Pemphigoid

Pemphigoid is a group of autoimmune subepithelial blistering conditions affecting the skin and mucous membranes. Autoantibodies are directed at various basement membrane components, with binding causing tissue separation and blister formation.

Mucous membrane pemphigoid

Mucous membrane pemphigoid is a rare, predominantly mucosal subepidermal blistering disorder. It is also called cicatricial pemphigoid and benign mucosal pemphigoid (but it is not very benign!)

- The incidence of mucous membrane pemphigoid is approximately 1.3–2 per million.
- It has a female predilection with a peak onset between 60 and 80 years.

Clinical features

Mucous membrane pemphigoid has a variable clinical presentation and disease severity with blistering in one or multiple sites.

- It usually starts in the mouth with the gradual appearance of clear vesicles or bullae that quickly form painful ulcers (see *Figs 7.10 a* and *b*). Desquamative gingivitis (see *Figs 7.10 c* and *d*) may cause bleeding and periodontitis.
- Mucous membrane pemphigoid may also affect ocular, nasal, nasopharyngeal, anogenital, laryngeal, and oesophageal mucosa.
- A positive Nikolsky sign is commonly observed.
- Up to 20% of patients have cutaneous blisters and ulcers.
- Skin and mucosal lesions may heal with scarring, although scarring is uncommon in the mouth.

Causes

Mucous membrane pemphigoid is an autoimmune bullous disease with autoantibodies directed against structural proteins in the basement membrane zone.

Identified target antigens include:
- bullous pemphigoid antigen 1 (BP230)
- bullous pemphigoid antigen 2 (BP180) / type XVII collagen
- laminin 332 (laminin 5) – associated with internal malignancy (controversial evidence)
- laminin 311 (laminin 6)
- integrin α6 and β4 subunits.

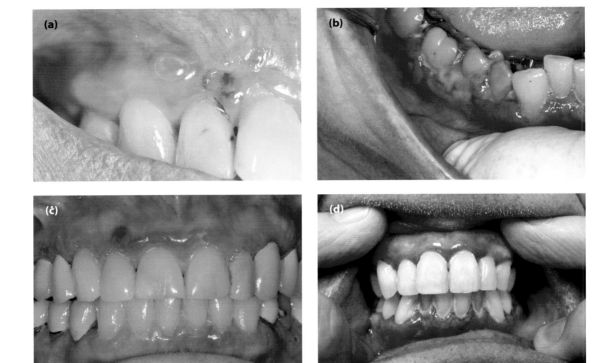

Figure 7.10 (a–d). Oral mucous membrane pemphigoid causing (a) blisters and (b) ulceration; (c) mild and (d) severe desquamative gingivitis.

(a and b) Reproduced with permission from Professor Nagamani Narayana, University of Nebraska Medical Centre, NE, USA; (c) reproduced with permission from Professor Yeshwant Rawal, University of Milwaukee School of Dentistry, Milwaukee. WI, USA; (d) reproduced from Health NZ – Waikato (www. waikatodhb.health.nz) with permission.

Diagnosis

A diagnosis of mucous membrane pemphigoid is made by history, clinical findings, histology, DIF, and serological investigations.

- Histopathological features of mucous membrane pemphigoid include subepithelial separation at the basement membrane zone, with minimal chronic inflammatory infiltrate in the lamina propria.
- DIF on fresh perilesional tissue demonstrates linear deposition of immunoreactants along the basement membrane zone (most commonly IgG, C3, or IgA).
- IgG localizes to the blister floor (the dermal side of split skin) in mucous membrane pemphigoid.
- Indirect immunofluorescence (IIF) or ELISA is usually negative but may reveal autoantibodies in the serum.

Treatment

Care of mucous membrane pemphigoid is often multidisciplinary, depending on the affected sites.

- Treatment is usually a combination of topical and systemic immunosuppressants.
- A topical corticosteroid, such as dexamethasone mouth rinse, may be sufficient to control mild oral disease.
- Most patients require oral medication, including doxycycline, dapsone, methotrexate, corticosteroids, azathioprine, mycophenolate mofetil, and cyclophosphamide.
- Rituximab (anti-CD20) has also been used effectively.

Prognosis

The prognosis of mucous membrane pemphigoid depends on the extent of disease activity, and it rarely goes into spontaneous remission. Conjunctival fibrosis (symblepharon) may lead to blindness in severe cases.

Bullous pemphigoid

Bullous pemphigoid is the most common subepidermal immunobullous disease.
- The reported incidence of bullous pemphigoid is 2.4–21.7 new cases per million population/year. This may be underestimated due to a recent association with vildagliptin, commonly used in type 2 diabetes mellitus.
- It affects males and females equally.
- Most patients with bullous pemphigoid are >70 years of age, but it may present at any age, including childhood.

Clinical features

The typical presentation of bullous pemphigoid is an older patient with an itchy rash and bullae. It can be localized or generalized.
- Patients often present with itchy, urticated erythematous plaques on the limbs, flexures, and trunk several weeks before tense fluid-filled bullae and erosions appear.
- 10–20% of patients develop blisters and erosions on any oral mucosa site, commonly the buccal mucosa (see *Fig. 7.11*), palate, and tongue. These tend to be mild and heal without scarring.

Causes

Bullous pemphigoid is an autoimmune bullous disease. The autoantibodies most often target the basement membrane proteins BP230 and BP180 and, less often, integrin α6 and laminin 332.

Diagnosis

The diagnosis of bullous pemphigoid is based on history, clinical findings, histology, DIF, and serological investigations.
- Histopathological features of bullous pemphigoid include subepithelial separation at the basement membrane zone, commonly filled with eosinophils. Urticarial and eczematous features may be present.
- DIF demonstrates the deposition of IgG antibodies and C3 in a linear band at the dermal–epidermal junction.

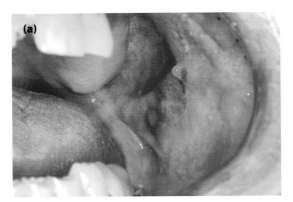

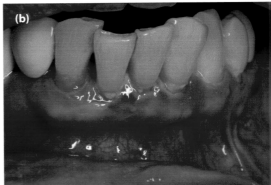

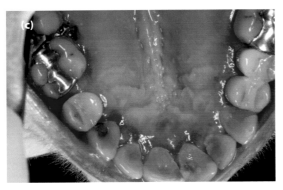

Figure 7.11 (a–c). Bullous pemphigoid on (a) the buccal mucosa and (b and c) the gingiva.

(a) Reproduced from Health NZ – Waikato (www.waikatodhb. health.nz) with permission; (b and c) reproduced with permission from Professor Nagamani Narayana, University of Nebraska Medical Centre, NE, USA.

- DIF on salt-split skin reveals IgG on the blister roof (the epidermal side of split skin) in bullous pemphigoid.
- IIF or ELISA may reveal a semi-quantitative assessment of pemphigoid autoantibodies in serum.

Treatment

Topical corticosteroid therapy and emollients may be sufficient for mild or localized bullous pemphigoid.
- Doxycycline plus nicotinamide may be effective.
- Treatment of more severe bullous pemphigoid requires oral corticosteroids, methotrexate, dapsone, mycophenolate mofetil, or azathioprine.
- Refractory bullous pemphigoid may be treated with rituximab or intravenous immunoglobulin.

Prognosis

Most patients affected with bullous pemphigoid achieve remission and should be maintained on treatment for 6 months to 5 years, after which many patients can stop treatment. Mortality associated with bullous pemphigoid is partly due to the medications used in treatment.

Pemphigoid gestationis

Pemphigoid gestationis is bullous pemphigoid arising in pregnancy. It has similar features to common bullous pemphigoid and may cause oral blisters and ulceration.

Linear IgA bullous dermatosis

Linear IgA bullous dermatosis, known in children as chronic bullous disorder of childhood, is a rare distinct subepidermal blistering disease in which characteristic annular plaques occur, studded with bullae (a string of beads). It may cause oral blisters and ulceration (see *Fig. 7.12*). IgA antibodies are found on direct immunofluorescence of a skin biopsy. Linear IgA bullous dermatosis often responds to dapsone.

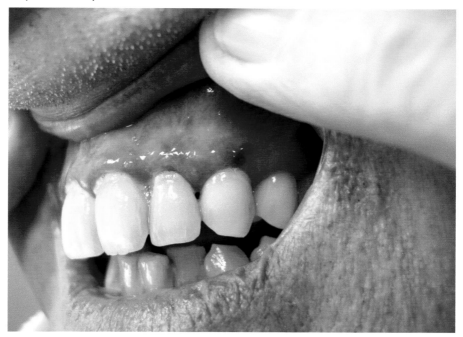

Figure 7.12. Blood-filled vesicle on the gingival margin due to linear IgA disease.

Reproduced from Health NZ – Waikato (www.waikatodhb.health.nz) with permission.

7.4.3 Pemphigus

Pemphigus is a group of rare chronic autoimmune blistering diseases affecting mucosal or cutaneous sites. Lesions result from autoantibodies binding to specific desmosomal proteins on the surface of the keratinocytes, resulting in loss of cell–cell adhesion (acantholysis).

Pemphigus vulgaris

Pemphigus vulgaris is the most common and clinically aggressive pemphigus variant.

- The incidence of pemphigus vulgaris varies from 0.1–0.5 patients per 100 000 per year.
- Pemphigus vulgaris is more common in the Ashkenazi Jew, Mediterranean and South Asian populations, associated with specific HLA subtypes.
- The mean age of onset is 50–60 years of age.

Causes

Pemphigus vulgaris is an autoimmune bullous disease.
- It is due to autoantibodies directed against intraepithelial adhesion proteins, the desmosomal cadherins (typically desmoglein-3 (DSG-3) and, in 50% of cases, DSG-1).
- DSG-3 is found primarily in the suprabasal layer of the epithelium.
- This antigen–antibody interaction activates complement, releasing inflammatory mediators and recruiting activated T cells.

Clinical features

A patient with pemphigus vulgaris complains of painful mouth ulcers and may also have flaccid blisters and erosions on their skin.
- Oral lesions affect up to 70% of cases and are usually the first sign of pemphigus vulgaris.
- Vesicles and bullae on the buccal and palatal mucosa rupture quickly to form tender, irregular mucosal erosions (see *Fig. 7.13*), ulcers, and desquamative gingivitis. A positive Nikolsky sign is often noted.

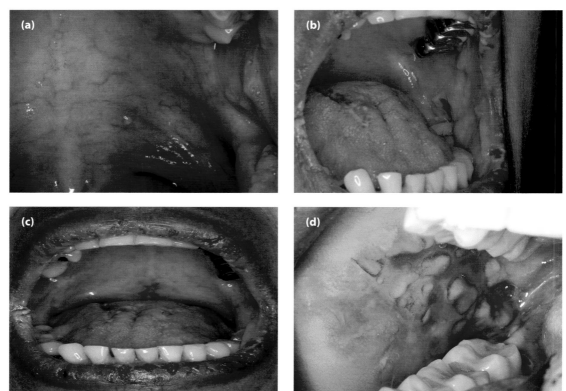

Figure 7.13 (a–d). Pemphigus vulgaris: (a) intact vesicle on the palate; (b) chronic erosion of the lip, (c) lip, tongue, and palate, and (d) buccal mucosa.

(a–c) Reproduced from Health NZ – Waikato (www.waikatodhb.health.nz) with permission; (d) reproduced with permission from Professor Yeshwant Rawal, University of Milwaukee School of Dentistry, Milwaukee, WI, USA.

- Pemphigus vulgaris may also affect the oropharynx, larynx, conjunctiva, oesophagus, and genitalia.
- Painful blisters, flaccid pustules, and erosions may affect any part of the skin surface, especially the scalp and trunk.

Diagnosis

Pemphigus vulgaris may be suspected clinically, but a biopsy of perilesional tissue is essential to confirm the diagnosis.

- Histopathological features are intraepithelial vesicles with intercellular oedema and acantholysis, clefting (separation of suprabasal keratinocytes from the basal cells), and a tombstone appearance of the remaining keratinocytes at the base of the blister.
- DIF performed on fresh tissue shows basket-weave staining of IgG, reflecting its deposition on the surface of the keratinocytes (see *Fig. 7.14*). IgM and complement components such as C3 are also often present.
- IIF is positive in 80–90% of patients with pemphigus vulgaris.
- ELISA using human recombinant DSG-1 and DSG-3 proteins also detects circulating autoantibodies.

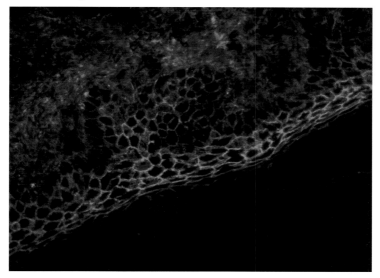

Figure 7.14. Pemphigus vulgaris. Direct immunofluorescent test shows basket-weave staining of IgG, reflecting its deposition on the surface of the keratinocytes.

Reproduced from Health NZ – Waikato (www.waikatodhb.health.nz) with permission.

Treatment

Treating pemphigus vulgaris can be challenging; it can take months to remission.

- Treatment relies primarily on oral corticosteroids and steroid-sparing agents such as azathioprine or mycophenolate.
- Rituximab suppresses pemphigus vulgaris and reduces dependence on high-dose corticosteroids.

- Other therapies for recalcitrant pemphigus vulgaris include intravenous immunoglobulin, immunoadsorption, plasmapheresis, and cyclophosphamide.

Prognosis

The natural course and disease severity of pemphigus vulgaris are variable.
- The mortality rate of pemphigus vulgaris ranges from 5–15%.
- Complications of immunosuppressive therapy may contribute to mortality.
- Serum levels of autoantibodies fluctuate with disease activity and can be used for monitoring.

Paraneoplastic pemphigus

Paraneoplastic pemphigus is a life-threatening, usually fatal, blistering autoimmune disease associated with an underlying malignancy, most commonly of lymphoproliferative origin.
- Paraneoplastic pemphigus is rare. Only twelve cases were found in a report of 100 000 adverse events in patients with non-Hodgkin lymphoma and chronic lymphocytic leukaemia.
- It most commonly affects adults aged 45–70 but may also affect children, particularly when associated with Castleman disease.
- No differences in incidence have been reported according to sex, race, or ethnicity.

Causes

Paraneoplastic pemphigus is an autoimmune bullous disease.
- Blistering is due to the immune recognition of antigens expressed by tumours that cross-react with epithelial antigens.
- Paraneoplastic pemphigus autoantibodies are directed against desmosomal and hemidesmosomal antigens, particularly periplakins and envoplakins.
- The most frequently reported associated malignancies are B-cell lymphoma, chronic lymphocytic leukaemia, Castleman disease, Waldenström macroglobulinaemia, and thymoma (with or without myasthenia gravis).

Clinical features

Paraneoplastic pemphigus presents with florid, painful, chronic oral ulcers that are recalcitrant to therapy. There may be an unusual rash with widespread cutaneous blistering and ulceration. At least five clinical variants of oral paraneoplastic pemphigus have been reported:
- Pemphigus-like superficial vesicles, flaccid vesicles, erosions, crusts, and erythema
- Bullous pemphigoid-like scaly erythematous papules and irregular ulceration
- Erythema multiforme-like polymorphic, erythematous, peeling plaques with erosions and ulcers
- GvHD-like disseminated dusky red, scaly papules.
- Lichen planus-like flat scaly papules and ulceration.

Paraneoplastic pemphigus may also cause a generalized polymorphous cutaneous eruption, conjunctivitis, and gastrointestinal or pulmonary disease.

Diagnosis

The diagnosis of paraneoplastic pemphigus is based on clinical, histological, and immunofluorescent findings. Investigations should include:
- skin or mucosal biopsies for histopathology and DIF
- serology for pemphigus antibodies
- blood tests and imaging to identify any underlying malignancy.

Treatment

Treatment of paraneoplastic pemphigus is difficult.
- The best outcomes have been reported after surgical excision of benign neoplasms.
- The first-line treatment is high-dose corticosteroids with the addition of steroid-sparing agents.
- Treatment failures are often managed with rituximab with or without concomitant intravenous immunoglobulin.

Prognosis

In general, the prognosis of paraneoplastic pemphigus is poor due to the progression of the underlying malignancy or infectious complications of immunosuppressive treatment.

7.4.4   Dermatitis herpetiformis

Dermatitis herpetiformis is an immunobullous skin disease in which IgA antibodies are directed against gliadin in gluten.
- Although dermatitis herpetiformis is associated with gluten-sensitive enteropathy (coeliac disease, see below), it rarely affects the oral mucosa.
- Dermatitis herpetiformis is twice as common in males as in females.
- The prevalence is estimated at 11–30 per 100 000.

Causes

Genetic and immunological factors contribute to the pathogenesis of dermatitis herpetiformis.
- Patients have an increased frequency of HLA DQ2 and DQ8.
- Intestinal intolerance to gluten leads to the activation of CD4$^+$ T cells in intestinal mucosa resulting in the production of B lymphocytes (IgA).
- IgA1 antibodies are directed against peptides present in gluten and against autoantigens such as the intestinal enzyme transglutaminase (TGT), which deposit in the skin.
- These antibodies cross-react with epidermal transglutaminase (transglutaminase 3, TG3).

Clinical features

Oral lesions are rarely seen in dermatitis herpetiformis. However, they may precede more typical intensively pruritic vesicles and plaques on extensor surfaces of the skin, such as the elbows, knees, shoulders, and buttocks.

- Oral mucosal lesions are commonly located in areas of occlusal trauma, especially on the buccal mucosa in line with the occlusal plane.
- They may be erythematous, vesicular, purpuric, or erosive.

Diagnosis

Diagnosis of dermatitis herpetiformis relies on history, clinical findings, and biopsy.

- Histopathology shows neutrophils and eosinophils at the tips of connective tissue papillae forming microabscesses with vesicles or bullae at the basement membrane.
- DIF on perilesional tissue shows IgA deposition in a granular pattern along the basement membrane, with some biopsies also displaying IgG, IgM, C3, C1q and fibrinogen.
- Serology for IgA antibody to TTG3 has high specificity but lower sensitivity than in coeliac disease.

Treatment

Dermatitis herpetiformis is usually treated with dapsone. Patients should follow a strict gluten-free diet.

7.5   Other inflammatory diseases localized to the mouth

7.5.1   Geographic tongue

Geographic tongue, also known as benign migratory glossitis and oral erythema migrans, is an inflammatory disorder of the dorsal and dorso-lateral surfaces of the tongue.

Causes

The cause of geographic tongue is unknown.

Clinical features

Geographic tongue is characterized by smooth, red areas of varying sizes surrounded by irregular white borders (see *Fig. 7.15*).

- Geographic tongue can occur suddenly and persist for months or longer and recur. Infrequently, lesions may appear on other mucosal sites in the mouth, particularly the palate.
- Some patients complain of burning or tongue irritation, mainly when consuming hot, spicy food and acidic beverages. Most often, there are no symptoms.

Treatment

No treatment is required for geographic tongue.

- Avoiding hot, spicy food and acidic beverages can reduce discomfort and burning sensations.
- Topical anaesthetic agents or benzydamine hydrochloride mouth rinse may be used to relieve symptoms.

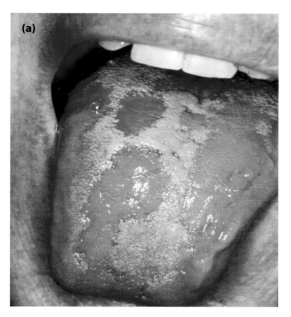
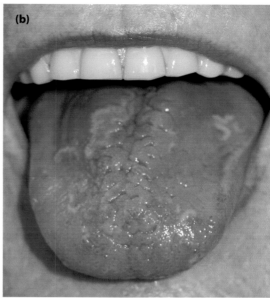

Figure 7.15 (a and b). Geographic tongue: smooth, red areas of varying sizes surrounded by irregular white borders.

Reproduced from Health NZ – Waikato (www.waikatodhb.health.nz) with permission.

7.5.2   Lingual papillitis

Eruptive or transient lingual papillitis (also known as lie bumps) describes a common acute stomatitis where there are one or multiple inflamed fungiform papillae on the dorsum of the tongue, particularly on its tip (see *Fig. 7.16*).

Causes

Transient lingual papillitis is thought to be a reaction to a viral infection, stress, trauma, or spicy or sugary foods.

Clinical features

Lingual papillitis commonly affects young children and may also arise in adults. The affected area stings, especially if consuming hot food or beverages, and the affected fungiform papillae are red and prominent. It usually resolves within 2 or 3 days.

Treatment

Treatment is usually unnecessary. People with recurrent lingual papillitis should undergo a dental check-up.
- Avoiding hot, spicy food and acidic beverages can reduce discomfort and burning sensations.
- Topical anaesthetic agents or benzydamine hydrochloride mouth rinse may be used to relieve symptoms.

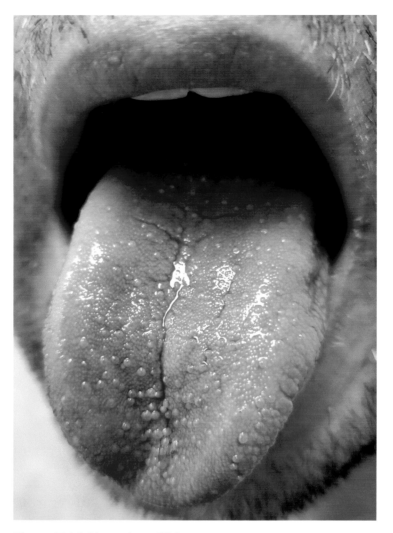

Figure 7.16. Lingual papillitis.

Reproduced from Health NZ – Waikato (www.waikatodhb.health.nz) with permission.

7.5.3   Glandular cheilitis

Glandular cheilitis, also called cheilitis glandularis, is an uncommon inflammatory disorder of the minor salivary glands of the lip.

- It is characterized by progressive enlargement and eversion of the lower labial mucosa.
- It results in the obliteration of the mucosal–vermilion interface.
- Glandular cheilitis most often occurs on the lower lip.
- It is more common in adult males than in females.

Causes

Glandular cheilitis is thought to be caused by actinic damage.

Clinical features

Glandular cheilitis presents as swelling and eversion of the lower lip (see *Fig. 7.17*).
- The orifices of the minor salivary gland ducts on the lower lip are dilated.
- Mucopurulent secretions can be expressed from the ductal openings.
- Occasional mucosal erosion, crusting, or ulceration may occur.
- In Caucasians, it is associated with squamous cell carcinoma of the lip.

Treatment

Glandular cheilitis can be treated by vermilionectomy (lip shave).

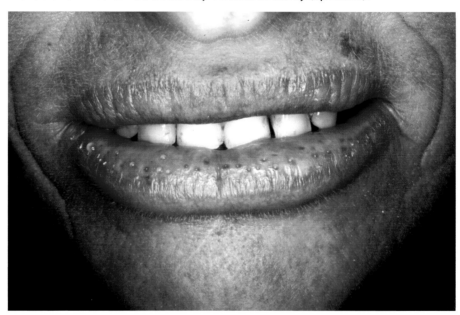

Figure 7.17. Glandular cheilitis.

Reproduced from Health NZ – Waikato (www.waikatodhb.health.nz) with permission.

7.5.4   Plasma cell gingivitis/cheilitis

Plasma cell gingivitis and plasma cell cheilitis are characterized by a dense chronic inflammatory infiltrate in the lamina propria, mostly non-neoplastic plasma cells. The average age of onset of plasma cell gingivitis/cheilitis has been reported as 45 years, and males have a higher prevalence.

Causes

The cause of plasma cell gingivitis and cheilitis is not fully understood.

In some cases, the disease may be due to a local contact reaction to an antigen such as cinnamaldehyde or cinnamon, used as flavouring agents in chewing gums, dentifrices, and toothpaste.

Clinical features

Plasma cell gingivitis/cheilitis presents as sharply demarcated erythematous and oedematous plaques, with or without erosions or ulcers (see *Fig. 7.18*).

- It affects the free and attached maxillary and mandibular gingiva or the vermilion of the lips.
- Rarely, plasma cell gingivitis may extend beyond the gingiva (plasma cell gingivostomatitis).
- Burning sensations and pain are often reported.

Treatment

Treatments reported effective for plasma cell gingivitis/cheilitis include corticosteroids, immunomodulators, antibiotics, plaque control, and mouthwashes.

If an allergen is detected by patch testing, it should be removed or avoided.

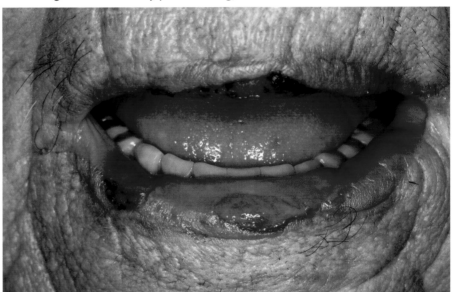

Figure 7.18. Plasma cell cheilitis.

Reproduced from Health NZ – Waikato (www.waikatodhb.health.nz) with permission.

CHAPTER 8

ORAL MUCOSAL NON-INFLAMMATORY DISORDERS AND CONDITIONS

See also:
- *Section 4.8.4: Postinflammatory pigmentation*
- *Section 5.2.10: Peutz–Jeghers syndrome; Section 5.3.3: Laugier–Hunziker syndrome; Section 5.2.8: McCune–Albright syndrome*

8.1 Endogenous pigmentation

8.1.1 Racial pigmentation

Racial pigmentation is also known as physiological pigmentation or melanoplakia. In the mouth, it usually occurs in non-white populations. It is often detected incidentally and is harmless.

- The most common site is a band-like brown–black pigmented zone at the junction of the attached gingiva and the alveolar mucosa (see *Fig. 1.2*).
- It may also affect the buccal mucosa, tongue, hard palate, and lips (see *Fig. 8.1*).

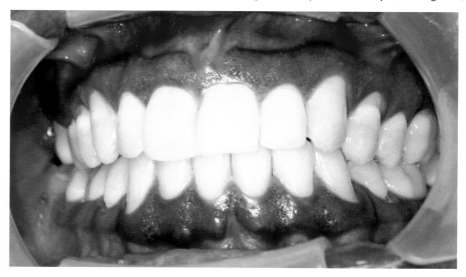

Figure 8.1. Physiological oral pigmentation on the gingiva presenting as bilateral, symmetrical, dark brown discolouration of the labial gingiva, including the marginal and papillary gingiva but not transgressing the mucogingival junction.

Reproduced from *Head Face Med.* 2014;10:8, under a CC BY 2.0 DEED licence.

8.1.2   Oral melanotic macule

Although melanotic macules are common on the vermilion of the lips, an intraoral melanotic macule is less common. Multiple melanotic macules are also known as melanosis.

- A melanotic macule is a brown or black well-circumscribed macule a few millimetres in diameter (see *Figs 8.2a* and *c*).
- Melanotic macules most often arise on the vermilion aspect of the lower lip or palate.
- Dermoscopy shows uniform curvilinear (see *Figs 8.2b* and *d*) or structureless pigmentation.
- Monitoring or biopsy is undertaken if the lesion is atypical, with asymmetry of structure and colours on dermoscopy/mucoscopy, or is changing.

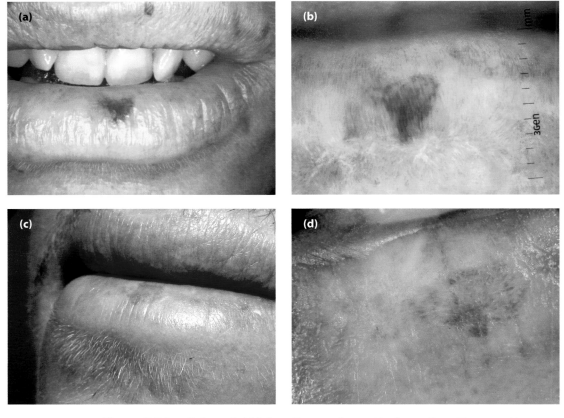

Figure 8.2 (a–d). (a and c) Melanotic macules on the lower lip with respective dermoscopy images (b and d). Dermoscopy of (b) shows curved thick parallel lines.

All images reproduced from Health NZ – Waikato (www.waikatodhb.health.nz) with permission.

8.1.3   Addison disease

Addison disease results from inadequate production of the steroid hormones cortisol and aldosterone by the adrenal cortex. Classic Addison disease causes primary adrenal insufficiency. It has an autoimmune cause in about 75% of cases.

Clinical features

The clinical manifestations of Addison disease are subtle.

- Oral hyperpigmented macules can be found diffusely on the tongue, gingiva (see *Fig. 8.3a*), buccal mucosa, and hard palate. The macules are blue–black or brown and can be spotty or streaked in configuration.
- Hyperpigmentation also affects the skin (see *Fig. 8.3b*), conjunctiva, and genital mucosa.
- Systemic features of Addison disease include fatigue, anorexia, orthostasis, nausea, muscle and joint pain, and salt craving.
- Addison disease is suspected after a thorough clinical evaluation, detailed patient history, and identification of characteristic findings.
- Primary adrenal insufficiency is diagnosed after confirming an elevated adrenocorticotrophic hormone (ACTH) level and an inability to stimulate cortisol levels with an ACTH (cosyntropin) stimulation test.

Treatment

Treatment of primary adrenal insufficiency requires the replacement of mineralocorticoids and glucocorticoids.

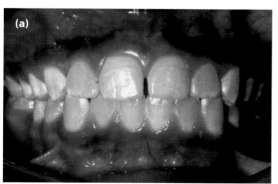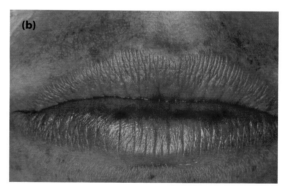

Figure 8.3 (a and b). Addison disease: (a) gingival pigmentation and (b) pigmentation of lower lip.

(a) Reproduced from *Color Atlas of Oral and Maxillofacial Diseases*, 2019; B.W. Neville, D.D. Damm, C.M. Allen & A.C. Chi, with permission from Elsevier; (b) reproduced from Health NZ – Waikato (www.waikatodhb.health.nz) with permission.

8.2 Cysts

8.2.1 Cysts of minor salivary glands

Pseudocysts arising from minor salivary gland ducts are common and are classified as extravasation cysts (90%) and mucus retention cysts. Local trauma from a tooth may contribute to their development.

- A mucocele (mucus retention cyst) describes a bluish, soft, fluctuant swelling (see *Figs 8.4a* and *b*) caused by occlusion or rupture of minor salivary gland duct.
- A ranula is a sublingual pseudocyst on the floor of the mouth (see *Fig. 8.4c*) due to obstruction to the salivary gland excretory duct and spillage of mucin.

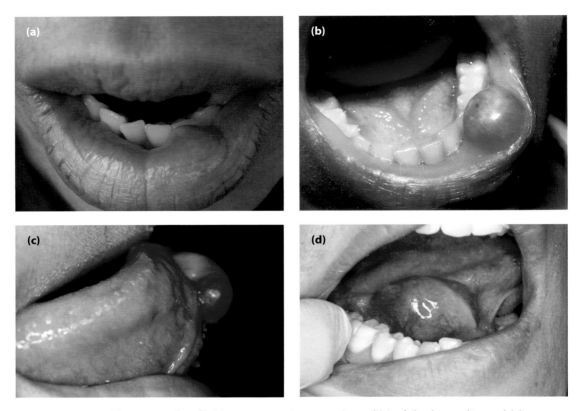

Figure 8.4 (a–d). Mucus retention cyst: (a and b) of the lower lip and (c) tongue (mucocele); (d) of the floor of the mouth (ranula).

(a and c) Reproduced from Health NZ – Waikato (www.waikatodhb.health.nz) with permission; (b) reproduced from *A Digital Manual for the Early Diagnosis of Oral Neoplasia*, International Agency for Research on Cancer, with permission; (d) Reproduced with permission from Professor Nagamani Narayana, University of Nebraska Medical Centre, NE, USA.

8.2.2   Gingival odontogenic cyst

Gingival cysts are rare.
- Gingival cysts of the newborn are small keratin-filled cysts on the alveolar mucosa crest.
- Gingival cysts in adults arise over the age of 40.

Causes

Gingival cysts are due to remnants of the dental lamina.

Clinical features

Gingival cysts of the newborn are solitary or multiple whitish nodules on the maxillary alveolus. They regress spontaneously within weeks.

The gingival cyst of the adult presents as a solitary well-circumscribed dome-shaped painless soft swelling up to 1cm in size in the mandibular canine or premolar region.

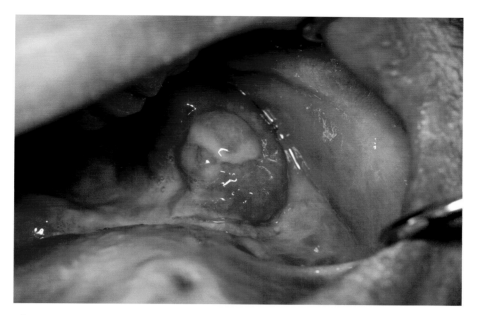

Figure 8.5. Dentinogenic ghost cell tumour with secondary aneurysmal bone cyst formation on histology.

Reproduced from Health NZ – Waikato (www.waikatodhb.health.nz) with permission.

A dentigerous cyst includes a tooth. A dentinogenic ghost cell tumour is a rare calcifying odontogenic cyst in which ameloblastoma-like epithelial islands, ghost cells, and dentinoid are found (see *Fig. 8.5*).

Treatment

Surgical removal is recommended for gingival cysts in an adult, and is curative.

8.2.3 Eruption cyst

A tooth eruption cyst is a soft-tissue cyst counterpart of a dentigerous cyst – both occur in the dental follicle surrounding an erupting deciduous or permanent tooth.

Clinical features

An eruption cyst is a soft, fluctuant, painless, blue or red swelling over an erupting tooth (see *Fig. 8.6*). The cyst usually ruptures spontaneously, exposing the erupting tooth.

Treatment

No treatment is required. Surgical or laser incision can be undertaken.

8.2.4 Dermoid and epidermoid cysts

Dermoid and epidermoid cysts are ectoderm-lined inclusion cysts representing fewer than 0.01% of all oral cavity cysts.

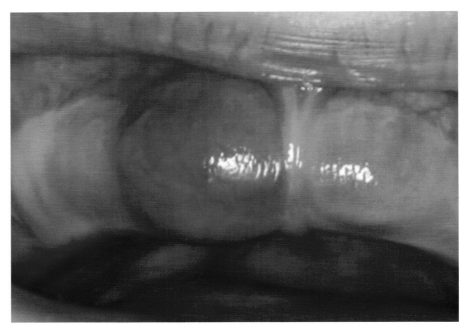

Figure 8.6. Eruption cyst.

Reproduced from *Color Atlas of Oral and Maxillofacial Diseases*, 2019; B.W. Neville, D.D. Damm, C.M. Allen & A.C. Chi, with permission from Elsevier.

- A dermoid cyst contains hair, sebaceous glands, sweat glands, and squamous epithelium.
- An epidermoid cyst has only squamous epithelium (mainly composed of keratin).
- Diagnosis may be made in infancy, childhood, or early adult life.

Causes

Dermoid and epidermoid cysts develop from the embryonic remnants of epithelium.

Clinical features

Dermoid and epidermoid cysts grow slowly and progressively on the floor of the mouth (see *Fig. 8.7*).
- Their size may vary from a few millimetres to 10cm in diameter.
- A cyst above the geniohyoid muscle displaces the tongue upwards, causing difficulty in mastication, speech, and swallowing.
- A cyst below the geniohyoid muscle may protrude in the submental region.

Treatment

Dermoid and epidermoid cysts are surgically removed.

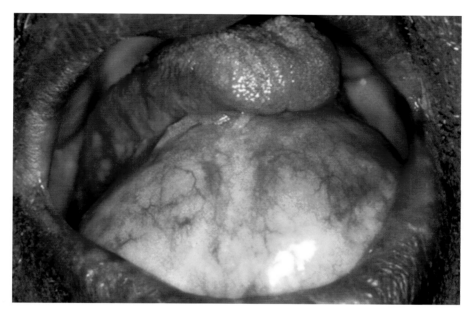

Figure 8.7. Epidermoid cyst presenting as a large swelling in the floor of the mouth, elevating the tongue.

Reproduced from *Color Atlas of Oral and Maxillofacial Diseases*, 2019; B.W. Neville, D.D. Damm, C.M. Allen & A.C. Chi, with permission from Elsevier.

8.2.5 **Lymphoepithelial cyst**

An oral lymphoepithelial cyst may rarely develop within oral lymphoid tissue. It usually occurs in young to middle-aged adults.

Causes

The origin of the cyst is ectopic foci of embryonic epithelium in lymphoid tissue.

Lymphoepithelial cysts have also been reported as a part of diffuse infiltrative lymphocytosis in patients infected with HIV.

Clinical features

A lymphoepithelial cyst is a submucosal mass usually <1.5cm in diameter.
- The most common sites are the floor of the mouth (70%), the lateral border of the tongue (10%), and the ventral surface of the tongue (7%).
- The cyst is white or yellow and asymptomatic.
- On histopathology, a lymphoepithelial cyst is characterized by a cyst covered by a parakeratinized stratified squamous epithelium, a capsule of dense fibrous connective tissue and keratinous content.

Treatment

The treatment of a lymphoepithelial cyst is conservative surgical removal.

8.2.6   Nasolabial cyst

A nasolabial cyst is a developmental non-odontogenic cyst in the soft tissues of the upper lip lateral to the midline.
- It is rare, representing <1% of jaw cysts and 2.5% of non-odontogenic cysts.
- The peak prevalence is in the fourth and fifth decades.
- It is more common in females.

Causes

The origin of a nasolabial cyst is a remnant of the embryonic nasolacrimal ridge or duct, or less likely, entrapped epithelium, along the fusion line of the medial nasal, lateral nasal, and maxillary processes.

Clinical features

A nasolabial cyst is slow-growing and usually <3cm in size.
- 10% are bilateral.
- A neonatal nasolabial cyst may resolve spontaneously during infancy.
- They are usually asymptomatic, rarely causing nasal obstruction or pain if infected.
- The cyst may cause distension of the nasolabial fold, elevation of the nasal ala extra-orally, and obliteration of the mucolabial fold intraorally.
- Diagnosis is based on clinical findings, CT scan, and histopathology.

Treatment

The treatment of a nasolabial cyst is surgical excision, performed intraorally.

8.2.7   Thyroglossal duct cyst

A thyroglossal duct cyst is in the midline of the neck, anywhere along the thyroid gland's route of migration between the tongue and the inferior neck. It is developmental, affecting 7% of the global population.

Causes

A thyroglossal duct cyst is due to the failure of the thyroglossal duct to close.

Clinical features

A thyroglossal duct cyst is an asymptomatic mobile midline neck mass, often near the hyoid bone.
- Rarely, it can present as an abscess or intermittently draining sinus.
- The mass will elevate with tongue protrusion or swallowing.
- Diagnosis is based on clinical examination and ultrasound imaging.
- Undertake thyroid function testing preoperatively if ectopic thyroid tissue is expected.

Treatment

Treatment for thyroglossal duct cysts is surgical removal. High recurrence rates (45–55%) have been reported. Fewer than 1% of thyroglossal duct cysts develop into carcinoma.

8.3   Oral mucinosis

Oral mucinosis is a rare benign degenerative disorder in which focal mucin deposition occurs in the skin or mucosa.
- A painless mass occurs within connective tissue.
- It most often affects the gingiva or palate.
- The surface colour of the mucosa is the same as the surrounding tissue.
- The diagnosis is usually made on histopathology.

CHAPTER 9

ORAL MUCOSAL MANIFESTATIONS OF SYSTEMIC DISEASES

See also:
- *Section 4.6: Adverse drug reaction*
- *Chapter 5: Oral mucosal diseases of developmental and genetic origin*
- *Chapter 6: Oral mucosal infections*
- *Section 7.1: Recurrent aphthous ulcer; Section 7.2.3: Desquamative gingivitis; Section 7.2.4: Graft-versus-host disease; Section 7.2.5: Lupus erythematosus; Section 7.3.3: Sarcoidosis*

9.1 Atrophic glossitis

Atrophic glossitis represents a partial or complete loss of filiform papillae and, to a lesser extent, fungiform papillae on the dorsal surface of the tongue. Atrophy usually accompanies inflammation of the tongue (glossitis).

Causes

Atrophic glossitis may be caused by nutritional deficiency or underlying systemic disease.
- Glossitis has been associated with deficiencies of riboflavin, niacin / nicotinic acid, pyridoxine (vitamin B6), biotin (vitamin B7), vitamin B12, folic acid, iron, zinc, and vitamin E.
- It has also been associated with protein-calorie malnutrition, candidosis, *Helicobacter pylori* colonization, xerostomia, and diabetes mellitus.

Clinical features

Atrophic glossitis presents with a smooth, glossy, red or pink tongue
(see *Fig. 9.1*). It may cause pain, burning sensation (glossodynia), numbness, or taste disturbance.

Treatment

Treatment of atrophic glossitis includes identifying and replacing the missing nutrient (e.g. by vitamin supplementation) or treating the underlying condition.

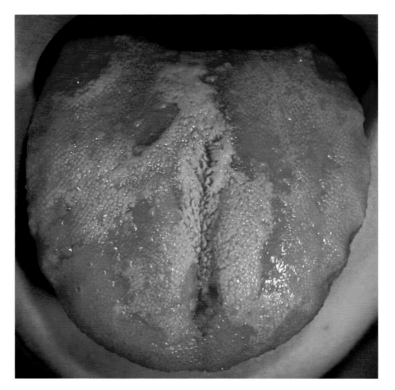

Figure 9.1. Atrophic glossitis (histological diagnosis).

Reproduced from *Open Dentistry Journal* (2016) 10:619–35, under a CC-BY 4.0 licence.

9.2   Vitamin deficiencies

Vitamin deficiency may be primary when caused by insufficient vitamin intake, or secondary when due to an underlying disorder such as malabsorption.

- Vitamin A, various B vitamins, folate, and vitamin D deficiencies are common in many countries.
- Scurvy (vitamin C deficiency) and pellagra (niacin deficiency) are rare.
- The B group of vitamins and vitamin C are water-soluble, whereas vitamins E and K are fat-soluble.
- Frequently, several vitamins are deficient in a patient with malnutrition and the precise cause of oral symptoms may be challenging (see *Fig. 9.2*).

9.2.1   Riboflavin (vitamin B2) deficiency

Oral symptoms of riboflavin deficiency are:

- painful atrophic glossitis
- sore throat
- chapped, cracked lips
- angular cheilitis.

Photophobia is characteristic of riboflavin deficiency.

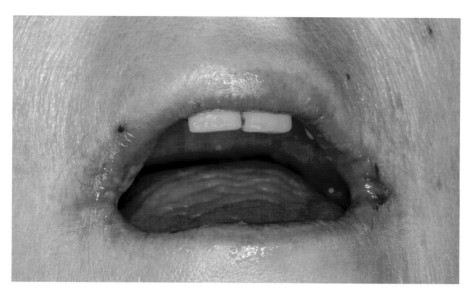

Figure 9.2. Oral signs of malnutrition: angular cheilitis and atrophic glossitis.

Reproduced from Health NZ – Waikato (www.waikatodhb.health.nz) with permission.

9.2.2 Niacin (vitamin B3) deficiency

Niacin deficiency or pellagra may result in atrophic glossitis.

Pellagra is characterized by:
- diarrhoea
- dermatitis – a peeling rash on sun-exposed sites such as the backs of hands and neck
- dementia.

9.2.3 Pyridoxine (vitamin B6) deficiency

Oral symptoms of pyridoxine deficiency include atrophic glossitis and angular cheilitis.

Other features of pyridoxine deficiency may include:
- seborrhoeic dermatitis
- conjunctivitis
- somnolence
- confusion
- neuropathy, including seizures.

Blood tests may reveal microcytic anaemia. Pyridoxine and riboflavin deficiency usually co-exist.

9.2.4 Biotin (vitamin B7) deficiency

Oral symptoms of biotin deficiency include atrophic glossitis and a perioral erythematous rash.

Other features of biotin deficiency may include:

- a rash in a seborrhoeic distribution
- fine, brittle scalp and eyebrow hair
- conjunctivitis
- mild depression
- fatigue, somnolence, and lethargy
- myalgia
- paraesthesia
- hallucinations.

9.2.5   Folate (vitamin B9) deficiency

Folate deficiency may cause painful atrophic glossitis and aphthous ulcers.

Other features of folate deficiency may include:
- loss of appetite
- weight loss
- weakness
- headaches
- palpitations
- behavioural disorders
- spina bifida due to maternal folate deficiency.

Blood tests may reveal megaloblastic macrocytic anaemia.

9.2.6   Cyanocobalamin (vitamin B12) deficiency

Vitamin B12 deficiency may cause glossitis and angular cheilitis.

Other features of cyanocobalamin deficiency may include:
- weakness, light-headedness, and dizziness
- headaches
- breathlessness
- low-grade fever
- hypotension and tachycardia
- easy bruising
- nausea, loss of appetite, and weight loss
- dyspepsia and heartburn
- paraesthesia of fingers and toes
- tinnitus
- hair loss
- adverse pregnancy outcomes.

Blood tests may reveal megaloblastic macrocytic anaemia.

9.2.7   Tocopherol (vitamin E) deficiency

Vitamin E deficiency may cause atrophic glossitis.

Other features of tocopherol deficiency are due to poor conduction of electrical impulses along nerves due to nerve membrane structure and function changes, such as peripheral neuropathy and ophthalmoplegia.

Blood tests may reveal haemolytic anaemia.

9.2.8   Vitamin K deficiency

There are two types of vitamin K – phylloquinone (K1) and menaquinones (K2). Vitamin K is essential for the synthesis of certain clotting factors.

Vitamin K deficiency causes bleeding gums.

Other features of vitamin K deficiency may include:
- spontaneous bruising
- nosebleeds
- heavy menstrual bleeding in women.

9.2.9   Ascorbic acid (vitamin C) deficiency

Vitamin C deficiency causes scurvy, characterized by weakness, weight loss, and general aches and pains.

Causes

Scurvy may result from a dietary lack of fruit and vegetables or malabsorption of vitamin C. It is more common in patients with chronic kidney disease, smokers, and alcoholics.

Lowered levels of ascorbic acid result in defective collagen and ground substance synthesis.

Clinical features

The first symptoms of scurvy are irritability and anorexia.
- Oral scurvy results in erythema, enlargement, petechiae, and spontaneous bleeding of the gingivae (see *Fig. 9.3*).
- Tooth decay, mobility, and loss occur with advanced disease.
- Cutaneous scurvy includes poor wound healing, easy bruising, hyperkeratosis, and petechiae.
- Perifollicular haemorrhages with corkscrew and swan-neck hairs on woody oedema affecting the lower legs.
- Nail findings include koilonychia and splinter haemorrhages.
- Other symptoms include anaemia, weakness, fatigue, epistaxis, haemorrhage into joints, myalgia, bone pain, and depression.

Diagnosis

The diagnosis of scurvy is made by assessing serum ascorbic acid levels and evaluating the response to treatment.

Treatment

Supplements of ascorbic acid will correct the condition, and the oral lesions will resolve spontaneously.

Vitamin C is found in citrus fruits, potatoes, onions, broccoli, strawberries and many other fruits and vegetables.

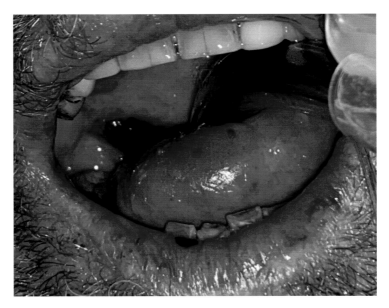

Figure 9.3. Patient with sepsis with intraoral bleeding. Extremely low serum ascorbic acid levels confirmed scurvy, with rapid recovery after supplementary vitamin C.

Reproduced from Health NZ – Waikato (www.waikatodhb.health.nz) with permission.

9.3 Angioedema

Angioedema is localized subcutaneous or submucosal swelling which results from the extravasation of fluid into the interstitial tissue. It is mediated by mast cells, histamine, or bradykinin release. It can affect the lips and mouth.

In most cases, angioedema accompanies urticaria. However, urticaria (which results in cutaneous weals) does not affect the oral mucosa.

Causes

Angioedema with urticaria can be due to allergic or non-allergic causes.
- An acute type 1 IgE-mediated allergic or hypersensitivity anaphylactic reaction may be triggered by medication (e.g. penicillin or sulfa drug, NSAID, or vaccine), food (peanuts, shellfish), insect venom (most often wasps, bees), and natural rubber latex.
- Acute urticaria and angioedema not associated with anaphylaxis are most often associated with a viral infection, vaccination, medication, or an unknown trigger.
- Chronic spontaneous urticaria and angioedema are due to autoimmune disease.
- Rarely, vibration or a cold stimulus may induce angioedema.

Angioedema without urticaria can rarely be due to inherited or acquired C1-esterase inhibitor deficiency.

- Angioedema is triggered by emotional stress, trauma such as a dental procedure, or hormonal factors such as exogenous oestrogen.
- Angioedema due to ACE inhibitors can occur several months after taking the medication.

Clinical features

The clinical features depend on the type of angioedema.
- The onset of allergic angioedema associated with anaphylaxis is abrupt. Sites of swelling include the face, lips (see *Fig. 9.4*), mouth, tongue, throat, larynx, uvula, extremities, and genitalia.
- Significant airway involvement in anaphylaxis results in dyspnoea, dysphagia, stridor, vocal changes, hoarseness, or drooling – this requires urgent management.
- Non-allergic forms of angioedema may have an abrupt or gradual onset.
- The lips or other affected sites are often oedematous without a colour change. There may be a burning sensation.
- Angioedema persists for 24–48 hours and then resolves spontaneously.

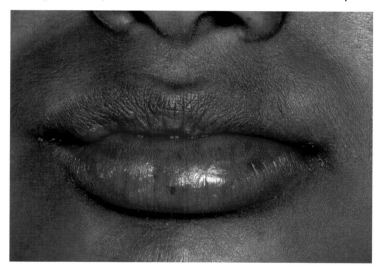

Figure 9.4. Angioedema of the lower lip.

Reproduced from Health NZ – Waikato (www.waikatodhb.health.nz) with permission.

Treatment

Treatment depends on the type of angioedema.
- Allergic angioedema associated with anaphylaxis is treated with adrenaline. Treatment in the hospital is often necessary.
- Like urticaria, mild angioedema is treated with non-sedating antihistamines. Triggers should be avoided.
- Occasionally, oral corticosteroids, ciclosporin, or tranexamic acid are needed to reduce swelling.

- Treatment-resistant chronic urticaria and angioedema may be treated with omalizumab.
- C1-INH replacement may be administered for angioedema due to C1-INH deficiency.

9.4 Hypothyroidism

Hypothyroidism can be primary, secondary, or tertiary.

Causes

Hypothyroidism results from acquired thyroid disease, genetic mechanisms, or abnormalities in the hypothalamic–pituitary axis.
- Primary hypothyroidism reflects the underproduction of thyroxine by the thyroid gland. It is usually due to iodine deficiency or excess, autoimmune Hashimoto thyroiditis, previous treatment for hyperthyroidism (radioiodine therapy, subtotal thyroidectomy), radiation therapy to the neck, or prolonged treatment with iodides.
- Congenital hypothyroidism is due to aplasia, hypoplasia, or defective thyroid hormone synthesis.
- Secondary hypothyroidism is due to pituitary disease causing a deficiency of thyroid-stimulating hormone due to dysfunction, postpartum necrosis, neoplasm, or infiltrative disease.
- Tertiary hypothyroidism is due to hypothalamic disease causing a deficiency of the thyrotropin-releasing hormone and is due to granuloma, neoplasm, or irradiation.
- Hereditary hypothyroidism, which is rare, is associated with a mutation in the beta form of the thyroid hormone receptor that renders it inactive.
- Children with trisomy 21, Turner syndrome, Klinefelter syndrome, coeliac disease, or type 1 diabetes mellitus are at higher risk for associated autoimmune thyroid disorder.

Clinical features

Hypothyroidism's most common clinical features include:
- dry skin
- cold intolerance
- weight gain
- constipation
- fatigue.

Common signs in patients with moderate to severe hypothyroidism (myxoedema) include:
- bradycardia
- ankle swelling
- periorbital puffiness
- coarse hair.

Untreated severe myxoedema may cause coma.

The common oral findings in hypothyroidism include:
- macroglossia
- dysgeusia
- delayed eruption of the teeth
- poor periodontal health
- altered tooth morphology
- delayed wound healing.

Diagnosis

Patients with suspected hypothyroidism should have thyroid-stimulating hormone (TSH) and thyroxine (T_4) measured, and thyroid antibodies confirms the diagnosis.

Treatment

The treatment of hypothyroidism is thyroid replacement for life.

9.5 Thrombocytopenic purpura

Thrombocytopenic purpura refers to purple discolouration of the skin and mucous membrane due to bleeding when there are abnormally low levels of platelets in the blood. An average platelet count is 150 000–450 000 platelets per microlitre of blood. Bleeding may occur if the count is less than 50 000 and becomes dangerous when less than 5000 or 10 000/mm³.

Causes

Thrombocytopenia is caused by decreased production of platelets by megakaryocytes in the bone marrow, increased destruction of platelets in the circulation, or abnormal sequestration of platelets in the spleen.
- Thrombocytopenic purpura may be disease- or drug-induced, immunological (autoimmune), or thrombotic.
- The most common causes of thrombocytopenia are bone marrow aplasia, fibrosis, or infiltration by malignant cells, the effect of alcohol or a cytotoxic drug, or an infective agent such as HIV.
- Thrombotic thrombocytopenic purpura is a rare disorder in which multiple blood clots occur in the blood vessels, using up the platelets and causing haemolytic anaemia.

Clinical features

Thrombocytopenic purpura presents as bleeding, petechiae, ecchymosis, haemorrhagic blisters, and haematoma.
- The first sign of thrombocytopenia may be spontaneous gingival bleeding or oral bleeding induced by minor trauma, such as during brushing or when using dental floss.
- Purpura occurs in trauma-prone regions such as vestibular mucosa, the junction between the hard and soft palate (see *Fig. 4.1*), the lateral edges of the tongue, and the floor of the mouth under the tongue.

- Bleeding may also include melaena, haematuria, epistaxis, or excessive menstrual flow. Intracranial bleeding caused by thrombocytopenia is life-threatening.

Diagnosis

A diagnosis of thrombocytopenic purpura can be made if a CBC and a peripheral blood smear reveal significant thrombocytopenia. Further tests are required to determine its cause.

Other disease entities that might be causing purpura should be excluded by medical history and physical examination.

Treatment

The treatment of thrombocytopenic purpura depends on its cause and is administered by a haematologist. Treatment is urgent if the platelet count is below 50 000/mm^3.

Treatment might include corticosteroids, immunosuppressive agents, chemotherapy, splenectomy, plasmapheresis, or platelet transfusions.

9.6 Leukaemia

Leukaemia is a large group of neoplastic diseases with a malignant proliferation of white blood cells. There are four main types of leukaemia:
- Acute myeloid (or myelogenous) leukaemia (AML)
- Chronic myeloid (or myelogenous) leukaemia (CML)
- Acute lymphocytic (or lymphoblastic) leukaemia (ALL)
- Chronic lymphocytic leukaemia (CLL).

Clinical features

Oral manifestations may occur in any leukaemia but are most common in acute myeloid leukaemia.
- Oral symptoms include gingival hyperplasia (see *Fig. 9.5a*), oral ulceration, bleeding and petechiae (see *Fig. 9.5b*), mucosal pallor, and infection.
- Oral manifestations may be primary (i.e. the result of direct infiltration by malignant cells) or secondary to thrombocytopenia, neutropenia, or impaired granulocyte function.
- General features of leukaemia include fatigue, fever, adenomegaly, persistent or recurrent infection, pallor, haematoma, petechiae, and unexpected bleeding from the skin and other mucous membranes.

Diagnosis

The diagnosis of leukaemia may be initially suspected due to the clinical symptoms and signs of the disease. Investigations may include the following tests:
- Complete blood count, differential, and peripheral blood film
- Needle biopsy and aspiration of bone marrow

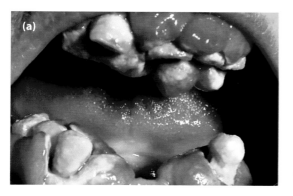

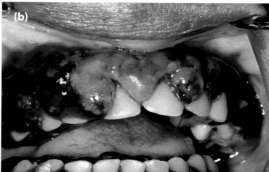

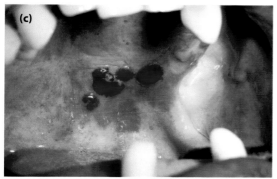

Figure 9.5 (a–c). (a) Infiltration of gingival tissue with leukaemia cells in a patient with acute myeloid leukaemia and (b) in monocytic leukaemia; (c) purpura and haemorrhagic bullae in a patient with unspecified leukaemia.

(a) Reproduced with permission from *Pocket Dentistry* (Chapter 11; www.pocketdentistry.com); (b) reproduced with permission from Professor Nagamani Narayana, University of Nebraska Medical Centre, NE, USA; (c) reproduced with permission from Professor Yeshwant Rawal, University of Milwaukee School of Dentistry, Milwaukee, WI, USA. All images included here after enhancement by AIPDerm (www.aipderm.com).

- Karyotyping
- Flow cytometry
- Molecular panel and mutation analysis
- Lymph node biopsy
- Lumbar puncture
- Imaging including X-rays, ultrasound, CT, PET, and MRI scans.

Treatment

The treatment of leukaemia is rapidly evolving and will depend on the type of leukaemia and its severity. It may include any of the following:
- Chemotherapy
- Targeted therapy
- Immunotherapy
- Radiation therapy
- Stem cell transplantation.

9.7   Coeliac disease

Coeliac disease is a chronic autoimmune disorder of the small intestine triggered by ingesting gluten and related prolamines in genetically predisposed patients.
- The prevalence of coeliac disease in western populations is 1–1.5%.
- This increases to 3–6% in patients with type 1 diabetes mellitus and up to 20% in first-degree relatives of patients with coeliac disease.

Clinical features

The clinical spectrum of coeliac disease is varied. Commonly, patients present with malabsorption and diarrhoea. Oral features may include:
- recurrent aphthous ulcers
- enamel hypoplasia or hypomineralization, most commonly affecting the permanent incisors of children with active or undiagnosed coeliac disease during odontogenesis. Enamel hypoplasia may compromise aesthetics, cause tooth sensitivity, and increase the risk of caries and tooth decay.

See also *Section 7.4.4*, dermatitis herpetiformis.

Diagnosis

The diagnosis of coeliac disease is confirmed by serological testing and small bowel biopsy.

Treatment
- A strict lifelong gluten-free diet is the only effective treatment for coeliac disease.
- Mouth ulcers improve or resolve with adherence to a gluten-free diet.
- Topical corticosteroids may provide symptomatic relief.
- Systemic medications for aphthous ulcers include doxycycline, zinc sulphate, colchicine, prednisone, and immunomodulating agents.
- Children with extensive enamel defects usually require interdisciplinary management, involving extraction, complex restorations, or orthodontics.

9.8   Inflammatory bowel disease

Inflammatory bowel disease (IBD) comprises the spectrum of Crohn disease and ulcerative colitis.
- The annual incidence of IBD is 1–20 per 100 000 population, and the prevalence is 25–300 per 100 000 (greater among Ashkenazi Jews).
- IBD may occur at any age with a bimodal peak onset of 20–40 and 60–70 years.
- There is no gender predilection.
- Up to 15% of patients with IBD have a first-degree relative who also has IBD.
- The estimated prevalence of oral lesions in patients with IBD is between 20% and 50%. Oral lesions are more common in children than in adults.

Causes

IBD involves a dysregulated inflammatory response in genetically predisposed individuals. It is postulated that an unknown environmental trigger interacts with the intestinal flora.

Clinical features of oral lesions

Any part of the gastrointestinal tract can be affected by IBD.

* Although intestinal involvement usually precedes oral lesions, oral lesions are the first sign of IBD in 5–10% of patients, and the IBD may be subclinical.
* Oral lesions tend to be more severe during active gastrointestinal disease, but up to 30% may continue to have oral lesions despite disease control at other sites.
* Oral lesions are more common in Crohn disease than ulcerative colitis, particularly in patients with proximal gastrointestinal tract or perianal involvement.

Oral lesions seen with inflammatory bowel conditions are classified as non-specific or specific. Specific lesions contain non-caseating granulomas on histological examination. Their activity is not correlated with bowel disease activity and can precede it.

9.8.1   Non-specific oral lesions

* Aphthous ulcers affect up to 10% of patients with ulcerative colitis and 20–30% of patients with Crohn disease (see *Fig. 9.6a*).
* Angular cheilitis (see *Fig. 9.6b*).
* Persistent submandibular lymphadenopathy.

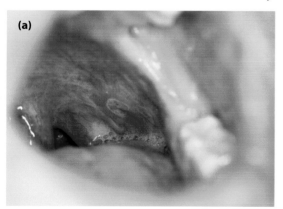
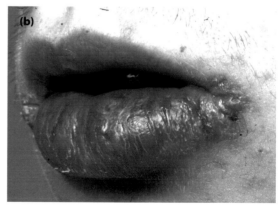

Figure 9.6 (a and b). Non-specific oral features of Crohn disease: (a) aphthous ulcer and (b) angular cheilitis (patient also has fissured granulomatous cheilitis of the lower lip).

Reproduced from Health NZ – Waikato (www.waikatodhb.health.nz) with permission.

9.8.2   Oral lesions specific to Crohn disease

* Mucosal tags on labial and buccal vestibules and retromolar region.
* Cobblestoning, fissuring, corrugation, and swelling of the posterior buccal mucosa (see *Fig. 9.7*).
* Mucogingivitis – oedematous, granular, hyperplastic gingiva that may ulcerate.
* Lip and facial swelling with vertical fissures, deep linear ulcerations in the buccal sulci and hyperplastic folds.
* Midline lip fissuring.

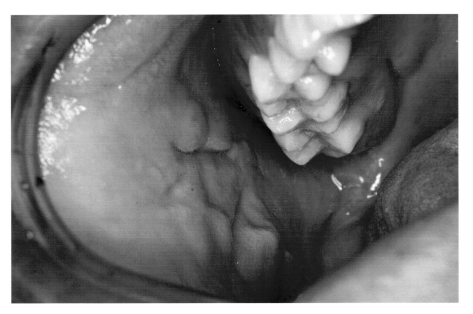

Figure 9.7. Oral lesions in Crohn disease.

Reproduced from Health NZ – Waikato (www.waikatodhb.health.nz) with permission.

Treatment of oral lesions

Treatment usually involves collaboration with the treating gastroenterologist.
- Oral lesions may require topical or systemic corticosteroids, immunosuppressive drugs such as azathioprine or methotrexate, and biological agents.

9.8.3 Pyostomatitis vegetans

Pyostomatitis vegetans is a chronic mucocutaneous ulcerative disorder. It is most prevalent in patients aged between 20 and 60 years, with an average age of 34. The male-to-female ratio is 2:3.

Pyostomatitis vegetans is associated with IBD, especially active ulcerative colitis.

Clinical features

Pyostomatitis vegetans usually affects the labial gingiva, labial mucosa, and buccal mucosa (see *Fig. 9.8*).
- Oral lesions consist of multiple miliary white/yellow pustules with an oedematous and erythematous base.
- Pustules commonly rupture and coalesce to form 'snail tracks'.
- Histopathology of a biopsy shows intraepithelial or subepithelial microabscesses with eosinophils and neutrophils. There may be hyperkeratosis, acanthosis, and acantholysis.

Treatment

Pyostomatitis vegetans responds to treatment of the underlying inflammatory bowel disease. Topical or systemic corticosteroids may be required.

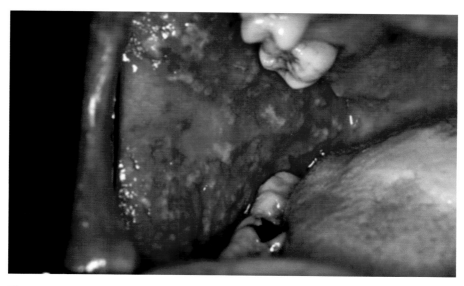

Figure 9.8. Pyostomatitis vegetans. Superficial pustules, some of which suggest a 'snail track' pattern.

Reproduced from *Color Atlas of Oral and Maxillofacial Diseases*, 2019; B.W. Neville, D.D. Damm, C.M. Allen & A.C. Chi, with permission from Elsevier.

9.9 Oral manifestations of diabetes mellitus

Diabetes mellitus is a common metabolic disease characterized by persistent hyperglycaemia due to defective insulin secretion, insulin resistance, or both. Hyperglycaemia leads to dysfunction and failure of various organs; the eyes, kidneys and cardiovascular systems may be irreversibly damaged.

Causes

Diabetes mellitus is classified as type 1 or type 2.
- Type 1 diabetes mellitus is due to loss of insulin production.
- Type 2 diabetes mellitus is due to impaired insulin production and function.

Clinical features

The extensive manifestations of diabetes mellitus are beyond the scope of this book.

The oral manifestations of poorly controlled diabetes may include:
- angular cheilitis and intraoral candidosis (see *Chapter 6*)
- oral dryness
- sialosis (sialadenosis), a chronic swelling of large salivary glands, particularly the parotid glands (see *Fig. 9.9a*)
- a predisposition to periodontal disease (see *Fig. 9.9b*).

Diagnosis

Diabetes mellitus is commonly diagnosed by random and fasting blood sugar levels and elevated glycosylated haemoglobin. An oral glucose tolerance test may be performed.

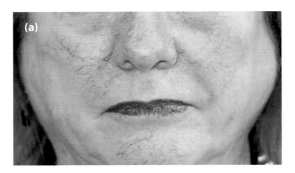
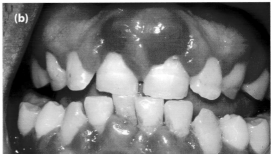

Figure 9.9 (a and b). Oral features of diabetes: (a) bilateral parotid enlargement; (b) gingivitis and gingival enlargement.

(a) Reproduced from Health NZ – Waikato (www.waikatodhb.health.nz) with permission; (b) reproduced with permission from Professor Yeshwant Rawal, University of Milwaukee School of Dentistry, Milwaukee, WI, USA, and included here after enhancement by AIPDerm (www.aipderm.com).

Treatment

Diabetic control relies on diet, exercise, and various medications.

9.10 Vasculitis

Vasculitis can present with intraoral lesions.

9.10.1 Cutaneous small vessel vasculitis

Small vessel or hypersensitivity vasculitis often presents with urticated papules and palpable purpura, commonly distributed on the lower legs. When vasculitis is

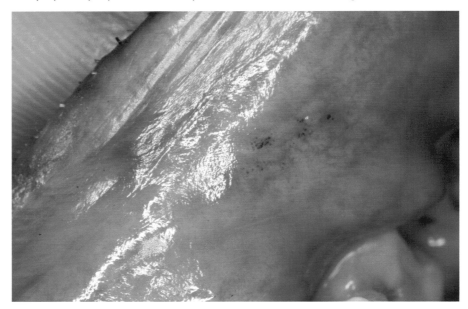

Figure 9.10. Intraoral petechiae in a patient with small vessel vasculitis.

Reproduced from Health NZ – Waikato (www.waikatodhb.health.nz) with permission.

more generalized or has systemic features, intraoral petechiae may be observed (see *Fig. 9.10*). These are often asymptomatic and resolve spontaneously or with systemic treatment with corticosteroids or immune-suppressive medications.

9.10.2   Giant cell arteritis

Giant cell arteritis is a medium to large vessel vasculitis that commonly affects the temporal arteries but can be more widespread.
- The mean age of onset of giant cell arteritis is 70.
- The female-to-male preponderance is 3:1.
- Giant cell arteritis may arise in association with polymyalgia rheumatica.

Causes

The inflammatory plaques and oedema are due to inflammation of the arterial vessel wall. Subsequent vessel occlusion causes local ischaemia.

Clinical features

Giant cell arteritis may cause pain when chewing or talking due to claudication of the masticatory muscles.
- Other orofacial manifestations include mucosal ischaemia or necrosis, facial swelling, orofacial pain, dysphagia or dysarthria, mental neuropathy, and a submandibular mass.
- Two-thirds of patients present with sudden onset headaches in the temporal area with scalp sensitivity.
- 25–50% of patients present with visual disturbance due to retinal ischaemia, with blindness in 6–10% of cases.
- The temporal artery is prominent, tender on palpation, and may be pulseless. It may develop a nodular or tortuous texture.
- Some patients will also experience fatigue, fever, and weight loss.
- Large vessel involvement may cause aortic arch symptoms or limb claudication.

Diagnosis

A patient is classified as having giant cell arteritis if three of the following five American College of Rheumatology classification criteria are present:
1. Age at onset >50 years
2. New onset or new type of headache with distinctive characteristics
3. Temporal artery tenderness or decreased pulsation
4. ESR >50mm/h
5. Arterial biopsy showing vasculitis with mononuclear cells or granulomatous inflammation with multinucleated giant cells.

Treatment

Treatment with high-dose corticosteroids should be commenced as soon as the diagnosis of giant cell arteritis is considered, to reduce the risk of blindness.
- The response to corticosteroid therapy is rapid, with symptoms dramatically decreasing within a few days.

- Many patients require a long course of high-dose corticosteroids.
- Relapses are common.

9.10.3   Granulomatosis with polyangiitis

Granulomatosis with polyangiitis, formerly known as Wegener granulomatosis, is a rare, life-threatening systemic disease that may involve every organ system. The mean age of presentation is the seventh decade, but it may present at any age.

Characteristic features of granulomatosis with polyangiitis are the following:
- Midline destructive lesion
- Histopathology showing necrotizing granulomatous vasculitis of small and medium-sized vessels
- Presence of antineutrophil cytoplasmic antibodies (ANCA).

Causes

The pathogenesis of granulomatosis with polyangiitis is uncertain, with genetic, environmental, autoimmune, and infectious factors implicated.

Clinical features

Granulomatosis with polyangiitis damages the kidneys, lungs, mucous membranes, and skin.
- Symptoms in the oral cavity, sinuses, ears, and throat are present in 70–100% of patients.
- The most common features are rhinitis and sinusitis with oedema of the nasal mucosa, purulent or bloody chronic nasal discharge, nasal crusting, and oral mucosa inflammation with ulcers.
- Strawberry gingivitis describes enlarged, friable, erythematous, or violaceous interdental gingiva with red or yellow spots (see Figs 9.11a and b).
- Oral mucosal petechiae may be present.
- Skin involvement results in ulcers, palpable purpura, papules, nodules, and vesicles.
- Other affected organs include the lungs, kidneys, nervous system, eyes, ears, and heart.

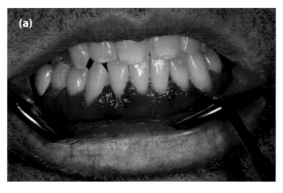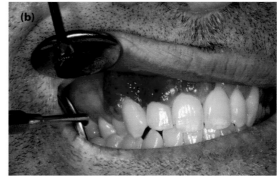

Figure 9.11 (a and b). Granulomatosis with polyangiitis: (a) lower gingiva and (b) upper gingiva.

Diagnosis

Current diagnostic criteria for granulomatosis with polyangiitis include identifying at least two of the following features:
- Nasal or oral inflammation
- Abnormal chest radiograph
- Abnormal urinary sediment
- Granulomas in a biopsy.

ANCA antibodies:
- c-ANCA targets proteinase-3 (PR-3) and is specific for granulomatosis with polyangiitis.
- p-ANCA targets protoplasmic perinuclear antibodies and is less clear.

Treatment

Standard therapy for granulomatosis with polyangiitis is oral or pulsed intravenous cyclophosphamide and high-dose corticosteroids. Rituximab, azathioprine, mycophenolate mofetil, and methotrexate are other drug options.

9.11 Cushing syndrome

Cushing syndrome or hypercortisolism is the result of endogenous or exogenous corticosteroids.

Causes
- Cushing disease is due to excess ACTH from a pituitary adenoma resulting in endogenous glucocorticoid secretion by the adrenal glands.
- Cushing syndrome may also be iatrogenic, following treatment with systemic corticosteroids or, rarely, excessive, prolonged use of topical corticosteroids.

Clinical features

Symptoms and signs of hypercortisolism may include:
- easy bruising of the skin
- weight gain with fat deposition of the mid–upper back
- rounded, reddened face
- excessive body and facial hair
- proximal myopathy
- diabetes mellitus
- hypertension
- gastric reflux
- osteoporosis
- psychiatric effects such as anxiety and depression.

Oral manifestations of hypercortisolism are common:
- Dry mouth
- Oral candidosis
- Tooth decay
- Gingival enlargement
- Poor wound healing.

Diagnosis

Cushing syndrome requires clinical suspicion and investigations, such as:
- 24-hour urinary cortisol
- dexamethasone suppression test
- CT or MRI imaging of adrenal glands and pituitary gland.

Treatment

The treatment of Cushing syndrome depends on its cause and is usually undertaken by or on the advice of an endocrinologist.

9.12 Acromegaly

Acromegaly (gigantism in adults) is due to pituitary growth hormone excess after the bony epiphyseal growth plates have fused.

Clinical features

Typical characteristics of acromegaly include:
- growth of hands and feet
- prominent nose and frontal bones

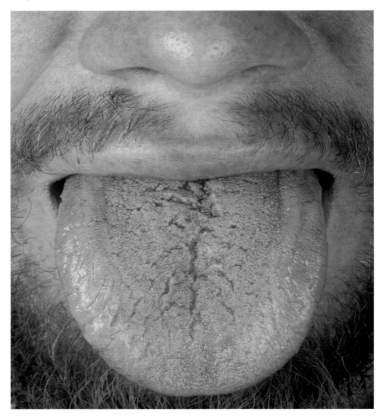

Figure 9.12. Macroglossia in a patient with acromegaly.

Reproduced from Health NZ – Waikato (www.waikatodhb.health.nz) with permission.

- the lower jaw enlarges and protrudes (macrognathia or prognathia)
- patients develop musculoskeletal problems and fatigue, and the voice may deepen.

Oral features of acromegaly include:
- macroglossia (see *Fig. 9.12*)
- enlarging diastemas (gaps between the teeth) or teeth crowding
- periodontal disease.

Cutaneous features of acromegaly include:
- thick doughy skin
- thick, hard nails
- hypertrichosis, hyperhidrosis, and seborrhoea
- skin tags and hyperpigmentation.

9.13 Parathyroid disease

Parathyroid disease can be primary or secondary.
- Primary hyperparathyroidism is due to excessive parathyroid hormone production by the parathyroid glands, due to parathyroid adenoma.
- Secondary hyperparathyroidism is due to parathyroid hyperplasia because of chronic hypercalcaemia from renal failure, inadequate vitamin D metabolism, or inadequate calcium intake or absorption, aggravating osteopenia, and osteoporosis.
- This can lead to tertiary hyperparathyroidism, with excessive PTH secretion from loss of inhibitory control of the parathyroid glands.

The consequences of hyperparathyroidism include brown tumours.
- Asymptomatic brown tumours in the mandible and maxilla affect about 1.5% of patients with secondary hyperparathyroidism.
- They are more common in females than in males.
- They are radiolucent well-demarcated uni- or multilocular nodules. If large enough to breach the bone cortex, localized jaw expansion and a slow-growing mass may be noted intraorally.

Brown tumours are managed surgically, along with the correction of hyperparathyroidism.

9.14 Sickle cell anaemia

Sickle cell anaemia is a genetic disease caused by the replacement of glutamic acid by valine in position six at the N-terminus of the beta-chain of globin, thus resulting in haemoglobin S. Under hypoxia conditions, erythrocytes that contain haemoglobin S take on a shape resembling a sickle.

Clinical features
- Oral mucosal manifestations of sickle cell anaemia include mucosal pallor and yellow discolouration.
- There may be delayed tooth eruption, enamel, and dentine mineralization defects, and hypercementosis.

- Radiographically, there may be radiopaque areas in the maxilla and mandible, representing repairs to bone infarction; loss of trabeculation and increased medullary space and resultant increased radiolucency; thinning of the lower border of the mandible; and loss of alveolar bone height.
- A coarse trabecular pattern resembling a staircase may be noted in the interproximal region due to horizontal rows of trabecular bone and bony projections.

9.15 Amyloidosis

Amyloidosis has systemic and localized forms in which insoluble fibrillar proteins are deposited. All forms of oral amyloid are rare. Localized deposits of amyloid present as non-specific masses and are benign. Systemic amyloidosis is a progressive metabolic disease that most often results in yellow, orange, red, blue, or purple inflamed papules, nodules, and ulcers in the mouth. The most common sign is a large, firm tongue (macroglossia) (see *Fig. 9.13*). Macroglossia can cause speech impairment and dysphagia.

The diagnosis of oral amyloidosis is made by biopsy with special stains. Amyloidosis can be hereditary, primary, or secondary to multiple myeloma, rheumatoid arthritis, Crohn disease, and other chronic inflammatory diseases. The prognosis is poor if there is renal or cardiac disease.

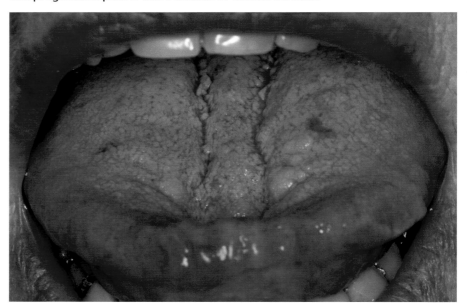

Figure 9.13. Acquired macroglossia in systemic amyloidosis.

Reproduced from Health NZ – Waikato (www.waikatodhb.health.nz) with permission.

9.16 Drug-induced osteonecrosis of the jaw

Osteoporosis is a systemic skeletal disease characterized by bone fragility and susceptibility to fracture. Osteonecrosis of the jaw is an occasional complication of its treatment.
- In Australia, 29% of women and 10% of men aged 75 and over have osteoporosis.
- They are often treated with bisphosphonates and denosumab.

Drug-induced osteonecrosis of the jaw is exposed bone or bone in the maxillofacial region that has persisted for more than 8 weeks.
- It is probed through an intraoral or extraoral fistula.
- It occurs in patients with current or previous treatment with anti-resorptive therapy alone or in combination with immune modulators or antiangiogenic medications.
- Patients should have no history of radiation therapy to the jaws or metastatic disease affecting the jaws.

Risk factors

Drug-induced osteonecrosis of the jaw is more common in oncological patients (<5%) than in osteoporotic patients (<0.05%). Other risk factors include:
- concomitant medications
- underlying systemic disease
- dental infections
- surgical procedures.

The risk of drug-induced osteonecrosis of the jaw depends on the type of drug, its potency and dosage, its administration route, and the treatment length. It is caused by:
- bisphosphonates
- anti-angiogenic medications
- systemic corticosteroids
- immunosuppressive agents such as ciclosporin and tacrolimus.

Causes

The pathogenesis of drug-induced osteonecrosis of the jaw is multifactorial and poorly understood. Anti-resorptive drugs inhibit osteoclastic activity, resulting in increased bone mineral density and reducing the risk of bone fractures.
- This alteration of bone turnover also affects bone healing processes.
- The newly formed bone may become ischaemic and necrotic due to insufficient blood supply.
- Corticosteroids may interfere with normal healing processes of the jawbone.

Clinical features

Drug-induced osteonecrosis of the jaw is classified into four clinical stages.

1. Stage 0 Non-exposed osteonecrosis of the jaw
   - Occurs in up to 25% of cases
   - Unexplained symptoms mimic odontalgia or loosening of teeth
2. Stage 1 Exposed and necrotic jawbone or fistula that connects to the bone
   - Absence of infection or symptoms
3. Stage 2 Clinical features of Stage 1, with infection and symptoms
4. Stage 3 Exposed necrotic bone extending beyond the alveolar bone.

Complications of drug-induced osteonecrosis of the jaw include pathological fracture, extra-oral fistulae, oroantral or oronasal communication, and osteolysis extending to the lower border of the mandible or floor of the sinus.

Diagnosis

Diagnosing drug-induced osteonecrosis of the jaw relies on clinical history and examination.
- Imaging, such as a CT scan, will aid diagnosis and staging.
- Radiographic features range from sclerosis and periodontal ligament widening to areas of osteolysis with or without sclerotic areas.

Treatment

Treatment of drug-induced osteonecrosis of the jaw includes non-surgical treatments and surgery.
- Topical antiseptics, systemic antibiotics and analgesia are prescribed to control infection, encourage spontaneous exfoliation of bony sequestrum, and reduce pain.
- Surgical debridement or resection may be indicated.
- Liaison with the endocrinology or oncology team is paramount to ensure continued fracture prevention in osteoporotic patients and continuation of oncologic treatment in cancer patients.

9.17 Psychogenic oral disease

Psychogenic and psychosomatic oral diseases may also be classified as medically unexplained oral symptoms and syndromes (MUOS), in which there are no accompanying clinical or laboratory findings. The most common presentations are:
- burning mouth syndrome
- atypical odontalgia
- oral dysaesthesia
- halitophobia
- phantom bite syndrome
- odontophobia.

9.17.1   Burning mouth syndrome

The term burning mouth or orodynia describes intermittent or constant burning pain, discomfort, or a tingling sensation in the mouth. Glossodynia is a burning discomfort localized to the tongue. By convention, the symptom is not accompanied by visible signs of a painful infection or inflammatory disease (see *Fig. 9.14*).

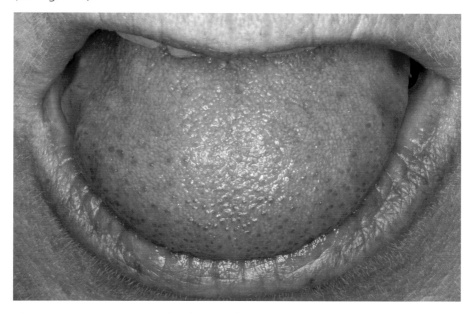

Figure 9.14. Burning mouth. The tip of the tongue was noted to be persistently speckled due to papillitis, but this did not account for the patient's generalized oral discomfort.

Reproduced from Health NZ – Waikato (www.waikatodhb.health.nz) with permission.

Causes

Causes of a burning mouth are usually speculative. Burning discomfort due to repetitive trauma, a dry mouth, infection, medication, or inflammation (e.g. lichen planus) should be excluded. Other possibilities include:
- a neuropathic origin within the mouth or trigeminal pathway – a minor form of glossopharyngeal neuralgia
- a nutritional deficiency.

A burning mouth is often a psychogenic symptom caused by psychological stress or anxiety.

Treatment

After excluding a specific pathology, treatment may include reassurance, an analgesic or anti-inflammatory, or a psychoactive medication such as a tricyclic antidepressant (e.g. amitriptyline), gabapentin, or pregabalin.

9.17.2   Atypical odontalgia

Atypical odontalgia is also known as atypical facial pain, phantom tooth pain, or orofacial neuropathic pain. It is characterized by chronic pain without an identifiable cause in a tooth or teeth or in a site where teeth have been extracted or following endodontic treatment.
- The pain of atypical odontalgia is described as a constant throbbing or aching.
- It is not significantly affected by exposure to hot or cold food or drink or by chewing or biting.
- The pain may or may not be relieved by injecting a local anaesthetic.

The most frequent treatment is tricyclic antidepressants such as amitriptyline.

9.17.3   Oral dysaesthesia

Oral dysaesthesia is characterized by pain or discomfort in the oral cavity for which no local or systemic cause can be identified.
- Oral dysaesthesia usually occurs in the fifth to seventh decade of life and is more common in females than males.
- Psychological and social co-morbidities such as anxiety and depression, somatization, hypochondria, cancer phobia, and insomnia have been reported in 85% of patients with oral dysaesthesia.
- Oral dysaesthesia often presents as a stinging sensation or pain affecting the tongue and lips. Other sites may be the hard palate, alveolar ridges, buccal mucosa, and floor of the mouth.
- The oral mucosa appears clinically normal.

Oral dysaesthesia is treated with antidepressants, analgesics, antiepileptics, anxiolytics, and antipsychotics.

9.17.4   Halitophobia

Halitophobia is also known as pseudohalitosis, psychosomatic halitosis, or delusional halitosis. It is a rare psychiatric condition characterized by an excessive preoccupation with the belief that one's exhaled breath has an unpleasant odour.
- Individuals with halitophobia cover their noses or stand back during a conversation.
- They do not acknowledge that their symptom is psychosomatic.
- In some patients, halitophobia is associated with olfactory reference syndrome, characterized by a person's stubborn belief that they have unpleasant body odour emanating from their skin, armpits, genitalia, or other body parts.
- Hypochondria can also trigger a flawed self-perception of their breath.

9.17.5   Phantom bite syndrome

Phantom bite syndrome is also known as occlusal dysaesthesia. It is characterized by a persistent uncomfortable bite sensation that does not correspond to any physical alteration related to occlusion, pulp, periodontium, muscle, or temporomandibular joint and causes significant functional impairment.

- These individuals have an erroneous and unshakable belief and demand bite correction.
- Treatment with antidepressants is reported to be of benefit.

9.17.6 Odontophobia

Odontophobia is often called dental fear, dental phobia, or dental anxiety. This extreme fear of receiving dental care may be a form of post-traumatic stress disorder due to previous adverse dental experiences.
- Dental phobia may be fear of pain, fear of the unknown, fear of injections, fear of cost, fear of the side-effects of anaesthesia, or fear of contracting germs.
- A patient with dental anxiety and an impending visit to the dentist becomes nervous and may have disturbed sleep as the appointment date comes closer.
- They feel uneasiness during the dental procedure and may suffer from extreme emotions, such as crying uncontrollably.

CHAPTER 10

ORAL NEOPLASTIC LESIONS: BENIGN, POTENTIALLY MALIGNANT, AND MALIGNANT

See also:
- *Section 5.1.3: Vascular malformation; Section 5.1.4: Lymphatic malformation*
- *Section 9.13: Parathyroid disease – brown tumours*

10.1 Benign lesions of the oral mucosa

Benign tumours of the oral mucosa are derived from mesenchymal cells. They are uncommon and rarely symptomatic.

10.1.1 Melanocytic naevus

Melanocytic naevi, commonly called moles, are hamartomas composed of focal collections of naevus cells in the epithelium or underlying connective tissue. Common on the skin, they rarely occur on the oral mucosa.

Clinical features
- The most common intraoral sites for melanocytic naevi are the hard palate (see *Fig. 10.1*) and buccal mucosa.
- A mucosal melanocytic naevus presents as a painless, solitary, well-circumscribed, dome-shaped macule or papule.
- Common naevi arise in childhood, whereas blue naevi may occur in childhood or adulthood. They then remain stable.
- Dermoscopy shows uniform, symmetrical structures and pigmentation arranged as a reticular pattern, clods, or structureless pigmented zones.
- Most melanocytic naevi are <5mm in diameter and brown, blue, or black.

Histopathology

The location of naevus cells classifies melanocytic naevi within the oral mucosa.
- Junctional naevus: the naevus cells are confined to the basal epithelium.
- Intramucosal naevus: the naevus cell nests are found within the lamina propria.
- Compound naevus: junctional and intramucosal naevus cells are both present.
- Blue naevus: intensely pigmented spindle-shaped naevus cells within the lamina propria.

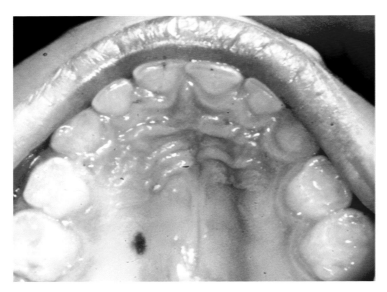

Figure 10.1. Melanocytic naevus presenting as a brown macule on the hard palate.

Reproduced with permission from Professor David Wilson, Adelaide, Australia, and included here after enhancement by AIPDerm (www.aipderm.com).

Treatment

Oral naevi are benign; however, they may be confused with melanoma, or melanoma may rarely arise within a naevus.

An excisional biopsy is recommended for a changing naevus or one with atypical features.

10.1.2   Melanotic neuroectodermal tumour of infancy

Melanotic neuroectodermal tumour of infancy is a rare, biphasic, neuroblastic and pigmented epithelial neoplasm. The tumour mainly arises in the craniofacial region, predominantly the maxilla, followed by the skull and mandible. It may also occur in the brain, epididymis, mediastinum, ovary, uterus, and peripheral bones.

Clinical features

Melanotic neuroectodermal tumour emerges within the first year of life, mostly under 6 months. It is never congenital.
- Although biologically benign, the tumour proliferates rapidly and is destructive.
- The infant presents with a painless, non-encapsulated, non-ulcerative, bluish-black gingival mass (*see Fig. 10.2*).
- In the maxilla, a melanotic neuroectodermal tumour usually carries one of the primary central incisors outward.
- Radiographs show local irregular resorption of bone and displacement of tooth buds.

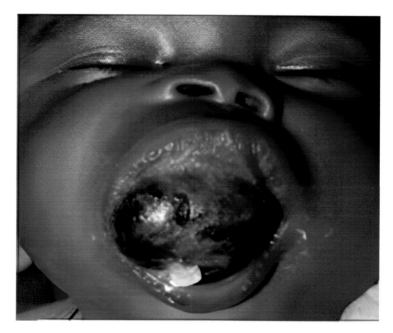

Figure 10.2. Melanotic neuroectodermal tumour of infancy presenting as a pigmented mass on the anterior maxilla.

Reproduced from https://en.wikipedia.org./wiki/Melanotic_neuroectodermal_tumuor_of_infancy under CC BY-SA 4.0 licence, and included here after enhancement by AIPDerm (www.aipderm.com).

- The diagnosis is based on clinical and radiographic findings and is confirmed by histopathology.
- 24-hour urine vanillylmandelic acid (VMA) is elevated in 10–15% of cases.

Peripheral surgical excision with 2–5mm margins is recommended. The overall incidence of local recurrence is 10–15%.

10.1.3   Lipoma

A lipoma is a benign adipose tissue tumour often occurring on the limbs or trunk.
- Lipomas are rare in the oral cavity.
- Oral lipoma usually arises over the age of 60 years.

Causes

Possible causes of lipoma include:
- fatty degeneration
- trauma to the site
- genetic factors
- hormonal abnormalities.

Clinical features

A lipoma is a slow-growing, soft, smooth, yellowish nodule.
- The most common site for lipoma within the oral cavity is the buccal mucosa.
- A lipoma occasionally arises on the tongue, lip, palate, or floor of the mouth.

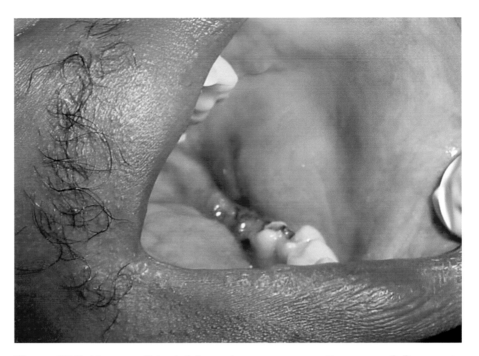

Figure 10.3. Lipoma of the left buccal mucosa presenting as a soft fluctuant mass.

Reproduced from *A Digital Manual for the Early Diagnosis of Oral Neoplasia*, 2008, International Agency for Research into Cancer, with permission, and included here after enhancement by AIPDerm (www.aipderm.com).

- It is generally asymptomatic.
- A lipoma may be fluctuant on palpation (see *Fig. 10.3*).

Diagnosis

A definitive diagnosis of lipoma may require a biopsy and histopathological examination.

Treatment

Lipoma is harmless, and treatment may not be necessary. It has a good prognosis, with no recurrence if completely excised.

10.1.4   Peripheral nerve sheath tumours

The peripheral nerve sheath tumours include several that may arise within the oral cavity.

The most common intraoral peripheral nerve sheath tumours are:
- Neurofibroma
- Schwannoma
- Mucosal neuroma
- Granular cell tumour.

Diagnosis is made by biopsy and histopathological examination with wide morphological variability. Hybrid tumours may occur.

Neurofibroma

A neurofibroma is a benign proliferation of Schwann cells, perineural cells, and fibroblasts.

- Neurofibroma may be solitary or multiple associated with neurofibromatosis type 1 (10%). Most patients with neurofibromatosis type 1 have intraoral lesions, which may be unrecognized as an association (e.g. dental caries).
- Neurofibromas are classified as dermal, originating from a single peripheral nerve, or plexiform, originating from multiple nerve bundles.
- Neurofibroma is rarely diagnosed within the oral cavity, although it is the most common benign intraoral neural tumour.

Clinical features

Intraoral dermal neurofibromas present as asymptomatic, smooth, submucosal nodules. Plexiform neurofibromas are poorly circumscribed and locally invasive.

- Solitary and multiple neurofibromas often occur on the tongue and lips, but may arise anywhere in the oral mucosa.
- Neurofibromatosis type 1 is characterized by café-au-lait macules, axillary freckling, iris Lisch nodules, and cutaneous neurofibromas, among other manifestations.
- Patients with neurofibromatosis may develop periodontitis, gingival hyperplasia, enamel defects, and dental and skeletal abnormalities.
- Neurofibromatosis type 1 can reduce life expectancy due to malignant transformation or vasculopathy.
- As ill-defined tumours have a high risk of recurrence, imaging with MRI is used to determine tumour extent before surgical excision.

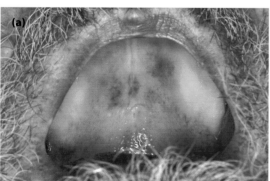 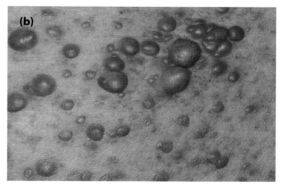

Figure 10.4 (a and b). Patient has neurofibromatosis type 1. (a) Biopsy-proven diffuse neurofibroma on hard palate presenting as telangiectases and yellowish papules; (b) cutaneous pedunculated neurofibromas.

Reproduced from Health NZ – Waikato (www.waikatodhb.health.nz) with permission.

Schwannoma

A schwannoma (neurilemmoma) is a benign encapsulated neoplasm of Schwann cells in the nerve sheath or perineurium. There are several histological variants.
- Up to 50% of schwannomas occur in the head and neck region, but they are rare in the mouth.
- A schwannoma usually involves a spinal root nerve, cervical, sympathetic, vagus, or ulnar nerve.
- Multiple schwannomas are associated with neurofibromatosis type 2.

Clinical features

Schwannoma presents as an asymptomatic, solitary, smooth, submucosal swelling.
- The most common oral sites for schwannoma are the tongue (see *Fig. 10.5*) and lips, but schwannoma may also affect other mucosal sites.

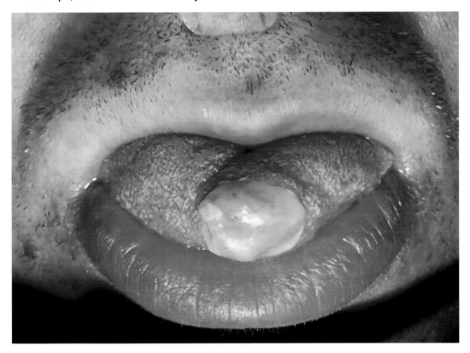

Figure 10.5. Schwannoma of the tip of the tongue. A partially ulcerated mass on the anterior tongue.

Reproduced from *Head and Neck Pathol.* 2020;14:571 (https://doi.org/10.1007/s12105-019-01071-9), with permission from Springer Nature, and included here after enhancement by AIPDerm (www.aipderm.com).

Treatment

Intraoral schwannoma is generally harmless, and treatment may not be necessary. It has a good prognosis, with no recurrence if completely excised.

Granular cell tumour

A granular cell tumour is diagnosed by histopathology, which reveals a mass of cells with eosinophilic cytoplasm and a granular appearance.

- Granular cell tumours are rare.
- Up to 65% occur in the head and neck region, with 70% in the oral cavity and 25% on the tongue.
- Others arise on the skin, in the gastrointestinal tract, or elsewhere.
- Granular cell tumours most often occur in the 2nd and 6th decades of life, but may occur at any age.
- Congenital cases have been reported.
- They are twice as common in women as in men.

Causes

Granular cell tumours are thought to originate from Schwann cells in the peripheral nerve sheath. Genetic mutations have been described.

Clinical features

Oral granular cell tumour presents as an asymptomatic yellow, brown, or pink nodule on the tongue (see *Fig. 10.6*), buccal mucosa, or hard palate. Although usually solitary, multiple lesions may occur.

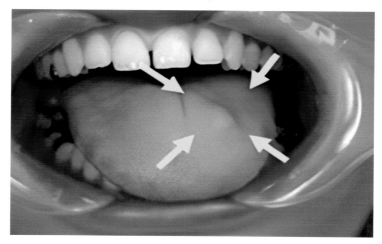

Figure 10.6. Granular cell tumour presenting as a nodule on the dorsum of the tongue (arrows).

Reproduced from *Head Face Med.* 2018;14:1 (https://doi.org/10.1186/s13005-017-0158-9), under a CC BY-4.0 licence, and included here after enhancement by AIPDerm (www.aipderm.com).

Diagnosis

A definitive diagnosis is made following a biopsy and histopathological examination. About 1–2% are classified as malignant.

Treatment

Local excision of a benign granular cell tumour with wide margins is curative with a good prognosis.

Mucosal neuroma

Mucosal neuroma is a cutaneous neural component of MEN 2B syndrome, an autosomal dominant disorder associated with thyroid carcinoma and phaeochromocytoma. See also *Section 5.2.11*.

- Mucosal neuroma presents with multiple tumours on the tongue (see *Fig. 10.7*), gingiva, and buccal mucosa and enlarged lips.
- Early diagnosis is crucial due to the poor prognosis of late diagnosis of MEN 2B in affected patients.
- Diagnosis is confirmed by molecular genetic testing.

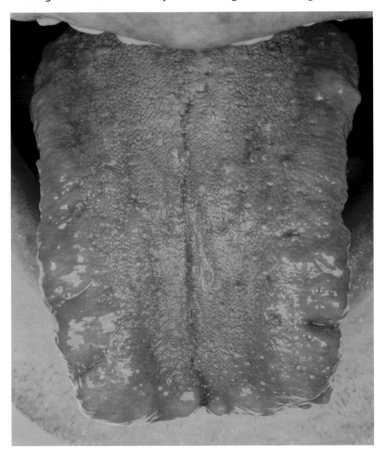

Figure 10.7. Multiple mucosal neuromas on the tongue of a patient with MEN 2B.

Reproduced from Health NZ – Waikato (www.waikatodhb.health.nz) with permission.

10.1.5   Haemangioma

Haemangioma describes a group of common benign blood vessel tumours. The classification of blood vessel tumours is complex, confusing, and evolving. Infantile proliferative haemangioma may rarely occur in the mouth. See also *Section 5.1.3* for additional information.

Capillary haemangiomas are due to small vessel proliferation, and cavernous haemangiomas affect larger, deeper vessels or sinusoids.

- Intraoral sites include tongue, lips, buccal mucosa, gingiva, and palatal mucosa.
- Typically, there is a single soft, solitary, flat or nodular (sessile) mass.
- Its surface can be smooth or lobulated, purple or deep red in colour (see *Fig. 10.8*).
- A haemangioma may or may not blanch on applying pressure using a transparent slide (diascopy).

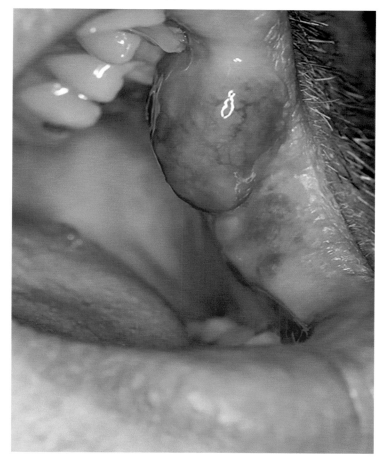

Figure 10.8. Unclassified vascular lesion on the inner lip.

Reproduced from Health NZ – Waikato (www.waikatodhb.health.nz) with permission.

Infantile haemangioma

Infantile proliferative haemangioma arises during the first 2 months of life. It usually proliferates for 6–12 months, and then involutes over 5–10 years.

- About 10% of infantile haemangiomas persist into adult life.
- About 6% of newborns develop one or more haemangiomas. They are more common in preterm infants, babies with low birth weight, and those with European ancestry compared to other races.
- There is a 3:1 female predilection.
- Although 60% of cases of infantile proliferative haemangioma occur in the head and neck region, it is rare in the oral cavity.
- A true congenital haemangioma is uncommon. It is usually stable, neither proliferating nor involuting.

Causes

Infantile haemangioma arises from the proliferation of endothelial cells. The cause is not fully understood, with contributions from genetic mutations, vascular endothelial growth factors, placental injury, and hormonal influences.

Clinical features

An infantile haemangioma is an enlarging soft or firm, red or purple nodule (see *Fig. 10.9*). It may blanch on pressure.

- The surface of an infantile haemangioma may be smooth or lobulated.
- Common intraoral sites are the tongue, lips, gingiva, palate, and buccal mucosa.
- Subtypes of infantile haemangioma include capillary, cavernous and mixed haemangioma. In the oral cavity, the bones and muscles may be affected as well as the mucosa and skin.
- Haemangiomas are associated with various syndromes.
- Complications include ulceration, bleeding, dysphagia, speech impairment, and airway compromise.

(a) 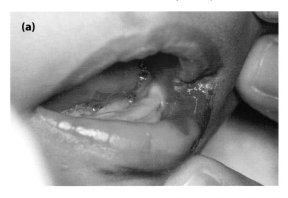 (b)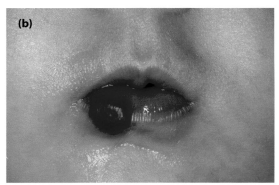

Figure 10.9 (a and b). Infantile proliferative haemangioma.

Reproduced from Health NZ – Waikato (www.waikatodhb.health.nz) with permission.

Diagnosis

The diagnosis of haemangioma is generally based on history and clinical findings. Biopsy is rarely necessary and may be complicated by bleeding.

Treatment

A small infantile haemangioma requires no intervention and will regress with time. A multidisciplinary team often manages a large lesion, especially if it interferes with feeding or other functions. Those requiring intervention may be treated by:
- topical or oral beta-blocker
- systemic steroids
- intralesional sclerosing injections
- laser therapy
- cryotherapy.

10.1.6 Angioleiomyoma

Angioleiomyoma is a benign tumour of vascular smooth muscle origin. Oral angioleiomyomas are rare.
- An angioleiomyoma presents as a firm asymptomatic dome-shaped nodule.
- Multiple lesions may occur.
- The tumour is often red like adjacent mucosa but may be bluish.
- The most common oral sites are the lips, palate, buccal mucosa, and tongue.
- The recommended management is local excision. Recurrence is uncommon.

10.1.7 Rhabdomyoma

Rhabdomyoma is a benign tumour derived from striated muscle. Oral rhabdomyomas are rare and tend to affect middle-aged or older patients.
- Rhabdomyoma presents as an asymptomatic nodule that can grow into a large tumour.
- Common oral sites are the soft palate, floor of the mouth, and base of the tongue.
- Surgical excision results in recurrence in up to 42% of cases.

10.1.8 Peripheral ameloblastoma

Peripheral ameloblastoma occurs exclusively in the soft tissues of the gingiva.
- Its most common site is the mandibular lingual gingiva in the premolar region.
- It is an ulcerated, exophytic or lobular, purple mass (see *Fig. 10.10*).
- The histology resembles intraosseous ameloblastoma.
- Peripheral ameloblastoma is less aggressive than intraosseous ameloblastoma and recurs less frequently after surgical excision.

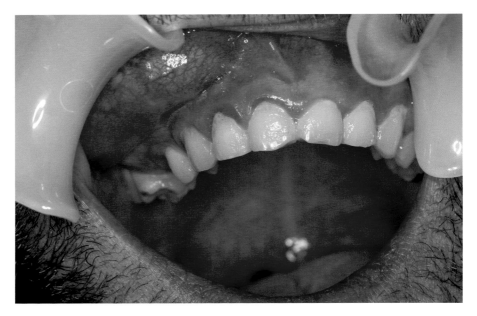

Figure 10.10. Peripheral ameloblastoma.

Reproduced from Health NZ – Waikato (www.waikatodhb.health.nz) with permission.

10.1.9   Rare odontogenic tumours

Other benign odontogenic tumours rarely occur peripherally without a bony component.

- Calcifying epithelial odontogenic tumour
- Adenomatoid odontogenic tumour
- Cementoblastoma
- Cemento-ossifying fibroma.

Non-neoplastic bone lesions such as fibrous dysplasia and osseous dysplasia may also present as a diffuse swelling of the alveolar bone.

10.2   Benign salivary gland tumours

The World Health Organization Histological Classification of Salivary Gland Tumours (4th edition, 2017) recognizes three common benign salivary gland tumours:

- Pleomorphic adenoma
- Warthin tumour
- Sialadenoma papilliferum.

10.2.1   Pleomorphic adenoma

Approximately two-thirds of all salivary gland tumours are pleomorphic adenomas, also known as 'mixed tumours' due to the derivation of cells from epithelial and myoepithelial origins. Pleomorphic adenomas occur in middle age, with a slight female predilection.

Pleomorphic adenomas comprise:
- 50–77% of parotid gland tumours
- 53–72% of submandibular gland tumours
- 33–41% of minor salivary gland tumours.

Causes

The cause of the pleomorphic adenoma is mainly unknown. Most tumours show cytogenetic aberrations, including chromosomal translocation, which activates one of the two genes: *PLAG1* or *HMGA2*.
- Other chromosomal abnormalities involve oncogenes and tumour suppressor genes.
- Prior radiation to the head and neck increases the risk of developing pleomorphic adenoma.

Clinical features

A pleomorphic adenoma is a slowly enlarging, painless, well-circumscribed, firm, rubbery mass (see *Fig. 10.11*).
- Intraoral sites include the palate, upper lip, and buccal mucosa.
- They are more commonly located unilaterally in the superficial lobe of the parotid gland in front of the ear. They may cause eversion of the ear lobe, if situated in the parotid tail.
- Rapid enlargement of the mass or facial nerve involvement should also raise a concern about malignant transformation.

Diagnosis

A definitive diagnosis is required to exclude a malignant tumour of the salivary gland.

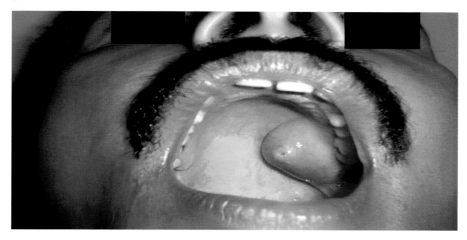

Figure 10.11. Pleomorphic adenoma of the palate; a firm, well-circumscribed, smooth swelling on the posterior aspect of the left half of the hard palate.

Reproduced from *A Digital Manual for the Early Diagnosis of Oral Neoplasia,* 2008, International Agency for Research on Cancer, with permission, and included here after enhancement by AIPDerm (www. aipderm.com).

- Imaging studies (ultrasound, CT scan, and MRI) may be used to gather information before the biopsy.
- Fine needle aspirate or incisional biopsy may be undertaken for histopathological examination.

Treatment

Pleomorphic adenoma is cured by surgical resection with an appropriate margin.
- Simple nucleation of the tumour is associated with a high risk of recurrence.
- The risk of recurrence is greatest within 18 months of resection and occurs in 7–15% of cases.
- There is a 5% chance of malignant transformation within the tumour.

10.2.2   Warthin tumour

A Warthin tumour is often called an adenolymphoma because it is composed of lymphoid tissue.
- It is an encapsulated tumour with unique histology.
- Warthin tumours comprise up to 25% of all salivary gland tumours.
- They almost always affect the parotid gland and comprise up to 30% of parotid tumours.
- They may be multifocal and are bilateral in up to 17% of patients.
- The tumour commonly occurs in middle age with a male predilection.
- It is eight times as common in smokers compared to non-smokers.

Causes

The Warthin tumour develops from heterotopic salivary ducts trapped within intra-parotid or para-parotid lymphoid tissue.

Clinical features

A Warthin tumour is a slowly enlarging, painless, firm, or fluctuating mass in the parotid gland (see *Fig. 10.12*).
- It rarely occurs within the oral cavity.
- Patients may experience pain, pressure, and acute parotitis if the mass ruptures.
- The tumour is frequently located near the tail of the parotid gland.

Diagnosis

The diagnosis of Warthin tumour is made by biopsy.
- Imaging studies (ultrasound, CT scan, and MRI) may be used to gather information before the biopsy.
- Fine needle aspirate or incisional biopsy for histopathological examination reveals a dense lymphoid stroma and a double layer of oncocytic epithelium with papillary and cystic architecture.

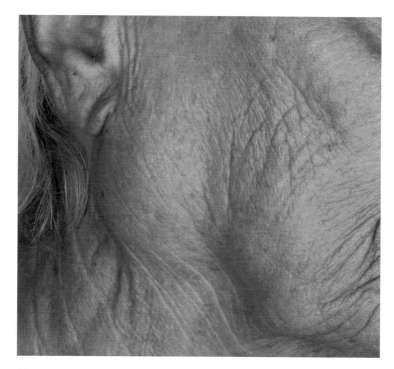

Figure 10.12. Warthin tumour in right parotid gland resulting in swelling over the right jawline.

Reproduced from Health NZ – Waikato (www.waikatodhb.health.nz) with permission.

Treatment

A Warthin tumour is removed by surgical resection, which is curative unless the tumour is multifocal.

- The risk of recurrence is up to 6%.
- Malignant transformation to lymphoma, adenocarcinoma, mucoepidermoid carcinoma, oncocytic carcinoma, salivary duct carcinoma, or Warthin adenocarcinoma is rare (0.3%).

10.2.3   Sialadenoma papilliferum

Sialadenoma papilliferum is a rare benign intraductal tumour found in older adults.

- It has an exophytic growth pattern with multiple papillary surface fronds and deeper duct-like structures, which may be continuous with the surface epithelium.
- It accounts for fewer than 1% of all minor salivary gland tumours and 3–5% of head and neck tumours.
- The peak incidence is in the fifth, sixth and seventh decades of life.

Causes

The origin of sialadenoma papilliferum is thought to be excretory duct reserve cells that can differentiate into either ductal or squamous cells.

Clinical features

Sialadenoma papilliferum occurs mainly in the hard palate and less commonly in the soft palate, buccal mucosa, nasal cavity, upper lip, parotid glands, and rarely in the bronchus and oesophagus.
- It is a slow-growing, painless, exophytic, round to oval, white papillary mass.
- Histology shows the fusion of the complex ductal component with the surface epithelium.

Treatment

Sialadenoma papilliferum is treated by conservative surgical resection with a good prognosis.

10.2.4 Other benign salivary gland tumours

The other benign salivary gland tumours are solitary, firm, but mobile nodules within the major or minor salivary glands. They are usually painless and slowly enlarging.
- Myoepithelioma
- Basal cell adenoma
- Oncocytoma
- Lymphadenoma
- Cystadenoma
- Ductal papilloma
- Sebaceous adenoma
- Canalicular adenoma and other ductal adenomas.

A definitive diagnosis is made on histology, either from a fine-needle aspirate, incisional biopsy, or excisional biopsy. Complete surgical excision is usually curative, with a good prognosis.

10.3 Oral potentially malignant disorders

Oral potentially malignant disorders (OPMDs) are associated with an increased risk of malignant transformation to squamous cell carcinoma (SCC) compared with normal oral mucosa. Factors affecting malignant transformation include:
- patient demographics
- risk factors for malignancy
- lesion appearance, size, and anatomical location
- the presence and grade of epithelial dysplasia at the time of biopsy.

See also:
- *Section 4.5.1: Submucous fibrosis and verrucous hyperplasia; Section 4.6.4: Lichenoid drug eruption; Section 4.9.1: Acanthosis nigricans; Section 4.9.2: Plummer–Vinson syndrome*
- *Section 5.2.2: Dyskeratosis congenita; Section 5.2.3: Epidermolysis bullosa; Section 5.2.4: Fanconi anaemia*
- *Section 7.2.1: Oral lichen planus; Section 7.2.2: Oral lichenoid reaction; Section 7.2.4: Graft-versus-host disease; Section 7.2.5: Lupus erythematosus*

10.3.1 Actinic keratosis of the lip

Actinic keratosis is the dysplastic keratinization of the vermilion of the lip due to chronic sun exposure.

It is also known as:
- solar keratosis of the lip
- solar cheilosis
- actinic cheilitis.

Actinic keratosis of the lip is common in white-skinned people living in the tropics or Australasia. It is rare in dark-skinned people or those living in the higher latitudes of the northern hemisphere. Prevalence ranges between 0.9% and 43.24% of the population, depending on the geographic region and skin colour.

Causes

Actinic keratosis of the lip is primarily due to exposure to ultraviolet (UV) B (wavelength 290–320nm) and UVA (320–400nm) in solar radiation.

Risk factors include:
- chronic exposure to sunlight
- previous keratinocyte cancer
- older age
- male sex
- fair skin
- smoking and alcohol abuse
- immunosuppression
- a genetic condition such as albinism or xeroderma pigmentosum.

Individuals with Fitzpatrick skin types I and II are most at risk. The vermilion has few melanocytes and is thinly keratinized, so it is poorly protected from UV.
- UV radiation damages DNA and releases hydroxyl and oxygen radicals, which contribute indirectly to DNA damage.
- UVB has been considered a complete carcinogen because of its ability to initiate the genetic alteration of epithelial cells, including the inactivation of *p53*, and promote the expansion of clones of transformed cells.
- UVA also causes DNA mutations and penetrates more deeply than UVB, impairing DNA repair and reducing immune surveillance.

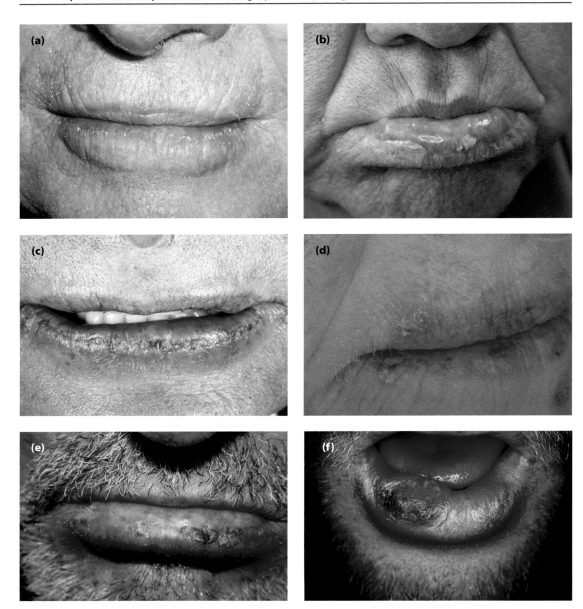

Figure 10.13 (a–f). Actinic cheilitis presenting with (a and b) keratotic white papules and plaques with adherent scale, (c) crusted hyperkeratotic erosions, (d) actinic keratoses on the cutaneous lip, (d) erythema, scale, and ulceration; (e and f) an ulcerated nodule indicates transformation to squamous cell carcinoma.

All images reproduced from Health NZ – Waikato (www.waikatodhb.health.nz) with permission.

Clinical features

The individual with actinic keratosis of the lip is typically a middle-aged or older fair-skinned male with a history of significant outdoor exposure who presents with focal or diffuse dryness and epithelial atrophy of the vermilion of the lower lip.

Other features:
- Adherent scale (see *Fig. 10.13a*), keratotic white plaques (see *Fig. 10.13b*), superficial erosions and vertical fissures (see *Fig. 10.13c*), and erythema or pallor
- Loss of demarcation between the vermilion border of the lip and its adjacent skin
- A fine, sandpapery texture on palpation
- There may be adjacent cutaneous actinic keratoses (see *Fig. 10.13d*)
- Palpable thickening, induration, and ulceration may indicate invasive SCC (see *Fig. 10.13e*). The risk of intraepidermal or invasive SCC is higher for actinic keratosis of the lip than for actinic keratosis on the skin.

Diagnosis

Actinic keratosis of the lip is diagnosed clinically supported by dermoscopy and, if available, *in vivo* reflectance confocal microscopy (RCM). Histopathology is confirmatory.
- Obtain a detailed history of outdoor lifestyle, smoking, and alcohol consumption.
- Photography is helpful for documentation and monitoring.
- A biopsy of any persistent thickened or persistently ulcerated area should be performed if malignant transformation is suspected.
- Histopathology of actinic keratosis ranges from atrophy to hyperplasia of the squamous cell epithelium of the vermilion border with varying degrees of keratinization, disordered maturation, increased mitotic activity, and cytological atypia.
- Drop-shaped epithelial rete pegs are often present, but the basement membrane is intact. The underlying connective tissue shows basophilic degeneration (solar elastosis) and perivascular inflammation.

Treatment

Patients should be advised to limit further sun exposure lifelong and year-round.
- Peak exposure to UV radiation is at solar noon. Danger to the skin is expressed as UV Index, which ranges from 0 to 25 (this maximum has been recorded in Altiplano in South America at a high altitude on a clear day). Exposure depends on latitude, altitude, and cloud cover. For example, in midsummer in Auckland, New Zealand, UV radiation remains high (UV Index ≥6) at sea level between 10 am and 5 pm if the sky is clear. On the same day in London, UK, the UV Index does not rise above 0.4 at noon in midwinter, even on a cloudless day.
- Patients can download a smartphone app to determine the risk of sunburn at the current time wherever they are (e.g. GlobalUV™).
- They should be advised to wear a protective broad-brimmed hat and apply sun protection factor (SPF) 50+ broad-spectrum sunscreen lip balm every morning, with re-application every 2 hours when outdoors.

Treatment options for actinic cheilitis:
- Emollient (lip balm)
- Cryotherapy

- 5-fluorouracil cream or imiquimod cream (the lip is an unapproved site in New Zealand and Australia)
- Photodynamic therapy
- Curettage and electrosurgery
- Excision, including vermilionectomy
- Laser ablation.

Treatment may need to be repeated due to high rates of relapse.

Patients with actinic keratosis require periodic follow-ups.
- The patient should present for reassessment if they develop any lip thickening or a sore that persists for more than 3 weeks.
- Smoking cessation and moderate alcohol consumption should be recommended.

10.3.2   Leukoplakia

The 11th edition of the International Classification of Diseases released by the World Health Organization in 2021* defines leukoplakia as "a predominantly white lesion of the oral mucosa that cannot be characterized as any other definable lesion".
- Leukoplakia is potentially malignant.
- The incidence and prevalence of leukoplakia vary throughout the world, with a reported prevalence of 0.2–5%.
- Leukoplakia most frequently affects middle-aged and older men.

Causes

Nearly 75% of leukoplakia lesions are associated with tobacco use. Alcohol may contribute. In a small percentage of cases, the cause is unknown (idiopathic leukoplakia).

Clinical features

Leukoplakia presents as persistent solitary or multiple white plaques within the oral cavity that cannot be explained by the other entities discussed in this chapter.
- The most common sites are buccal mucosa, alveolar mucosa, and the floor of the mouth, tongue, lips, and palate.
- There is a fixed plaque that cannot be wiped off with gauze.

Two clinical types of leukoplakia are recognized: homogeneous and non-homogeneous leukoplakia.

Homogeneous leukoplakia
- Homogeneous leukoplakia is a uniform, predominantly white, flat, thin plaque with shallow fissures.

(* 'Leukoplakia', ICD-11 Coding Tool, Mortality and Morbidity Statistics (MMS) 2021-05 at https://icd.who.int/ct11/icd11_mms/en/release).

- The surface is consistently smooth, wrinkled, or corrugated (see *Figs. 10.14a* and *b*).
- It is usually asymptomatic and incidentally detected during a routine oral examination.

Non-homogeneous leukoplakia
- Non-homogeneous leukoplakia is an irregular, predominantly white (see *Fig. 10.14c*) or white-and-red plaque (erythroleukoplakia) (see *Fig. 10.14d*).
- It may be flat, nodular (speckled leukoplakia), or exophytic with papules (exophytic or verrucous leukoplakia) (see *Fig. 10.14e*). It often causes mild localized pain or discomfort.
- Proliferative verrucous leukoplakia is a multifocal verrucous aggressive lesion that carries high malignant potential (see *Fig. 10.14f*).

Diagnosis

Leukoplakia is diagnosed by taking a detailed history and conducting an examination. The exclusion of other definable white lesions establishes the diagnosis of leukoplakia. Leukoplakia should undergo a biopsy.
- Toluidine blue 1% stains tissues rich in DNA and can be applied directly to a lesion to screen for epithelial dysplasia, reveal the margins of a lesion, and guide a biopsy site.
- Histopathology of oral leukoplakia includes orthokeratosis with a prominent granular cell layer, parakeratosis, and acanthosis. Between 20% and 50% of lesions will show dysplasia.
- Epithelial dysplasia is identified by nuclear hyperchromatism, loss of polarity, mitotic figures, nuclear pleomorphism, altered nuclear-to-cytoplasmic ratio, deep cell keratinization, and the loss of differentiation and intercellular adherence.
- The degree of epithelial dysplasia may be mild, moderate, or severe. Total thickness epithelial dysplasia changes the diagnosis to carcinoma *in situ*.

Treatment
- Surgical excision
- Cryotherapy
- Carbon dioxide laser ablation
- Topical or intralesional bleomycin
- Systemic retinoid
- Systemic lycopene.

Tobacco cessation and avoiding alcohol are aimed to minimize further epithelial dysplasia and progression to SCC.
- Leukoplakia with mild dysplasia can regress spontaneously.
- The risk of SCC arising within leukoplakia ranges from 0.12–17.51%.
- Smoking cessation after surgical removal of oral leukoplakia reduces the risk of malignant transformation.

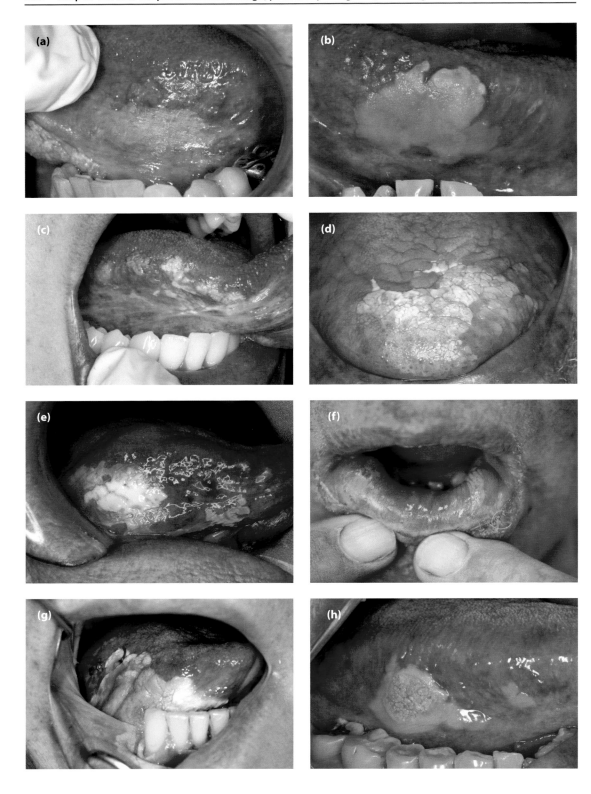

◄ **Figure 10.14 (a–h).** (a–d) Homogeneous leukoplakia (benign hyperkeratosis on biopsy); (e and f) non-homogeneous leukoplakia with intraepithelial neoplasia on biopsy; (g and h) verrucous leukoplakia.

Reproduced with permission from: (a) Professor Isaac Vander Waal, VU Medical Center, Amsterdam, The Netherlands; (b and h) Professor Kobkan Thongprasom, Faculty of Dentistry, Chulalongkorn University, Bangkok, Thailand; (c) Professor Nagamani Narayana, University of Nebraska Medical Centre, NE, USA; (d–f) Health NZ – Waikato (www.waikatodhb.health.nz); (g) Professor Yeshwant Rawal, University of Milwaukee School of Dentistry, Milwaukee, WI, USA.

10.3.3   Erythroplakia

Erythroplakia of the oral mucosa is an uncommon red plaque that cannot be clinically or pathologically diagnosed as any other definable disease. It is usually diagnosed in middle-aged to elderly patients with a male preponderance.

Causes

Risk factors for erythroplakia include tobacco use, excessive alcohol consumption, and betel quid chewing.

Clinical features

Erythroplakia presents as persistent solitary irregular, well-defined, smooth, or granular, velvety-red atrophic and non-indurated plaque (see *Fig. 10.15a* and *b*). Multiple plaques occur occasionally.
- Erythroplakia is often asymptomatic.
- The most common sites are the floor of the mouth, the tongue, the soft palate, and the buccal mucosa.
- A mixed red and white irregular plaque is called erythroleukoplakia.

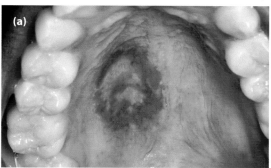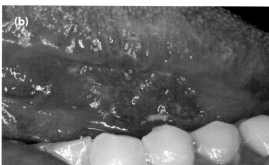

Figure 10.15 (a and b). Erythroplakia of (a) palate and (b) tongue.

Reproduced with permission from Professor Yeshwant Rawal, University of Milwaukee School of Dentistry, Milwaukee, WI, USA.

Diagnosis

A definitive diagnosis of erythroplakia requires a biopsy. Once inflammatory and infective causes of the red plaque are excluded, 70–90% are carcinoma *in situ* or invasive SCC on histopathology.

Dermoscopy of a carcinoma *in situ* reveals irregularly distributed, polymorphous, dot and clod vessels.

Treatment

The treatment of erythroplakia is dependent on histology.
- Smoking cessation reduces the risk of malignant transformation.
- Surgical excision is usually indicated for carcinoma *in situ*.
- Oral SCC may require single or multimodal treatment.

10.3.4   Reverse smoker's palate

Reverse smoking refers to smoking with the burning end of the smoking device inside the mouth. This practice occurs in some communities in India, the Philippines, South America, and the Caribbean.

The hard palate and tongue are damaged by the combustion products of tobacco and extreme heat.

Clinical features

Reverse smoker's palate may be hypopigmented (see *Fig. 10.16*) or present with irregular elevated white, red, hyperpigmented and hypopigmented patches and plaques on the hard palate and tongue. Lesions are not removable by scraping.
- Reverse smoker's palate may be asymptomatic or symptomatic.
- Ulceration is suspicious of malignancy.

Diagnosis

The diagnosis depends on a history of reverse smoking. A biopsy is essential if any features suggest non-healing ulceration or SCC.

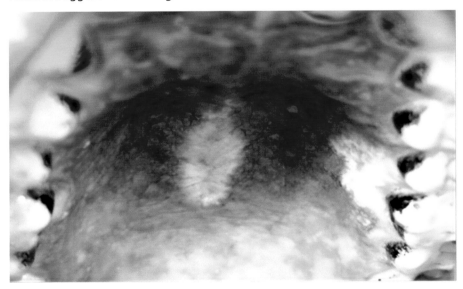

Figure 10.16. Reverse smoker's palate showing a hypopigmented patch.

Reproduced with permission from *Pocket Dentistry* (Smoker's palate; www.pocketdentistry.com), and included here after enhancement by AIPDerm (www.aipderm.com).

Histopathology may reveal any of the following features:
- Orthokeratosis or parakeratosis
- Melanin pigmentation in or below the basal cell layer
- An inflammatory cell infiltrate in the connective tissue
- Mild, moderate, or severe epithelial dysplasia (SCC *in situ*)
- Invasive SCC.

Treatment

Treatment of reverse smoker's palate depends on the clinical and histopathologic findings. It should include the following:
- Cessation of any form of tobacco use
- Surgical excision of malignancy
- Periodic follow-up.

10.4 Malignant lesions of the oral mucosa

Oral malignancies include squamous cell carcinoma and salivary gland malignancies, among others. Their management and prognosis depend on staging, i.e. the extent of the tumour locoregionally and at distant sites.

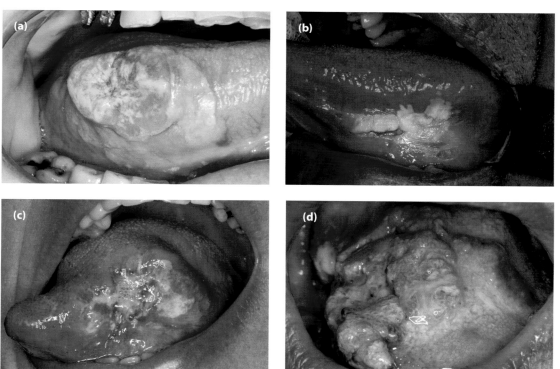

Figure 10.17 (a–d). Squamous cell carcinoma of the tongue.

(a) Reproduced with permission from Professor Yeshwant Rawal, University of Milwaukee School of Dentistry, Milwaukee, WI, USA; (b–d) reproduced from Health NZ – Waikato (www.waikatodhb.health.nz) with permission.

10.4.1   Squamous cell carcinoma

Oral SCC is the most common malignant epithelial neoplasm of the oral cavity (90% of all oral neoplasms), with an annual incidence of 300 000 cases globally.
- Increasing age is a significant risk factor for oral SCC, with the male-to-female ratio approximately 2:1.
- Recently, there has been a rise in incidence among females aged 18–44.
- An asymptomatic OPMD precedes most cases.

Causes

Risk factors for oral SCC:
- Tobacco use
- Excessive alcohol consumption
- Betel quid use
- High-risk human papillomavirus infection (HPV-16 and 18).

An oral potentially malignant disorder predisposes to oral SCC.

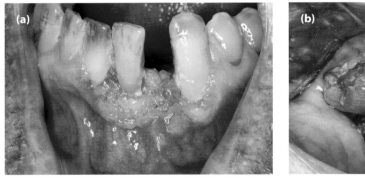
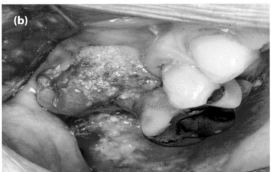
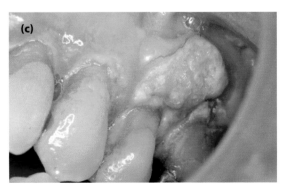
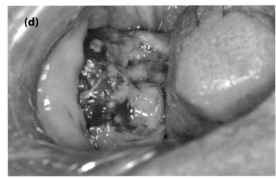

Figure 10.18 (a–d). Squamous cell carcinoma: (a and b) alveolar, (c) associated with lichen planus, and (d) retromolar.

(a and c) Reproduced from Health NZ – Waikato (www.waikatodhb.health.nz) with permission; (b) reproduced with permission from Professor Nagamani Narayana, University of Nebraska Medical Centre, NE, USA; (d) reproduced with permission from Professor Kobkan Thongprasom, Faculty of Dentistry, Chulalongkorn University, Bangkok, Thailand.

Clinical features

Oral SCC most commonly presents as a red or white nodule (see *Figs 10.17–19*).

- Common sites for oral SCC include the floor of the mouth, lateral/ventral tongue, and retromolar trigone.
- Ulceration and induration are frequently observed.
- Oral SCC may have an exophytic fungating (cauliflower-like) growth mass or have a verrucous hyperkeratotic or papillary surface.
- 3% of oral SCCs are classified as verrucous carcinoma (see *Fig. 10.20*).
- Early oral SCC may be asymptomatic. Pain, paraesthesia, and tethering / reduced tissue mobility may indicate advanced disease.

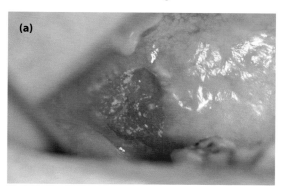

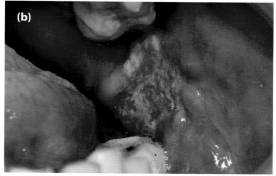

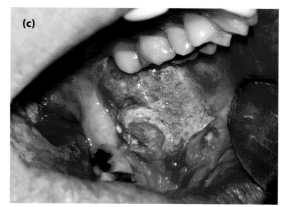

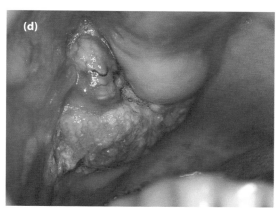

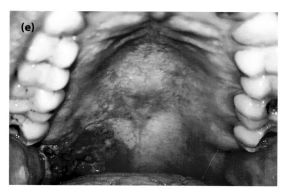

Figure 10.19 (a–e). Squamous cell carcinoma: (a–d) buccal and (e) palatal.

(a) Reproduced with permission from Professor Kobkan Thongprasom, Faculty of Dentistry, Chulalongkorn University, Bangkok, Thailand; (b and d) reproduced from Health NZ – Waikato (www.waikatodhb.health.nz) with permission; (c) reproduced with permission from Professor Nagamani Narayana, University of Nebraska Medical Centre, NE, USA; (e) reproduced with permission from Professor Yeshwant Rawal, University of Milwaukee School of Dentistry, Milwaukee, WI, USA.

Diagnosis

Dermoscopy may show irregular keratinization and polymorphous vessels. A definitive diagnosis of oral SCC requires a biopsy.
- The histopathology reveals invasive tumour islands in the connective tissue arising from a dysplastic epithelium with varying surface keratinization.
- A verrucous carcinoma shows papillomatosis, marked hyperkeratosis and parakeratosis, and a broad 'pushing' deep tumour margin.

Treatment

Staging requires evaluation of the neck for regional lymphadenopathy; head, neck, and chest CT scan; and PET scanning to check for distant disease.
- Most oral SCCs are managed surgically, with adjuvant radiation or chemoradiation for suspected or confirmed locoregional or distant spread.
- The 5-year survival after diagnosis of oral SCC is 40–50%.
- Locoregional spread to lymph nodes is a poor prognostic feature, reducing the survival rate by 50%.
- Metastases initially affect the regional lymph nodes and, later, the lungs.
- Verrucous carcinoma has a high tendency for local invasion and a low propensity for dissemination, resulting in a better prognosis than the more common types of oral SCC.

Oral verrucous carcinoma

Oral verrucous carcinoma is a locally aggressive, exophytic, low-grade, slow-growing variant of well-differentiated SCC. It has low metastatic potential.
- Oral verrucous carcinoma shows geographic variation in its incidence.
- It is mainly diagnosed in older men, usually around the age of 60.

Causes

Oral verrucous carcinoma is strongly associated with smoking or chewing tobacco. Other potential causes are:
- betel quid (paan) and areca nut chewing
- alcohol
- HPV.

Precursors include leukoplakia, oral verrucous hyperplasia (see *Section 4.5.1*), and oral lichenoid reaction (see *Chapter 6*).

Clinical features

Oral verrucous carcinoma presents as a painless, thick white plaque or mass with blunt (*see Figs 10.20a* and *b*) or pointed surface projections.

The most common sites of oral mucosal verrucous carcinoma are the buccal mucosa, the mandibular alveolar crest, the gingiva, the tongue, and the lips.

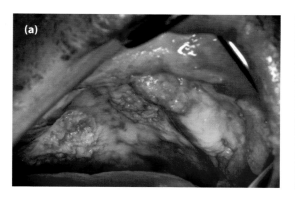
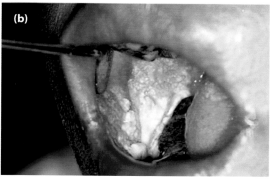

Figure 10.20 (a and b). (a) Multiple verrucous carcinomas within intraoral proliferative verrucous leukoplakia and (b) in a betel nut chewer.

(a) Reproduced from Health NZ – Waikato (www.waikatodhb.health.nz) with permission; (b) reproduced from *A Digital Manual for the Early Diagnosis of Oral Neoplasia*, 2008, International Agency for Research on Cancer, with permission, and included here after enhancement by AIPDerm (www.aipderm.com).

Treatment

The primary treatment for verrucous carcinoma is surgical excision. The 5-year survival rate is 80–90%. Irradiation alone or in combination with surgery is rarely performed.

Oral carcinoma cuniculatum

Oral carcinoma cuniculatum is a variant of verrucous squamous cell carcinoma.

Causes

Carcinoma cuniculatum has been associated with:
- tobacco
- alcohol
- trauma
- HPV infection.

Clinical features

Oral carcinoma cuniculatum is a locally aggressive tumour with multiple, branching, keratin-filled crypts known as rabbit burrows or cuniculi. It has a white to pink, slightly pebbly or papillary surface.
- Oral carcinoma cuniculatum occurs most commonly on the mucoperiosteum of the mandibular gingiva, where it may invade bone. It may also appear on the tongue.
- It is usually symptomatic, causing localized pain and swelling.
- Carcinoma cuniculatum may also arise on the face, abdomen, palm, leg, foot, oesophagus, penis, and cervix.

Diagnosis

The diagnosis of oral carcinoma cuniculatum is made by clinical, histological, and radiographic correlation.

Treatment

Oral carcinoma cuniculatum is treated by surgical resection with a wide margin.

It has a good prognosis following appropriate surgical treatment, with a low recurrence rate.

10.4.2 Melanoma

Melanoma is a malignant melanocytic neoplasm. Cutaneous melanoma is common in the skin of white sun-exposed individuals, especially those residing in Australia and New Zealand.
- Primary oral melanoma is rare and behaves aggressively.
- The average age at diagnosis is 60 years.
- It is more frequently diagnosed in Japanese, black, and Indian populations.

Causes

The cause or causes of oral melanoma are unknown.
- Many cutaneous melanomas are induced by solar irradiation. However, the oral mucosa is protected from sun exposure.
- Many genes are implicated in the development of melanoma. Oral melanoma is associated with mutations in *c-KIT* (CD117) in about 20% of patients. About 10% have mutations in *BRAF*, compared with 40–59% of cutaneous melanomas.

Clinical features

Oral melanoma may be *in situ* (in 15% of patients), resembling cutaneous lentigo maligna, invasive (in 30%), or both (in 55%).
- Melanoma may develop in or near an existing naevus, within mucosal melanosis, or in healthy-appearing skin or mucosa.
- Melanomas tend to occur on the hard palate and gingiva. Intraoral melanomas may be primary (*de novo*) or secondary (metastatic) lesions.
- Melanomas usually present as irregular dark blue–black macules (see *Fig. 10.21a*) or plaques but may be light brown, red, or, more often, variable colours.
- Advanced tumours present as irregular nodules and plaques. Mucosal ulceration may be present (see *Figs 10.21b* and *c*).
- Lymph node metastases are detected in about 30% of oral melanoma patients at the time of diagnosis.

Diagnosis

The first steps in the diagnostic process are a complete medical and dental history and a clinical examination of the lesion, including dermoscopy. Regional lymph nodes should also be evaluated.
- Dermoscopy of melanoma shows asymmetry of structure, colour, and border abruptness, with multiple colours including grey structures and thickened lines.

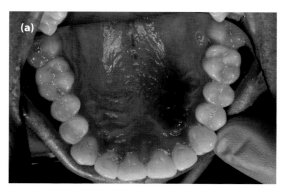

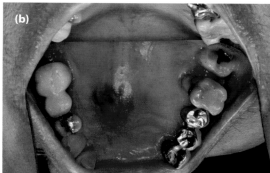

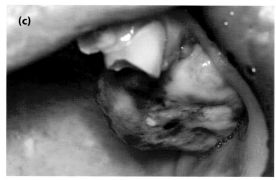

Figure 10.21 (a–c). Melanoma of the palate: (a and b) early and (c) advanced.

(c) Reproduced from Health NZ – Waikato (www.waikatodhb. health.nz) with permission.

- Where possible, a suspicious oral pigmented lesion should undergo an excisional biopsy for histopathological examination, including special stains such as S-100, HMB-45, and fatty acid synthase, which are positive in nearly all oral melanomas.
- Imaging studies, such as ultrasound scans or CT, may be used to determine the extent of melanoma.
- Tumour staging for mucosal melanoma differs from cutaneous melanoma in that there is no T1 or T2 stage.

Treatment

Multidisciplinary care is usually arranged for oral mucosal melanoma.
- Aggressive surgery for primary mucosal melanoma is often necessary but may result in significant surgical side-effects and complications. The local recurrence rate is high.
- Immunotherapy is rapidly becoming the treatment of choice for advanced melanoma. However, it is less successful for oral melanoma than for cutaneous melanoma. Some patients have had durable significant responses.
- Close follow-up is required.

Prognosis

The prognosis for patients with oral melanoma is poor, with a 5-year survival rate of around 25%.

After surgical ablation, recurrence and metastasis are frequent, and most patients die of the disease within 2 years.

10.4.3 Kaposi sarcoma

Kaposi sarcoma is a locally aggressive mucocutaneous vascular malignancy of endothelial origin. There are four main clinicopathological types.
- Oral disease is most frequently due to acquired immunodeficiency syndrome disseminated Kaposi sarcoma (AIDS-KS).
- Kaposi sarcoma may also arise in the oral cavity in patients with well-controlled HIV infection and, very rarely, in non-HIV-infected and non-immune-suppressed individuals.
- Oral Kaposi sarcoma is estimated to occur in almost 20% of HIV-1-positive subjects aged 30–50.

Causes

Kaposi sarcoma is due to disseminated infection with human herpesvirus type 8 (HHV-8).

Clinical features

Kaposi sarcoma usually causes multiple pink, red, purple, or brown macules, nodules, or plaques (see *Fig. 10.22a*).
- Lesions are most often found on the hard palate and gingiva.
- They may be unifocal or multifocal.
- Kaposi sarcoma may manifest at any stage of HIV infection, but it is most often diagnosed in patients with low CD4$^+$ T-cell count with disseminated lesions and visceral involvement.

Diagnosis

Oral Kaposi sarcoma may be suspected by finding multiple irregular vascular tumours. Dermoscopy shows polymorphous vessels, various white structures, and sometimes, polychromasia. Definitive diagnosis of Kaposi sarcoma requires biopsy.
- Histopathology shows blood-filled slit spaces and pleomorphic spindle cells.

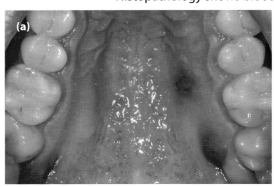
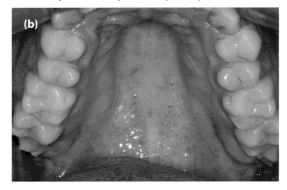

Figure 10.22 (a and b). Kaposi sarcoma before (a) and (b) after 6 months' treatment with a diode laser.

Reproduced from *J. Oral Med. Oral Surg.*, 2021;27:31 (https://doi.org/10.1051/mbcb/2021005) under a CC BY-4.0 licence.

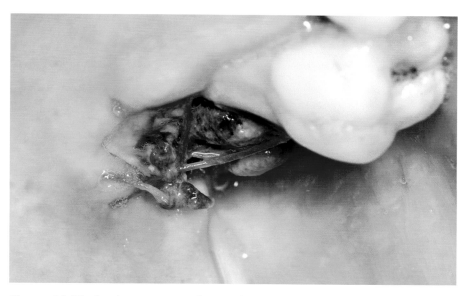

Figure 10.23. Angiosarcoma in the tooth socket of a wisdom tooth, which was extracted several months earlier.

Reproduced from Health NZ – Waikato (www.waikatodhb.health.nz) with permission.

- Further investigations for staging and treatment planning include MRI, CT, and PET scans.
- The differential diagnosis of Kaposi sarcoma includes angiosarcoma, an aggressive vascular tumour rarely detected in the oral cavity (see *Fig. 10.23*).

Treatment

Treatment relies on a combination of anti-retroviral therapy (cART) and chemotherapy if Kaposi sarcoma is multifocal and progressive.
- Treatment may include various forms of surgery, laser therapy (see *Fig. 10.22b*), or radiation therapy.
- Oral Kaposi sarcoma has a poor prognosis and a high fatality rate.

10.4.4 Lymphoma

Oral lymphoma represents 3.5% of all oral malignancies, most commonly B-cell non-Hodgkin lymphoma (NHL), mainly diffuse large B-cell NHL.

Clinical features

The most frequent oropharyngeal site for intraoral lymphoma is the lymphoid tissue of the Waldeyer ring (the oropharynx, lateral tongue, soft palate, and the floor of the mouth).
- Typically, a non-tender nodule appears, with or without surface ulceration.
- Gingival lymphoma may be associated with alveolar bone loss, oedema, and pain mimicking dental periapical or periodontal infection.

Diagnosis is by histopathology and immunohistochemistry with a panel of appropriate antibodies, and molecular investigations for various translocations. Flow cytometry may assist.

Treatment

Management of oral lymphomas is dependent on subtype and stage and often requires a multidisciplinary approach. The prognosis is grade-dependent and ranges from sustained long-term survival to a 5-year mortality rate of approximately 60%.

10.4.5   Leukaemia

Intraoral leukaemia is rare but oral symptoms are occasionally the first sign of the disease.
- Leukaemic cells may infiltrate the gingival soft tissues causing diffuse gingival swelling.
- Neutropenia leads to increased susceptibility to infection and ulceration.
- Thrombocytopenia causes petechial haemorrhages and spontaneous and prolonged bleeding.

10.4.6   Other primary malignant tumours

Other primary oral malignant neoplasms may rarely involve the gingivae.
- Fibrosarcoma
- Leiomyosarcoma
- Rhabdomyosarcoma
- Haematolymphoid tumours: D30-positive T-cell lymphoproliferative disorder, plasmablastic lymphoma, Langerhans cell histiocytosis, extramedullary myeloid sarcoma.

10.4.7   Metastases

Metastases in the oral cavity are rare. The primary malignancies most likely to metastasize to the oral cavity are the lung, kidney, liver, prostate, breast, female genital organs, and colorectum.
- Bony metastases may arise in the mandible.
- Soft tissue metastases can occur in the mouth, usually in the gingivae.

Clinical features

Metastases usually present as painful swelling with or without ulceration.
- The tumours often increase in size rapidly.
- Dermoscopy shows polymorphous vessels.
- Perineural spread manifests as paraesthesia in the distribution of the affected nerve.
- Bony metastases may be visible on dental radiographs, showing areas of radiolucency with poorly defined margins.

10.5   Malignant salivary gland tumours

10.5.1   Acinic cell carcinoma

Acinic cell carcinoma is a slow-growing salivary gland tumour that has unpredictable behaviour and can metastasize.
- Acinic cell carcinoma most commonly affects the parotid gland.
- It affects a wide age range, with a mean age of 50 years at diagnosis.
- The male-to-female ratio is 3:2.
- Acinic cell carcinoma is the second most common malignant salivary gland tumour in children.

Causes

Acinic cell carcinoma originates from reserve cells or pluripotent stem cells that reside at the junction of acini and the intercalated duct or within intercalated duct cells in mature salivary glands.

Clinical features

Acinic cell carcinoma presents as a solitary asymptomatic mass. It may resemble a benign encapsulated tumour.

Diagnosis

Definitive diagnosis of acinic cell carcinoma is usually made on fine-needle aspirate or biopsy. Histopathology shows acinar-like cells with a variety of other features.

Treatment

Acinic cell carcinoma is usually surgically excised.
- The tumour recurs in 30% of cases and metastasizes in 15%.
- The overall 5-year survival rate after surgery is over 80% but below 65% at 10 years.

10.5.2   Mucoepidermoid carcinoma

Mucoepidermoid carcinoma is the most common salivary gland malignancy (12–29%).
- It accounts for about 15% of all salivary gland tumours.
- It is diagnosed in children and adults with a female predilection.

Causes

Mucoepidermoid carcinoma is associated with translocations of *METC1* and *MAML2* genes, which create a new fusion gene that promotes neoplastic proliferation.

Clinical features

Mucoepidermal carcinoma is usually a slow-growing, asymptomatic mass in the parotid gland.
- It may also arise within a submandibular or sublingual gland.
- When located within the parotid gland, the facial nerve may be involved.
- Mucoepidermal carcinoma of minor salivary glands most often involves the palate (see *Fig. 10.24*).
- An extensive cystic component may result in a bluish fluctuant nodule.

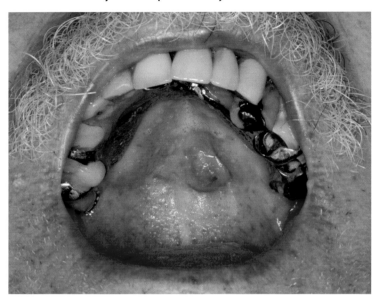

Figure 10.24. Mucoepidermoid carcinoma of the palate.

Diagnosis

A definitive diagnosis of mucoepidermal carcinoma is made on fine-needle aspirate and biopsy.
- The detection of gene translocation may support the diagnosis.
- An epithelial and mucus-secreting glandular component characterizes histopathology.

Treatment

Mucoepidermal carcinoma is usually treated surgically.
- Radiotherapy or chemotherapy is indicated when surgery is not feasible.
- Up to 40% of high-grade mucoepidermal carcinomas metastasize.
- It has a mortality rate of about 30%.

10.5.3   Adenoid cystic carcinoma

Adenoid cystic carcinoma is the second most common salivary gland malignancy, accounting for a third of malignancies in the minor salivary glands.

- The tumour may arise in any salivary gland.
- It most commonly occurs in individuals aged 40–60 years.
- There is a slight female predilection.

Causes

Adenoid cystic carcinoma is thought to be caused by activation of the oncogenic transcription factor gene *MYB*.

Clinical features

Adenoid cystic carcinoma is a slow-growing, painless or painful mass (see *Fig. 10.25*).
- Surface ulceration may occur.
- A plain X-ray may detect underlying bony destruction.
- If located within the parotid gland, facial nerve involvement may occur.
- Perineural spread is common and may be seen on an MRI.
- The tumour tends to be locally invasive and has a high likelihood of local recurrence and distant metastasis.

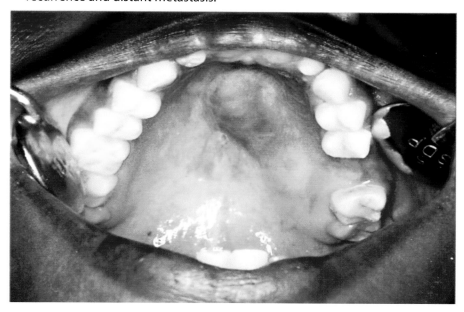

Figure 10.25. Adenoid cystic carcinoma presenting as a palatal slow-growing mass.

Reproduced from *Pan Africa Med. J.*, 2016;24:106 (doi: 10.11604/pamj.2016.24.106.8596) under a CC BY-4.0 licence, and included here after enhancement by AIPDerm (www.aipderm.com).

Diagnosis

A definitive diagnosis of adenoid cystic carcinoma is usually made on fine needle aspirate and biopsy. The histopathology shows:
- An unencapsulated lesion with an infiltrative destructive growth pattern.
- Groups of myoepithelial and ductal cells with three distinct patterns; cribriform, tubular, and solid.

- The solid or trabecular patterns predominate.
- The cribriform or 'Swiss cheese' pattern describes multiple cystic spaces surrounded by darkly staining cells without cytological atypia.

Treatment

Adenoid cystic carcinoma is usually excised surgically, with or without adjuvant radiotherapy.

- Some tumours are resistant to radiotherapy.
- The 5-year survival rate is fair; however, the long-term survival rate is abysmal.
- Lymph node metastasis is uncommon.
- A third of patients develop blood-borne lung, liver, or bone metastases.

10.5.4   Other malignant salivary gland tumours

- Polymorphous low-grade adenocarcinoma (see *Fig. 10.26*)
- Epithelial-myoepithelial carcinoma
- Clear cell adenocarcinoma NOS
- Basal cell adenocarcinoma
- Sebaceous carcinoma
- Sebaceous lymphadenocarcinoma
- Cystadenocarcinoma
- Low-grade cribriform cystadenocarcinoma
- Mucinous adenocarcinoma
- Oncocytic carcinoma
- Salivary duct carcinoma
- Adenocarcinoma NOS
- Myoepithelial carcinoma
- Carcinoma ex pleomorphic adenoma
- Carcinosarcoma NOS
- Metastasizing pleomorphic adenoma
- Squamous cell carcinoma
- Small cell carcinoma
- Large cell carcinoma
- Lymphoepithelial carcinoma
- Sialoblastoma
- Hodgkin lymphoma
- Diffuse B-cell lymphoma
- Extranodal marginal zone B-cell lymphoma
- Salivary gland metastases.

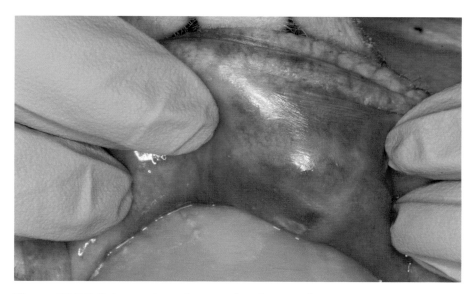

Figure 10.26. Polymorphous low-grade adenocarcinoma.

Reproduced from Health NZ – Waikato (www.waikatodhb.health.nz) with permission.

INDEX

Abscess, gingival and periodontal, 169–70
Acanthosis nigricans, 93–4
Acinic cell carcinoma, 281
Acquired immunodeficiency syndrome disseminated Kaposi sarcoma (AIDS-KS), 278
Acromegaly, 238–9
Actinic cheilitis, 263–6
Actinic keratosis of the lip, 39, 263–6
Acute graft-versus-host disease (GvHD), 186
Acute injury, 54–63
Acute lymphocytic (or lymphoblastic) leukaemia (ALL), 228
Acute myeloid (or myelogenous) leukaemia (AML), 228
Addison disease, 210–11
Adenocarcinoma NOS, 284
Adenoid cystic carcinoma, 282–4
Adenomatoid odontogenic tumour, 258
Adverse drug reaction, 80–8
Allergic contact stomatitis, 71–3
Alveolar ridge keratosis, 69
Amalgam tattoo, 90–1
Ameloblastoma, peripheral, 257
Amphotericin B, 131
Amputation neuroma, 62
Amyloidosis, 240
Angina bullosa haemorrhagica, 56
Angioedema, 224–6
Angiogranuloma, 62–3
Angioleiomyoma, 257
Angiosarcoma, 279
Angular cheilitis, 38, 174–5
Angular stomatitis, 174–5
Ankyloglossia (tongue-tie), 44
Aphthous ulcer, recurrent, 177–9
Aphthous-like ulceration (drug-induced), 83
Areca nut, 73–6
Argyrosis, focal, 90–1
Arteritis, giant cell, 235–6
Arteriovenous fistulas, 100
Ascorbic acid (vitamin C) deficiency, 223–4
Aspergillosis, 139
Aspergillus, 139
Atrophic glossitis, 44, 219–20
Atypical facial pain, 244
Atypical mycobacteria, 173
Atypical odontalgia, 242, 244

Bacterial infections, 161–74
    dental plaque biofilm, 166–70
    gonococcal stomatitis, 170–1
    staphylococcal infections, 161–4
    strawberry tongue, 171
    streptococcal infections, 164–6
    syphilis, 171–3
    tuberculosis, 173–4
    see also Viral infections
Basal cell adenocarcinoma, 284
Basal cell adenoma, 262
Behçet disease, 49
Benign lesions of the oral mucosa, 247–58
    angioleiomyoma, 257
    haemangioma, 255–7
    lipoma, 249–50
    melanocytic naevus, 247–8
    melanotic neuroectodermal tumour of infancy, 248–9
    peripheral ameloblastoma, 257
    peripheral nerve sheath tumours, 250–4
    rare odontogenic tumours, 258
    rhabdomyoma, 257
Benign migratory glossitis, 204
Benign mucosal pemphigoid, 195
Benign odontogenic tumours, 258
Benign, potentially malignant, and malignant, 247–85
    benign lesions, 247–58
    benign salivary gland tumours, 258–62
    malignant lesions, 271–80
    malignant salivary gland tumours, 281–5
    oral potentially malignant disorders, 262–71
    see also Cysts
Benign salivary gland tumours, 258–62
    other benign salivary gland tumours, 262
    pleomorphic adenoma, 258–60
    sialadenoma papilliferum, 261–2
    Warthin tumour, 260–1
Benign verrucous lesions, 156
Betel quid, 73–5
Biochemistry, 21–2
Biofilm, 166–70
Biopsy, 19
Biotin (vitamin B7) deficiency, 221–2
Biting, cheek/lip/tongue, 69
Blastomyces dermatitidis, 139, 140
Blastomycosis, 140

Bleeding, 54–6
Blue naevi, 247
Blue rubber bleb naevus syndrome, 100
Blunt verrucous hyperplasia, 76
Bowel disease, mouth ulcers due to, 95
Brush cytology, 19
Bruxism, 69
Bulla, xx
    haemorrhagic, 56
Bullous adverse reaction, 84
Bullous pemphigoid, 197–8, 198
Burn, mucosal, 57–60
    chemical burn, 58, 82
    thermal burn, 57
Burning mouth syndrome, 242–3

C. albicans, 129
Calcifying epithelial odontogenic tumour, 258
Calcifying fibroma, 67–8
Canalicular adenoma, 262
Candida albicans infections, 129–39
Candida leukoplakia, 134
Candidiasis, 129–39
Candidosis, 129–39
    chronic hyperplastic, 134–6
    chronic mucocutaneous, 136–8
    denture-related, 132–4
    erythematous, 132
    median rhomboid glossitis, 138–9
    pseudomembranous, 129
Cannon disease, 98–100
Capillary haemangiomas, 255
Capillary malformation, 100
Carcinoma cuniculatum, 275–6
Carcinoma ex pleomorphic adenoma, 284
Carcinosarcoma NOS, 284
Cementifying fibroma, 67–8
Cementoblastoma, 258
Cemento-ossifying fibroma, 258
Cheek biting, chronic, 68
Cheilitis glandularis, 206–7
Chemical burn, 58–9, 82
Chemicals, or radiation, 57
Chemotherapy-induced oral mucositis, 59–60
Chickenpox, 144–5
Chronic bullous disorder of childhood, 199
Chronic cheek biting, 68
Chronic hyperplastic candidosis, 134–6
Chronic inflammatory gingival enlargement, 42
Chronic lymphocytic leukaemia (CLL), 228
Chronic mucocutaneous candidosis, 136–8
Chronic myeloid (or myelogenous) leukaemia (CML),
    228
Chronic oral graft-versus-host disease (GvHD),
    186–7
Chronic repetitive injury, 63–73

Chronic ulcerative stomatitis, 189–90
Cicatricial pemphigoid, 195
Clear cell adenocarcinoma NOS, 284
CLOVES, 100
CMV, 147–8
Coeliac disease, 230
Common naevi, 247
Condyloma acuminatum, 156–8
Congenital disorders, 97–105
Congenital haemangioma, 256
Congenital hypothyroidism, 226
Congenital macroglossia, 97–8
Contact stomatitis, 71–3
Cosmetic tattoo, 91
Cowden syndrome, 121–2
Coxsackievirus, 148
Crohn disease, 230–3
    oral lesions specific to, 231–2
Cryotherapy burn, 57–8
Cryptococcosis, 139
Cryptococcus neoformans, 139
Cushing syndrome, 237–8
Cutaneous small vessel vasculitis, 234–5
Cyanocobalamin (vitamin B12) deficiency, 222
Cystadenocarcinoma, 284
Cystadenoma, 262
Cystic fibrosis, 105
Cysts, 211–16
    dermoid cysts, 213–15
    epidermoid cysts, 213–15
    eruption cyst, 213
    gingival odontogenic cyst, 212–13
    minor salivary glands, cysts of, 211–12
    nasolabial cyst, 216
    oral mucinosis, 217
    thyroglossal duct cyst, 216
Cytomegalovirus (CMV or HHV-5), 147–8

D30-positive T-cell lymphoproliferative disorder, 280
Darier disease, 105–8
Debris, 52–4
Deep mycoses, 139–40
    aspergillosis, 139
    blastomycosis, 140
    cryptococcosis, 139
    histoplasmosis, 139
    mucormycosis, 139
    paracoccidioidomycosis, 140
Delusional halitosis, 244
Dental and oral hygiene, 51–2
Dental anxiety, 245
Dental calculus, 166
Dental caries, 166
Dental fear / phobia, 245
Dental plaque / biofilm, 166–70
Denture granuloma, 66

Denture-induced hyperplasia, 66
Denture-related stomatitis, 132–4
Denture sore mouth, 66–7, 132–3
Denture stomatitis, 66–7
Dermatitis herpetiformis, 203–4
Dermoid cysts, 213–15
Dermoscopy, 17
Desquamative gingivitis, 41, 184–5
Destructive membranous periodontal disease, 114–15
Diabetes mellitus, oral manifestations of, 233–4
Diagnostic imaging, 22–3
    oral soft tissues, 22–3
    sialography, 23
Diascopy, 18
DIF, 20
Differential diagnosis of oral mucosal lesions, 25–50
    diseases affecting the gingivae, 41
    diseases affecting the lips, 38
    diseases affecting the tongue, 43
    dry mouth, 36
    halitosis, 37
    mucocutaneous disorders, 46
    non-neoplastic oral soft tissue swellings, 31
    oral diseases associated with systemic disorders, 49
    oral erosions and ulcers, 34
    oral vesicles and bullae, 33
    papillary and verrucous lesions of the oral mucosa, 30
    pigmented lesions of the oral mucosa, 29
    red and purple lesions of the oral mucosa, 27
    white lesions of the oral mucosa, 25
Diffuse B-cell lymphoma, salivary, 284
Digital mucoscopy, 17
Direct immunofluorescence (DIF), 20
Diseases affecting the lips, 38–40
Diseases affecting the gingivae, 41–3
Diseases affecting the tongue, 43–6
Disorders usually diagnosed in adult life, 123–7
Disorders usually diagnosed in childhood, 105–23
Drug eruption, 83–5
    fixed, 83
    immunobullous, 84–5
    lichenoid, 83–4
    lupus-like, 84
Drug-induced cheilitis, 39
Drug-induced gingival hyperplasia, 85–6
Drug-induced oral mucosal ulceration, 81–2
Drug-induced osteonecrosis of the jaw, 241–2
Drug-induced pigmentation, 91–2
Dry mouth, 36–7
Ductal adenoma, 262
Ductal papilloma, 262
Dyskeratosis congenita, 108–10
Dystrophic EB, 111

EB simplex, 111
EBV, 146
Echinocandins, 137
Ectodermal dysplasia, 103
Eczematous cheilitis, 38
EM, 88–90
Encephalotrigeminal angiomatosis, 100
Endogenous pigmentation, 209–11
Enteroviral vesicular pharyngitis, 149–50
Enterovirus, 148–50
Epidermoid cysts, 213–5
Epidermolysis bullosa (EB), 110–2
Epidermolysis bullosa acquisita (EBA), 193–4
Epithelial-myoepithelial carcinoma, 284
Epstein–Barr virus (EBV or HHV-4), 146
Epulis
    fibrous, 64–5
    fissuratum, 66
    giant cell, 65
    vascular, 62–3
Erosions and ulcers, xx, 34–6
Eruption cyst, 213
Eruptive lingual papillitis, 205
Erythema multiforme (EM), 88–90
    EM major, 88
    EM minor, 88
Erythroplakia, 269–70
Excessive tooth brushing, 69
Exfoliative cytology, 19
Exfoliative leukoedema, 98
Exostosis, 11
Extramedullary myeloid sarcoma, 280
Extranodal marginal zone B-cell lymphoma, salivary, 284
Extravasation cysts, 211
Extravascular blood, 54–6

False gingival enlargement, 42
Familial white folded gingivostomatitis, 98
Fanconi anaemia, 112
Fast-flow arteriovenous malformations, 100
Fibroepithelial polyp, 64–5
Fibroma of the gingiva, peripheral ossifying, 67–8
Fibrosarcoma, 280
Fibrous epulis, 64
    giant cell epulis, 65
Fine-needle aspiration (FNA), 19
Fissured tongue, 8–9
Fixed drug eruption, 83
Fluconazole, 137
Fluorescent in situ hybridization (FISH), 21
Focal argyrosis, 90–1
Focal dermal hypoplasia, 103–5
Folate (vitamin B9) deficiency, 222
Foliate papillae, 9
Fordyce granules, 123

Fordyce spots, 123
Frictional keratosis, 68–71
    alveolar ridge keratosis, 69
    chronic cheek biting, 68
    excessive tooth brushing, 68
    linea alba, 69
Frostbite or cryotherapy burn, 57
Frozen section, 20
Fungal infections, 129–40
    Candida albicans infections, 129–39
    deep mycoses, 139–40

Geographic tongue (migratory glossitis, erythema
        migrans), 44, 204–5
Giant cell arteritis, 235–6
Giant cell epulis, 65
Gigantism, 238–9
Gingivae, diseases affecting, 41–3
Gingival abscesses, 42, 169
Gingival and periodontal abscess, 169–70
Gingival cyst, 212–13
Gingival enlargement, 42–3
Gingival fibromatosis, 42
Gingival odontogenic cyst, 212–13
Gingivitis and periodontitis, 166–9
    hormone-related, 95
    ligneous, 114
Glandular cheilitis, 206–7
Glandular fever, 146–7
Glossal papillae, 7–8
Glossitis, 43–4
    with hyperplastic fungiform papillae, 171
Glossodynia (burning tongue), 44
Goltz / Goltz–Gorlin syndrome, 103–5
Gonococcal stomatitis, 170–1
Graft-versus-host disease (GvHD), 186–7
Granular cell tumour, 253–4
Granuloma, pyogenic, 62–3
Granulomatosis with polyangiitis, 236–7
Granulomatous cheilitis, 39
Granulomatous disorders, 190–3
    granulomatous gingivitis, 190
    orofacial granulomatosis, 191
    sarcoidosis, 193
Granulomatous gingivitis, 190
Gum abscesses, 169
Gums, diseases affecting, 41–3
Gumma, 172
GvHD, 186–7

Haemangioma, 255–6
    infantile, 256
Haematological disorders, 21
Haematolymphoid tumours, 280
Haemorrhagic bulla, 56
Hairy leukoplakia, 153–4

Hairy tongue, 44, 52–4
Halitophobia, 242, 244
Halitosis, 37–8
Hamartomas, 120
Hand, foot, and mouth disease, 148–9
Hard palate, 10
Heavy metal pigmentation, 92
Heck disease, 159
Hereditary benign intraepithelial dyskeratosis, 113
Hereditary gingival fibromatosis, 114
Hereditary haemorrhagic telangiectasia, 123–5
Hereditary hypothyroidism, 226
Hereditary leukokeratosis, 98
Herpangina, 149–50
Herpes labialis, 142–3
Herpes simplex virus (HSV), 140
Herpes simplex, 140–4
    herpes labialis, 142–3
    primary herpetic gingivostomatitis, 140–2
    recurrent oral mucosal herpes, 143–4
Herpes zoster, 145–6
Herpetiform aphthous ulcer, 178–9
HHT, 123–5
Histopathology, 20
Histoplasma capsulatum, 139
Histoplasmosis, 139
HIV-associated oral melanotic hyperpigmentation,
        155–6
Hodgkin lymphoma, salivary, 284
Homogeneous leukoplakia, 266–7
Hormone-related gingivitis, 95
HSV, 140
    type 1 (human herpesvirus-1), 140
    type 2 (human herpesvirus-2), 140
Human immunodeficiency virus, 153–6
Human papillomavirus, 156–60
Hygiene, dental and oral, 51–2
    adults, 51–2
    children, 52
    patients with oral mucositis due to radiotherapy or
        chemotherapy, 52
Hypercortisolism, 237–8
Hypersensitivity vasculitis, 234
Hypothyroidism, 226–7

IHC, 20–1
IIF, 20
Immunobullous diseases, 193–204
    dermatitis herpetiformis, 203–4
    epidermolysis bullosa acquisita (EBA), 193–4
    pemphigoid, 195–9
    pemphigus, 199–203
Immunobullous reaction, 84–5
Immunofluorescence, 20
Immunohistochemistry (IHC), 20–1
Immunology, 22

Impetigo, 161–2
In situ hybridization (ISH), 21
Incisional biopsy, 19
Indirect immunofluorescence (IIF), 20
Infancy, melanotic neuroectodermal tumour of, 248–9
Infantile haemangioma, 256–7
Infantile proliferative haemangioma, 256–7
Infection-related mucositis, 88
Infectious mononucleosis, 146–7
Inflammatory bowel disease (IBD), 230–3
    non-specific oral lesions, 231
    oral lesions specific to Crohn disease, 231–2
    pyostomatitis vegetans, 232
Inflammatory fibroepithelial hyperplasia, 66
Injury
    acute, 54
    chronic repetitive, 63–73
Intraoral leukaemia, 280
Irritant contact stomatitis, 71–3
ISH, 21

Jaw
    drug-induced osteonecrosis of, 241–2
    osteonecrosis of, 241
Junctional EB, 111
Juvenile spongiotic gingival hyperplasia, 95

Kaposi sarcoma, 278–9
Kawasaki disease, 171
    multisystem inflammatory syndrome in children, 171
Keratosis follicularis, 105–8
Kindler EB, 111
Klippel–Trenaunay syndrome, 100
Koplik spots, 150

Langerhans cell histiocytosis, 280
Large B-cell NHL, 279
Large cell carcinoma, salivary, 284
Latent syphilis, 172
Laugier–Hunziker syndrome, 125–6
LE, 188–9
Leiomyosarcoma, 280
Leukaemia, 228–9, 280
Leukoedema, 2, 126
Leukokeratosis nicotina palati, 78–9
Leukoplakia, 44, 266–8
    homogeneous, 266–7
    non-homogeneous, 267
Lichen planus, 44, 183
Lichenoid contact stomatitis, 61–3
Lichenoid disorders, 179–90
Lichenoid drug eruption, 83–4
Lie bumps, 205
Ligneous gingivitis, 114–15

Linea alba, 44, 69
Linear gingival erythema, 154–5
Linear IgA bullous dermatosis, 199
Lingua plicata, 8–9
Lingual papillitis, 44, 205–6
Lingual thyroid, 44
Lipoid proteinosis, 122–3
Lipoma, 249–50
Liposomal amphotericin B, 137
Lips, actinic keratosis of, 263–6
Lips, diseases affecting
    cheilitis, 38–40
Localized juvenile spongiotic gingival hyperplasia, 95
Low-grade cribriform cystadenocarcinoma, 284
Lupus erythematosus (LE), 188–9
Lupus-like reaction, 84
Lymph nodes, 14
Lymphadenoma, 262
Lymphangioma, 100–1
Lymphatic malformations, 100–3
Lymphoepithelial carcinoma, 284
Lymphoepithelial cyst, 215
Lymphoid tissue, 14–15
Lymphoma, 279–80

Macroglossia, 44, 239, 240
Macrognathia, 239
Macule, xx
Major aphthous ulcer, 178
Malignancies, 49
Malignant lesions, 271–6
    Kaposi sarcoma, 278–9
    leukaemia, 280
    lymphoma, 279–80
    melanoma, 276–7
    metastases, 280
    other primary malignant tumours, 280
    squamous cell carcinoma, 272–6
Malignant salivary gland tumours, 281–5
    acinic cell carcinoma, 281
    adenoid cystic carcinoma, 282–3
    mucoepidermoid carcinoma, 281–2
    other malignant salivary gland tumours, 284
Materia alba, 54
McCune–Albright syndrome, 115
Measles, 150–2
Median rhomboid glossitis, 44, 138–9
Medically unexplained oral symptoms and syndromes (MUOS), 242
Melanocytic naevus, 247–8
Melanoma, 276–7
Melanoplakia, 209
Melanosis, 210
Melanotic neuroectodermal tumour of infancy, 248–9
Melkersson–Rosenthal syndrome, 192

MEN type 3, 118–19
Menaquinones, 223
Metastases, 280
Metastasizing pleomorphic adenoma, 284
Miconazole, 131
Microbial culture, 18–19
Minor aphthous ulcer, 178
Minor salivary glands, cysts of, 211–12
Mixed infections, 174–5
Molecular pathology, 21
Moles, 247–8
Molluscum contagiosum, 160–1
Morsicatio buccarum, 68
Mouth ulcers, 177–99
Mucinous adenocarcinoma, 284
Mucinosis, oral, 217
Mucocele, 211
Mucocutaneous disorders, 46–8
Mucoepidermoid carcinoma, 281–2
Mucormycetes, 139
Mucosal burn, 57
    chemical, 58
    chemotherapy-induced mucositis, 59–60
    radiation-induced mucositis, 60–2
    thermal, 57
Mucosal neuroma, 254
Mucosal neuroma syndrome, 118–19
Mucoscopy, 17
Mucositis
    chemotherapy-induced, 59
    infection-related, 88
    radiation-induced, 60–2
Mucous membrane pemphigoid, 195–7
Mucus retention cysts, 211
Multifocal epithelial hyperplasia, 159–60
Multiple endocrine neoplasia type 2B, 118–19
Multiple hamartoma syndrome, 121–2
Multiple mucosal neuromas, 119
Mumps, 152
Mycobacterium bovis, 173
Mycobacterium tuberculosis, 173
Mycoplasma pneumoniae-induced rash and mucositis
    (MIRM), 89
Myeloid sarcoma, *280*
Myoepithelial carcinoma, 284
Myoepithelioma, 262

Naevus flammeus, 100
Nasolabial cyst, 216
Necrotizing periodontal diseases, 168–9
    necrotizing gingivitis, 168
    necrotizing periodontitis, 168
    necrotizing stomatitis, 168
Neisseria gonorrhoeae, 170–1
Neurofibroma, 251
Neuroma mucosal syndrome, 118–19

Neuroma
    mucosal, 254
    traumatic, 62
Niacin (vitamin B3) deficiency, 221
Nicotine palatinus, 78
Nicotine / nicotinic stomatitis, 78
Nikolsky sign, 18
Nodule, xx
Noma (cancrum oris), 168
Non-Hodgkin lymphoma (NHL), 279
Non-homogeneous leukoplakia, 267–8
Non-neoplastic oral soft tissue swellings, 31–3
Non-specific oral lesions, 231
Nutritional deficiency, 219
Nystatin, 131

Occlusal dysaesthesia, 245
Odontalgia, atypical, 244
Odontogenic tumours, 258
Odontophobia, 242
Oncocytic carcinoma, 284
Oncocytoma, 262
OPMDs, 262
Oral carcinoma cuniculatum, 275–6
Oral cavity, anatomical features and variants
    cheeks, 5–7
    hard palate, soft palate, and uvula, 10
    lips, 3–5
    lymph nodes, 14
    lymphoid tissue, 14–15
    maxilla and mandible, 11–13
    oral mucosa, 1–2
    temporomandibular joint (TMJ), 13
    tongue and mouth's floor, 7–9
Oral diseases associated with systemic disorders, 49–50
Oral dysaesthesia, 242, 244
Oral erosions and ulcers, 34–6
Oral erythema migrans, 204
Oral erythematous candidosis, 132
Oral hairy leukoplakia, 44
Oral hygiene, 51–2
Oral lichen planus (OLP), 179–83
Oral lichenoid reaction, 183–4
Oral lymphoid aggregates, 15
Oral manifestations of diabetes mellitus, 233–4
Oral melanotic macule, 210
Oral mucinosis, 217
Oral mucosa, 1–2
Oral mucosa to local or exogenous factors, reactions of
    debris, 52–4
    dental and oral hygiene, 51–2
Oral mucosal diseases of developmental and genetic
        origin, 97–128
    congenital disorders, 97–105
    disorders usually diagnosed in adult life, 122–7
    disorders usually diagnosed in childhood, 105–22

Oral mucosal infections, 129–75
Oral mucosal inflammatory diseases and conditions, 177–208
   granulomatous disorders, 190–3
   immunobullous diseases, 193–204
   lichenoid disorders, 179–90
   recurrent aphthous ulcer, 177–9
Oral mucosal lesions, differential diagnosis
   dry mouth, 36–7
   halitosis, 37–8
   non-neoplastic oral soft tissue swellings, 31–3
   oral erosions and ulcers, 34–6
   oral vesicles and bullae, 33–4
   papillary and verrucous lesions, 30–1
   pigmented lesions, 29–30
   red and purple lesions, 27–9
   white lesions, 25–7
Oral mucosal manifestations of systemic diseases, 219–45
   acromegaly, 238–9
   amyloidosis, 240
   angioedema, 224–6
   atrophic glossitis, 219–20
   coeliac disease, 230
   Cushing syndrome, 237–8
   diabetes mellitus, oral manifestations of, 233–4
   drug-induced osteonecrosis of the jaw, 241–2
   hypothyroidism, 226–7
   inflammatory bowel disease, 230–3
   leukaemia, 228–9
   parathyroid disease, 239
   psychogenic oral disease, 242–5
   sickle cell anaemia, 239–40
   thrombocytopenic purpura, 227–8
   vasculitis, 234
   vitamin deficiencies, 220–4
Oral mucosal non-inflammatory disorders and conditions, 209–17
   cysts, 211–16
   endogenous pigmentation, 209–11
   oral mucinosis, 217
Oral neoplastic lesions, 247–85
   benign, 247–62
   malignant, 271–85
   potentially malignant, 262–71
Oral potentially malignant disorders (OPMDs), 262
   actinic keratosis of the lip, 262–6
   erythroplakia, 269–70
   leukoplakia, 266
   reverse smoker's palate, 270–1
Oral submucous fibrosis, 73–5
Oral ulcers, 177
Oral verrucous carcinoma, 274–5
Oral verrucous hyperplasia, 75–6
Oral vesicles and bullae, 33
Orofacial granulomatosis, 191–3

Orofacial neuropathic pain, 244
Osler–Weber–Rendu syndrome, 100, 123–5
Ossifying fibroma of the gingiva, peripheral, 67–8
Osteonecrosis of the jaw, drug-induced, 241–2
Osteoporosis, 241
Other inflammatory diseases localized to the mouth, 204–8
   geographic tongue, 204
   glandular cheilitis, 206–7
   lingual papillitis, 205
   plasma cell gingivitis/cheilitis, 207–8
Other primary malignant tumours, 280

Paan, 73–5
Pachyonychia congenita, 115–17
Palatal leukokeratosis, 78
Papillary and verrucous lesions, 30–1
Papillary hyperplasia, 66–7
Papillary lesions of the oral mucosa, 156
Papilloma, 44
Papule, xx
Paracoccidioides brasiliensis, 140
Paracoccidioidomycosis, 140
Parathyroid disease, 239
Parkes–Weber syndrome, 100
Parulis, 169
Paterson–Kelly syndrome, 94
PCR, 21
Pellagra, 221
Pemphigoid, 195–9
   bullous pemphigoid, 197–8
   linear IgA bullous dermatosis, 199
   mucous membrane pemphigoid, 195–7
   pemphigoid gestationis, 198
Pemphigus, 199–203
   paraneoplastic pemphigus, 202–3
   pemphigus vulgaris, 199–202
Periodontal abscess, 42, 169
Periodontal diseases, 166
   necrotizing, 168–9
Periodontitis, 166–8
Peripheral ameloblastoma, 257–8
Peripheral giant cell granuloma, 65
Peripheral nerve sheath tumours, 250–4
   granular cell tumour, 253
   mucosal neuroma, 254
   neurofibroma, 251
   schwannoma, 252
Peripheral ossifying fibroma of the gingiva, 67–8
Peritonsillar abscess (quinsy), 166
Perleche, 174–5
Peutz–Jeghers syndrome, 117–18
Phantom bite syndrome, 242, 244–5
Phantom tooth pain, 244
Pharyngitis, streptococcal, 164–5
Phylloquinone, 223

Physiological pigmentation, 209
Pigment, 90–2
Pigmentation
    drug-induced, 91–2
    heavy metal, 92
    HIV-associated oral melanotic, 155–6
    postinflammatory, 92
    racial, 209
Pigmented lesions, 29–30
Plaque, xx
Plasma cell cheilitis, 207–8
Plasma cell gingivitis, 207–8
Plasmablastic lymphoma, 280
Pleomorphic adenoma, 258–60
Plicated tongue, 8–9
Plummer–Vinson syndrome, 94
Polymerase chain reaction (PCR), 21
Polymorphous low-grade adenocarcinoma, 284
Port wine stain (capillary malformation), 100
Posaconazole, 137
Postinflammatory pigmentation, 92
Pregnancy, 198
Pregnancy tumour or epulis, 62
Primary adrenal insufficiency, 210
Primary herpetic gingivostomatitis, 140–2
Primary hypothyroidism, 226
Primary oral melanoma, 276
Primary syphilis, 172
Prognathia, 239
Proteus syndrome, 100
Pseudocysts, 211
Pseudohalitosis, 244
Pseudomembranous candidosis, 129–32
Psychogenic oral disease, 242–5
    atypical odontalgia, 244
    burning mouth syndrome, 243
    halitophobia, 244
    odontophobia, 245
    oral dysaesthesia, 244
    phantom bite syndrome, 244
Psychosomatic halitosis, 244
Psychosomatic oral diseases, 242
PTEN hamartoma tumour syndrome, 120–1
Punch biopsy, 19
Purpura, xx, 54–6
    thrombocytopenic, 227–8
Pustule, xx
Pyogenic granuloma / vascular epulis, 62–3
Pyostomatitis vegetans, 232–3
Pyridoxine (vitamin B6) deficiency, 221

Racial pigmentation, 2, 209
Radiation mucositis, 60–2
Radiation-induced oral mucositis, 60–2
Radiotherapy or chemotherapy, oral mucositis due
    to, 52

Ramsay Hunt syndrome, 145
Ranula, 211
Rare odontogenic tumours, 258–60
Reaction to an underlying disease, 93–5
Reaction to infection or vaccination, 88–90
Reactions of the oral mucosa to local or exogenous
    factors, 51–96
Reactive gingival hyperplasia, 95
    hormone-related gingivitis, 95
    localized juvenile spongiotic gingival hyperplasia,
        95
Recurrent aphthous stomatitis, 177–9
Recurrent aphthous ulcer, 177–9
Recurrent herpes labialis, 140–3
Recurrent intraoral herpes, 143
Recurrent oral mucosal herpes, 143–4
Red and purple lesions, 27–9
Red strawberry tongue, 171
Reverse smoker's palate, 270–1
Reverse smoking, 270
Rhabdomyoma, 257
Rhabdomyosarcoma, 280
Riboflavin (vitamin B2) deficiency, 220–1
Rubeola, 150–2

Salivary diagnostic tests, 22
Salivary duct carcinoma, 284
Salivary gland metastases, 284
Salivary squamous cell carcinoma, 284
Sarcoidosis, 193
SCAR (severe cutaneous adverse reaction), 84
Scarlet fever, 171
SCC, 271–2
Schwannoma, 252
Scurvy, 223
Sebaceous adenoma, 262
Sebaceous carcinoma, 284
Sebaceous lymphadenocarcinoma, 284
Secondary hypothyroidism, 226
Secondary syphilis, 172
Serology, 22
Sharp verrucous hyperplasia, 76
Shingles, 145–6
Sialadenoma papilliferum, 261–2
Sialoblastoma, 284
Sialography, 23
Sickle cell anaemia, 239–40
Sjögren syndrome, 49
SJS, 86–8
Slow-flow venous malformation, 100
Small cell carcinoma, salivary, 284
Small vessel vasculitis, 234
Smear for cytology, 19
Smokeless tobacco keratosis, 76–8
Smoker's keratosis, 78
Smoker's melanosis, 79–80

Smoker's palate, 78
'Snail track' ulcers, 172
Snuff dipper's keratosis, 77
Soft palate, 10
Solar cheilosis, 263
Solar keratosis, 263
Squamous cell carcinoma (SCC), 272–6
    carcinoma cuniculatum, 275–6
    salivary, 284
    verrucous carcinoma, 274–5
Squamous papilloma, 156–8
Staphylococcal infections, 161–4
Staphylococcal scalded skin syndrome (SSSS), 161,
    163–4
Stevens–Johnson syndrome (SJS), 86–8
Stevens–Johnson syndrome / toxic epidermal
    necrolysis (SJS/TEN), 86–8
Stomatitis, chronic ulcerative, 189–90
Stomatitis palatini, 78
Strawberry tongue, 171
Streptococcal infections, 164–6
Streptococcal pharyngitis, 165–6
Submucous fibrosis, 73–5
Syphilis, 171–3
Syphilitic leukoplakia, 173
Systemic aciclovir, 141
Systemic disorders, oral diseases associated with,
    49–50
Systemic lupus erythematosus, 49

Target lesions, 89
Tattoo
    amalgam, 90–1
    cosmetic, 91
TB, 173–4
Teeth grinding, 69
Temporomandibular joint (TMJ), 13
TEN, 86–8
Terbinafine, 137
Tertiary hypothyroidism, 226
Tertiary syphilis, 172
Thermal burn, 57–8
Thrombocytopenia, 227
Thrombocytopenic purpura, 227–8
Thrombotic thrombocytopenic purpura, 227
Thyroglossal duct cyst, 216
Tobacco, smokeless, 76–8
Tobacco pouch keratosis, 77
Tobacco smoking, 78–80
Tocopherol (vitamin E) deficiency, 222
Toluidine blue, 18
Tongue and mouth's floor, 7–9
Tongue
    diseases affecting, 43–6
    hairy, 52–4
Tooth brushing, excessive, 69

Topical antifungal treatment, 131
Torus mandibularis, 12
Torus palatinus, 11
Toxic epidermal necrolysis (TEN), 86
Toxic shock syndrome, 171
Toxins, 73–80
Transient lingual papillitis, 205
Traumatic fibroma (irritational fibroma, fibroepithelial
    polyp), 44
Traumatic haemorrhagic bulla, 56–7
Traumatic neuroma, 62
Traumatic ulceration, 54
Treponema pallidum, 171–3
Tuberculosis (TB), 173–4
Type A reactions, 81
Type B reactions, 81
Tzanck smear / test, 19, 141

Ulcerative colitis, 230–3
Ulcerative stomatitis, chronic, 189–90
Ulcers, xx
    due to underlying bowel disease, 95
    erosions and, 34–6
    recurrent aphthous, 177–9
    traumatic, 54
Uvula, 10

Valaciclovir, 141
Varicella, 144–5
Varicella-zoster infection, 144–6
Vascular malformation, 100
Vasculitis, 234–7
    cutaneous small vessel vasculitis 234–5
    giant cell arteritis, 235–6
    granulomatosis with polyangiitis, 236–7
Venous lake, 126–7
Verruca vulgaris, 156–8
Verruciform xanthoma, 71
Verrucous carcinoma, 274–5
Verrucous hyperplasia, 75–6
Verrucous xanthoma, 71
Vesicles and bullae, xx, 33
Viral infections, 140–61
    cytomegalovirus, 147–8
    enterovirus, 148–50
    herpes simplex, 140–4
    human immunodeficiency virus, 153–6
    human papillomavirus, 156–60
    infectious mononucleosis, 146–7
    measles, 150–2
    molluscum contagiosum, 160–1
    mumps, 152
    varicella-zoster infection, 144–6
Viral swab, 141
Viral warts, 156–8
Vitamin deficiency, 220–4

ascorbic acid (vitamin C) deficiency, 223–4
biotin (vitamin B7) deficiency, 221–2
cyanocobalamin (vitamin B12) deficiency, 222
folate (vitamin B9) deficiency, 222
niacin (vitamin B3) deficiency, 221
pyridoxine (vitamin B6) deficiency, 221
riboflavin (vitamin B2) deficiency, 220–1
tocopherol (vitamin E) deficiency, 222
vitamin K deficiency, 223
Voriconazole, 137

Warthin tumour, 260–1
Wegener granulomatosis, 236–7
White gingivostomatitis, 98
White lesions, 25–7
White sponge naevus, 98–100
White strawberry tongue, 171

Xerostomia, 36–7

Zoster, 145–6